AF344502

CONTROL OF THE THYROID GLAND

Regulation of Its Normal Function and Growth

ADVANCES IN EXPERIMENTAL MEDICINE AND BIOLOGY

Editorial Board:

NATHAN BACK, *State University of New York at Buffalo*

IRUN R. COHEN, *The Weizmann Institute of Science*

DAVID KRITCHEVSKY, *Wistar Institute*

ABEL LAJTHA, *N. S. Kline Institute for Psychiatric Research*

RODOLFO PAOLETTI, *University of Milan*

Recent Volumes in this Series

Volume 254
MECHANISMS OF LYMPHOCYTE ACTIVATION AND IMMUNE REGULATION II
Edited by Sudhir Gupta and William E. Paul

Volume 255
CALCIUM PROTEIN SIGNALING
Edited by H. Hidaka

Volume 256
ENDOTOXIN
Edited by Herman Friedman, T. W. Klein, Masayasu Nakano, and Alois Nowotny

Volume 257
THE IMMUNE RESPONSE TO VIRAL INFECTIONS
Edited by B. A. Askonas, B. Moss, G. Torrigiani, and S. Gorini

Volume 258
COPPER BIOAVAILABILITY AND METABOLISM
Edited by Constance Kies

Volume 259
RENAL EICOSANOIDS
Edited by Michael J. Dunn, Carlo Patrono, and Giulio A. Cinotti

Volume 260
NEW PERSPECTIVES IN HEMODIALYSIS, PERITONEAL DIALYSIS, ARTERIOVENOUS HEMOFILTRATION, AND PLASMAPHERESIS
Edited by W. H. Hörl and P. J. Schollmeyer

Volume 261
CONTROL OF THE THYROID GLAND: Regulation of Its Normal Function and Growth
Edited by Ragnar Ekholm, Leonard D. Kohn, and Seymour H. Wollman

---

A Continuation Order Plan is available for this series. A continuation order will bring delivery of each new volume immediately upon publication. Volumes are billed only upon actual shipment. For further information please contact the publisher.

CONTROL OF THE THYROID GLAND

Regulation of Its Normal Function and Growth

Edited by

Ragnar Ekholm

University of Göteborg
Göteborg, Sweden

**Leonard D. Kohn
and Seymour H. Wollman**

National Institutes of Health
Bethesda, Maryland

PLENUM PRESS • NEW YORK AND LONDON

Library of Congress Cataloging in Publication Data

Control of the thyroid gland: regulation of its normal function and growth / edited by Ragnar Ekholm, Leonard D. Kohn, and Seymour H. Wollman.
p. cm. (Advances in experimental medicine and biology; v. 261)
Proceedings of a symposium held Mar. 20–21, 1989, in Bethesda, Md.
Includes bibliographical references.
ISBN 0-306-43380-X
1. Thyroid gland—Physiology—Congresses. 2. Thyroid gland—Growth—Congresses. 3. Growth factors—Physiological effect—Congresses. I. Ekholm, Ragnar. II. Kohn, Leonard D. III. Wollman, Seymour H.
[DNLM: 1. Receptors, Thyroid Hormone—physiology—congresses. 2. Thyroid Gland—physiology—congresses. 3. Thyroid Hormones—physiology—congresses. WK 202 C764 1989]
QP188.T54C66 1989
612.4'4—dc20
DNLM/DLC 89-23075
for Library of Congress CIP

Proceedings of a symposium on the Control of the Thyroid Gland: Regulation of Its Normal Function and Growth, held March 20–21, 1989, at the National Institutes of Health, in Bethesda, Maryland

© 1989 Plenum Press, New York
A Division of Plenum Publishing Corporation
233 Spring Street, New York, N.Y. 10013

All rights reserved

No part of this book may be reproduced, stored in a retrieval system, or transmitted in any form or by any means, electronic, mechanical, photocopying, microfilming, recording, or otherwise, without written permission from the Publisher

Printed in the United States of America

PREFACE

This volume presents the proceedings of a symposium on the "Control of the thyroid gland; regulation of its normal function and growth," held at the National Institutes of Health, Bethesda, Maryland on March 20 and 21, 1989.

Our motivation for the organization of this symposium was the fast development in recent years of our understanding of the regulation of the thyroid - and the progress in the field of cell regulation in general - which have led to profound modifications of our view of the control of the thyroid. Not so many years ago the thyroid was thought to be controlled by one regulator, the pituitary TSH, which with cyclic AMP in the role of second messenger was considered to express or regulate most or all processes in the gland. In the last several years it has been well documented that hormones other than TSH and various growth factors are involved in thyroid growth control and it has been increasingly clear that several hormones and neurogenic agents are obligate participants in the regulation of thyroid function. In addition, not only new agonists acting on the thyroid have been revealed, but new transducer and second messenger systems have been discovered. In particular the interest has been - and is - focused on the signals emanating from the hydrolysis of the inositol phospholipids, comprising the inositol trisphosphate/Ca^{2+} pathway and the diacylglycerol/protein kinase C pathway. Since these new signal systems must be coordinated with the "old" systems, the regulatory network has become very complex. Parallel with the development of these new areas in the field of thyroid regulation our understanding of the TSH system has been modified and essentially improved with respect to the pituitary - thyroid interrelation, the structure and function of TSH and the structure and function of the TSH receptor.

The proceedings deal with almost all aspects of thyroid regulation and summarizes the current state of our understanding of this biologically and clinically important issue. We think that this volume will be a valuable source of information not only to thyroidologists and endocrinologists in general, but also to researchers in other fields who are interested in cell regulation.

The Editors

CONTENTS

SIGNALS AND TRANSDUCTION

REGULATION OF GROWTH AND FUNCTION

THE THYROID AS A MODEL ENDOCRINE SYSTEM

Jacob Robbins

National Institutes of Health, Bethesda, Maryland 20892

The focus of this conference is on the regulation of growth and differentiated function of the thyroid gland. Our expectation is that the information and the insight that will be developed can serve as a model for other endocrine organs and, even more broadly, might contribute to an understanding of the growth and function of any specialized group of cells in a multi-cellular organism. In the vernacular of our time, we speak of communication between cells by chemical means. We know that this form of communication occurs at all levels of the plant and animal kingdoms, from sex factors exchanged between single yeast cells, to pheromones exchanged between insects, and on to endocrine organs of higher animals whose chemical signals are called hormones, and are transported to distant targets through a circulatory system.

The boundary that separates endocrine signals from other types of chemical communication is certainly arbitrary and constantly open to redefinition. Classical endocrine systems, however, are of two general types. The first are those that consist of a group of cells that send and receive signals without the interposition of another regulatory organ. Examples are the parathyroids and the pancreatic islets whose secretory products are polypeptide hormones. A subcategory consists of endocrine organs closely allied to the nervous system. They include the posterior pituitary, which is composed of neurons that secrete the neuropeptides, oxytocin and vasopressin, and the chromaffin cells of the adrenal medulla that secrete epinephrine and norepinephrine. The latter are analogous to sympathetic post-ganglionic cells and have their embryonic origin in the neural crest. Also derived from the neural crest are the thyroid parafollicular cells, whose secretory product is calcitonin. Although the thyroid could thus serve as a model neuroendocrine organ, this will not be our concern in this symposium.

The second type of endocrine system, to which the thyroid follicular cells belong, does have an interposed regulatory organ. Besides the thyroid, these include the ovary, the testis and the adrenal cortex and they have a number of features in common. First, they are all under the control of hormones secreted by the anterior pituitary gland, that are themselves regulated by neuropeptide hormones derived from the central nervous system. Second, the thyroid stimulating hormone and the gonadotropins (but not ACTH) are glycoproteins with extensive sequence homology. Third, the hormones that these glands secrete have relatively slow actions on growth and development, actions that are mediated through effects on protein synthesis. All of these hormones are small molecules - either steroids or, uniquely in the case of the thyroid, amino acids. Their effects on the cell nucleus are achieved through an homologous set of DNA-binding receptor proteins that are the products of genes related to the erb-A protooncogene.

The evolutionary implications of these homologies are still a mystery and extend beyond these particular endocrine systems. Thus, the pituitary gonadotropic hormones are also related to the chorionic gonadotropin of the placenta. All of the glycoprotein hormones, including TSH, are dimeric molecules that share an identical α subunit but have distinct β subunits that account for their individuality. It has been suggested that this protein family arose by gene duplication of a primitive α chain with subsequent duplications and sequence divergence of the β-chains during vertebrate evolution.

The extensive erb-A related protein family includes, in addition to the receptors for all the steroid hormones and the thyroid hormone, the receptors for vitamin D and retinoic acid as well. These receptor molecules share a common DNA-binding region but diverge in their hormone-binding domains. Clearly they must have a common origin. The mystery of these kinds of relationships is certainly not unique to endocrinology and continues to deepen as the lexicon of protein and gene sequences expands geometrically. It motivates us to search for analogies in previously unrecognized relationships and is certain to lead to new insight that might not otherwise have reached a conscious level. Hopefully this symposium will provide us with some flashes of recognition.

The complexity of the thyroid system ensures that the subjects to be discussed will be wide ranging. Although we are not concerned here with the action of thyroid hormone at its distant targets, the negative feedback at the pituitary is an important aspect of thyroid regulation. Is the mechanism of thyroid hormone action on the pituitary thyrotrophs analogous to its action in the periphery? There are reasons to believe that multiple mechanisms for thyroid hormone action might exist and hopefully this aspect will be explored. An interesting aspect of the negative feed-back by thyroid hormone is that it is accomplished not by the hormone that is secreted (mainly thyroxine) but by a metabolite (triiodothyronine) that is produced within the pituitary cell. In this respect, although differing in particulars, the thyroid resembles at least one other endocrine system: testosterone must first be converted in its target cell to dihydrotestosterone in order to exert its action. And like vitamin D, which undergoes processing (i.e., hydroxylations) in organs other than where it originates (i.e., in the liver and kidney) deiodination of thyroxine also takes place in these tissues, and triiodothyronine returns to the circulation for delivery to the target organs.

At the pituitary level we are also concerned with the complex interplay of the negative feedback by thyroid hormone, the positive influence of the hypothalamus mediated through TRH, and still other neuropeptide modulators. The striking contrast between the relatively steady stimulation of the thyroid gland and the more highly oscillatory control of the ovary and testis by GnRH and the gonadotropins, and of the adrenal by CRH and corticotropin, presumably is related to the role of the thyroid in maintaining the status quo.

This brings us to a consideration of how TSH regulates the growth and function of the thyroid gland. Here the thyroid can serve as a good model for the action of glycoprotein and other polypeptide hormones since the patterns of plasma membrane receptors and signal transduction mechanisms have much in common. But again, we should look not only for commonality but for differences that might extend our understanding of biological controls. Even in the case of TSH itself, the relatively rapid action leading to thyroid hormone secretion needs to be distinguished from the slow action that results in thyroid cell growth. Do these different actions stem from the same receptor? If so, are there different signaling mechanisms or different responses to the same signal in different intracellular loci?

In our concern for analogies between the thyroid and other endocrine systems we must not lose sight of the ways in which the thyroid gland is unique and thus may be a model only for itself. Indeed, it is this specialization that makes the thyroid gland an essential component of the vertebrate organism. A central feature of this gland is its requirement for the trace dietary element, iodine. This raises a new set of mysteries in evolution which still await a solution. Iodine incorporation into proteins of algae and lower marine animals such as sponges is widespread, but no function for this is known. Somewhat later in evolution, thyroxine and triiodothyronine made their appearance but their utilization as hormones evolved gradually. In tunicates they have no known biological role. In amphibia they are essential for metamorphosis, but are apparently not required for early fetal development in man. In teleosts, their function in migratory behavior is quite different from that in higher vertebrates where they assumed key roles in growth and development of the young animal, in energy metabolism, and in a variety of other metabolic processes. In these animal species, including the human, homeostatic mechanisms developed to ensure the steady availability of thyroid hormone to the organism. These mechanisms include a trapping system for iodide by the thyroid cell, a protein (thyroglobulin) that can efficiently form thyroid hormone at low iodine levels, a unique storage system in which the hormone in protein linkage is secreted into lacunae for later utilization, and a hormone secretion mechanism that begins with the ingestion of the stored thyroglobulin by the same cells in which it had been formed. In addition to the pituitary feedback system that we have already discussed, the thyroid cell developed an important autoregulatory mechanism that depends on iodine, and this also will be a subject for this symposium.

Thus we look forward to an illuminating program in which knowledge about one endocrine system, the thyroid gland, will be integrated into the general state of our understanding of how specialized organs are regulated in their growth, development and function.

WHAT CONTROLS THYROID GROWTH -- THAT IS, THYROID SIZE?

Leslie J. DeGroot

Thyroid Study Unit
The University of Chicago
5841 South Maryland Avenue
Chicago, IL 60637

INTRODUCTION

As an introduction to this conference, a physiologically oriented summary of factors controling thyroid size may be of interest, before analysis of factors controling growth at the molecular level. I have conceived of this as a series of levels of controls layered one on top of the other, in what might be called the cortex-hypothalamus-pituitary-thyroid-peripheral tissue axis.

1. Surely the first level of control is the intrinsic capacity of the thyroid gland to produce hormone, a function of the number of cells multiplied by their hormone production rate. Genetically determined functional differences in thyroid peroxidase, thyroglobulin, and no doubt many other proteins, must set the baseline synthetic capacity of the "naive" thyroid gland.

2. The next important and independent factor is the "set-point" of the pituitary thyrotroph. The pituitary and the thyroid develop together during ontogeny, and the pituitary clearly controls thyroid gland function through a hormonal feedback relationship. But the question which intrigues me, and for which I have no immediate answer, is: What determines the pituitary "set-point"? The amount of hormone that the thyroid gland produces, if possible, is the amount required to keep the pituitary equilibrated at its "set point". Why do we function with an FTI of 8 and TSH of 1.6 μU/ml, rather than an FTI of 28? Perhaps this set point represents some evolutionary compromise between the level of metabolic activity convenient for a certain size animal, and the food supply

required to maintain the animal's mass. It is to some extent an inverse function of size. Perhaps the set-point is related to thermal adjustment in a generally temperate climate. Although we can describe the phenomenon, we do not know the reason for the particular TSH-FTI set-point.

3. The next important element in this system must be iodide supply, since thyroid size definitely varies inversely in proportion to the dietary iodide available for trapping and biosynthesis of thyroid hormone.[1]

4. The pituitary-TSH-thyroid-T_4-T_3 feedback system is the major level of control. We would immediately agree that feedback control is regulated through intrapituitary cell conversion of T_4 to T_3, hormone occupancy of nuclear receptors, and binding of thyroid hormone receptors to response elements in the alpha and beta TSH subunit genes.[2,3] In the absence of the pituitary, thyroid growth and function are very restricted. However, feedback control, in a broad sense, must include a variety of factors that we rarely worry much about. For example, the T_4 available to control the pituitary must depend upon T_4 fractional loss in the gut, T_4 degradation in tissues throughout the body, efficiency of intrapituitary conversion to T_3, and function of the T_3 receptors inside the pituitary cell, including down-regulation of TRH receptors. Likewise, the efficiency of TSH stimulation of the thyroid will depend upon a host of factors, many of which will be discussed in this meeting, affecting the thyroid after TSH binds to its membrane receptors.

5. Hypothalamic control is added to the pituitary-thyroid system via TRH. Again there appears to be an "intrinsic" set-point for TRH secretion, and we know nothing about the how or why of this. T_4 and T_3 may feed back upon the hypothalamus to suppress TRH formation.[4] In addition to the positive stimulus to TSH synthesis and secretion by TRH,[5] negative regulation occurs through hypothalamic production of dopamine[6] and somatostatin.[7] It is not clear that these factors are controlled in any feedback relationship to thyroid hormone supply. Somatostatin is presumably regulated in a feedback loop with growth hormone and its metabolic effectors.[8]

6. Short loop feedback control systems also are thought to exist. For example, TSH may feed back directly on the hypothalamus and regulate TRH production, in the kind of "short-loop" shown for gonadotropins.[9] T_4 probably does feed back directly on the thyroid. Some biochemical evidence supports this hypothesis, and thyroid hormone receptors are abundant in thyroid tissue.[10] This may involve autocrine, paracrine, or endocrine loops, and we do not know for certain whether the signals are positive or negative.

7. Neural control is the next level in this progressive sophistication of systems. A variety of "neural" factors impinge to some extent upon thyroid function. Often the evidence for this is best found in animal experiments. Cold stress activates the thyroid.[11] Psychiatric stress may activate the thyroid.[12] High altitude causes stimulation of human thyroid function.[13] Stress may, by neural[14] or adrenal loops,[15] activate the thyroid. Thyroid function diminishes with age.[16] Is this a neural, hypothalamic, or pituitary change? An independent circadian rhythm of TSH supply, and thus thyroid activity, is superimposed on other controls through neural mechanisms.[17]

8. The adrenal cortex, through the circadian variation in cortisol secretion may play a role in controling thyroid circadian rhythm, although this is unproven. Excessive adrenal steroids clearly suppress the ability of TRH to stimulate the pituitary, and may directly suppress TRH secretion.[18,19]

9. Secretory products of the adrenal medulla have not been shown in man to have a significant direct influence on thyroid function, although sympathomimetic agonists can directly cause hormone secretion in animal thyroids.[20] There is also evidence that cervical sympathetic nerve stimulation can induce thyroid activation.[21] However, catecholamines activate 5' deiodinase in brown fat, inducing thermogenesis, and thus clearly affect body metabolism and thyroxine disposal.[22]

10. The role of the ovary and its main secretory product, estradiol, is unclear, although it is obvious that goitrogenesis is much more easily induced in females than in males. No clear explanation for this has ever been put forward, and it is not known to be related to the important changes in TBG caused by estradiol. Possibly recent observations of the similarity of estrogen receptor response elements and thyroid hormone receptor response elements in certain genes may offer a new approach.[23] It has been shown that TR can bind to the ERE.[24] Possibly estrogen receptors can bind to thyroid hormone response elements and activate or inactivate the same set of genes, although this has not been shown.

11. The main object of this workshop will be to survey another set of control elements which are primarily, at least so far as I understand, systems which do not provide "regulated" control of thyroid function. EGF,[25] insulin,[26] and IGF,[27] among other hormones, can stimulate the thyroid cell to grow or function. In "normal" circumstances, presumably their levels are relatively constant and probably form a base on which the other regulated systems impose their controls. Their importance, however, may be great in terms of overall thyroid growth and function.

12. After this list of physiological principles comes an array of factors including diet, drugs, and disease, which clearly can affect thyroid size. For example, thiocyanate may occur in the diet and is a goitrogen. Lithium is an important drug affecting thyroid size. Starvation, illness, diabetes, acromegaly, nephrotic syndrome, and autoimmunity affect thyroid hormone economy, thyroid gland size, or thyroid gland secretion.

One thing I will not do is try to put all of these factors together in one diagram. But I do wish to make the point that there is a hierarchy of control systems which affect thyroid growth and ultimate size, and that an impressive array of factors help control this process.

REFERENCES

1. L.J. DeGroot, P.R. Larsen, S. Refetoff and J.B. Stanbury, eds., Endemic Goiter and Related Disorders, in: "The Thyroid and Its Diseases," John Wiley & Sons, New York (1984).
2. D.S. Darling and J. Burnside, Binding of c-erbAβ to specific sequences of the rat thyrotropin β-subunit gene, 63rd Meeting of the American Thyroid Association, 1988, abstract no. 110.
3. J. Burnside and W.W. Chin, Thyroid hormone receptor binds to a region of the rat alpha subunit gene, 63rd Meeting of the American Thyroid Association, 1988, abstract no. 112.
4. E.M. Dyess, M.M. Kaplan, P. Wu, and R.M. Lechan, Pro-TRH transcription in the rat paraventricular nucleus (PVN) is directly regulated by triiodothyronine (T_3), 70th Meeting of the Endocrine Society, 1988, abstract no. 438.
5. I. Jackson, Thyrotropin-releasing hormone, N. Engl. J. Med. 306:145 (1982).
6. G. Delitala, Dopamine and TSH secretion in man, Lancet 2:760 (1977).
7. T.M. Siler, S.S. Yen, and R. Guillemin, Inhibition by somatostatin on the release of TSH induced in man by thyrotropin-releasing factor, J. Clin. Endocrinol. Metab. 38:742 (1974).
8. M. Berelowitz, S.L. Firestone, and L.A. Frohman, Effects of growth hormone excess and deficiency on hypothalamic somatostatin content and release and on tissue somatostatin distribution, Endocrinology 109:714 (1981).
9. J.M. Boeynaems, N. Galand, and J.E. Dumont, Inhibition by iodide of the cholinergic stimulation of prostaglandin synthesis in dog thyroid, Endocrinology 105:996 (1979).
10. A. Sakurai, A. Nakai, and L.J. DeGroot, Expression of three forms of thyroid hormone receptor in human tissues, Molecul. Endocrinol. in press (1988).
11. J.F. Wilber and D. Baum, Elevation of plasma TSH during surgical hypothermia, J. Clin. Endocrinol. 31:372 (1970).
12. D.I. Spratt, A. Pont, M.B. Miller, I.R. McDougall, M.F. Bayer,

and W.T. McLaughlin, Hyperthyroxinemia in patients with acute psychiatric disorders, Am. J. Med. 73:41 (1982).
13. F. Moncloa, R. Guerra-Garcia, C. Subauste, L.A. Sobrevilla, and J. Donayre, Endocrine studies at high altitude. I. Thyroid function in sea level natives exposed for two weeks to an altitude of 4,300 meters, J. Clin. Endocrinol. Metab. 26:1237(1966).
14. I.R. Falconer and B.S. Hetzel, Effect of emotional stress and TSH on thyroid vein hormone level in sheep with exteriorized thyroids, Endocrinology 75:42 (1964).
15. M. Taguchi and J.B. Field, Effects of thyroid-stimulating hormone, carbachol, norephinephrine, and adenosine 3', 5'-monophosphate on polyphosphatidylinositol phosphate hydrolysis in dog thyroid slices, Endocrinology 123:2019 (1988).
16. T.H. Oddie, J.H. Meade Jr, and D. Fisher, An analysis of published data on thyroxine turnover in human subjects, J. Clin. Endocrinol. Metab. 26:425 (1966).
17. E. Van Cauter, R. Leclercq, L. Vanhaelst, and J. Golstein, Effects of oral contraceptive therapy on the circadian patterns of cortisol and thyrotropin (TSH), Eur. J. Clin. Invest. 5:115 (1975).
18. J.R. Sowers, H.E. Carlson, N. Brautbar, and J.M. Hershman, Effect of dexamethasone on prolactin and TSH responses to TRH and metoclopramide in man, J. Clin. Endocrinol. Metab. 44:237 (1977).
19. J.E. Morley, Neuroendocrine control of thyrotropin secretion, Endocrine Reviews 2:396 (1981).
20. N.B. Ackerman and W.L. Arons, The effect of epinephrine and norepinephrine on acute thyroid release of thyroid hormones, Endocrinology 62:723 (1958).
21. L.J. DeGroot, P.R. Larsen, S. Refetoff, and J.B. Stanbury, eds., Physiology of the Hypothalamus, Pituitary, and Thyroid, in: "The Thyroid and Its Diseases," John Wiley & Sons, New York (1984).
22. J.E. Silva and P.R. Larsen, Adrenergic activation of triiodothyronine production in brown adipose tissue, Nature 305:712 (1983).
23. C.K. Glass, R. Franco, C. Weinberger, V.R. Albert, R.M. Evans, and M.G. Rosenfeld, A c-erbA binding site in rat growth hormone gene mediates trans-activation by thyroid hormone, Nature 329:738 (1987).
24. C.K. Glass, J.M. Holloway, O.V. Devary, and M.G. Rosenfeld, The thyroid hormone receptor binds with opposite transcriptional effects to a common sequence motif in thyroid hormone and estrogen response elements, Cell 54:313 (1988).
25. Y.L. Tseng, R.P. Schaudies, A. Ahmann, J. D'Avis, G.W. Geelhoed, K.D. Burman, and L. Wartofsky, Effects of epidermal growth factor (EGF) on thyroglobulin (Tg) and cyclic AMP (cAMP) production by human thyrocytes in long-term culture. 63rd Meeting of the American Thyroid Association, 1988, abstract no. 114.

26. L. Brenner-Gati, K. Berg, and M.C. Gershengorn, Insulin enhances thyroid-stimulating hormone (TSH)-induced cyclic AMP accumulation in FRTL-5 cells, 63rd Meeting of the American Thyroid Association, 1988, abstract no. 119.
27. K. Tahara, S.M. Aloj, E.F. Grollman, and L.D. Kohn, Effects of thyrotropin (TSH) and insulin/insulin-like growth factor-I (IGF-I) on arachidonic acid metabolism in FRTL-5 cells. 63rd Meeting of the American Thyroid Association, 1988, abstract no. 54.

THE PITUITARY-THYROID REGULATORY SYSTEM

P. Reed Larsen

Howard Hughes Medical Institute and
The Thyroid Division
Department of Medicine
Brigham and Women's Hospital
Harvard Medical School
Boston, Massachusetts

INTRODUCTION

The pituitary thyroid regulatory system is a classical example of a hypothalamic-pituitary-endocrine gland feedback loop. As one of the earliest such systems recognized and one which has proven to be so useful clinically, it has been widely studied. The critical elements in the system are shown in the diagram in Figure 1. The best recognized level of feedback regulation is that of thyroid hormone on pituitary thyrotropin (TSH) production. However, results of recent studies reviewed below demonstrate conclusively that there is also feedback regulation of thyrotropin-releasing hormone (TRH) synthesis by thyroid hormone. This complex system is exquisitely sensitive to changes in ambient thyroid hormone levels and serves to maintain the serum hormone concentration in an extremely narrow range in a given individual.

THYROID HORMONE HYPOTHALAMIC INTERRELATIONSHIPS

It is clear that normal function of the pituitary thyrotroph requires the secretion of TRH. TRH is widely distributed in the central nervous system as well as in extraneural tissues. However it is the TRH specifically

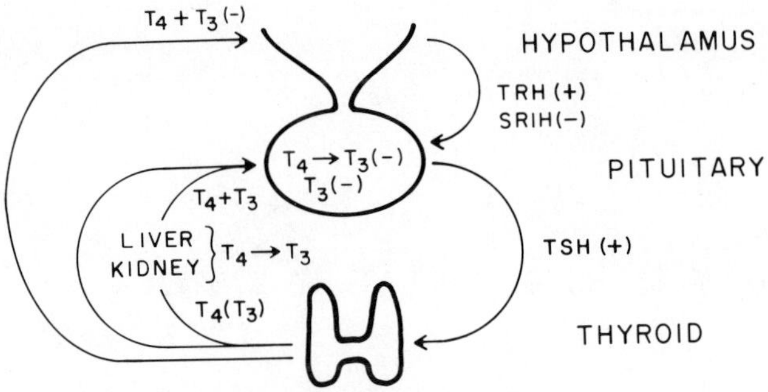

Figure 1. Critical elements of the hypothalmic-pituitary thyroid regulatory system.

synthesized in the medial parvocellular portion of the paraventricular nuclei which regulates thyrotroph, and therefore thyroid function. The critical role played by TRH has been demonstrated in many ways. For example, TSH concentrations can be measured following passive immunization with anti-TRH antisera (1-3). One such study is shown in Table 1 where greater than a 50%

Table 1

TRH-Ab inhibits basal TSH secretion but has little effect on TSH secretion in hypothyroid rats

	Serum TSH μU/ml					
	Normal			5 Days p Tx		
Time (h)	0	0.5	2	0	0.5	2
TRH Ab	135	57	45	640	420	510
NRS	147	160	163	660	590	640

Harris et al, JCI 61:441, 1978 (2).

decrease in serum TSH is found which persists at least two hours after anti-TRH antiserum administration (2). Normal rabbit serum has no effect. Also shown is the fact that in the thyroidectomized rat basal TSH levels are elevated but the infusion of TRH antisera has little if any effect on serum TSH concentrations. Such findings suggest that there are changes in the relative importance of hypothalamic and pituitary factors which are influenced by thyroid status.

One of the most exciting new developments in the field of thyroid pituitary regulatory physiology has been the cloning of the rat TRH structural gene and its promoter (4). The transcribed unit of this gene is 2.6 kb and contains 3 exons. The third exon encodes five copies of the TRH sequence and the carboxy terminal region of the pro-TRH molecule. Each copy of the TRH sequence, gln-his-pro-gly, is flanked by paired basic amino acid cleavage sites thus facilitating the release of the TRH peptide by post-translational processing. The availability of the cDNA coding for pro-TRH allowed studies of the effects of thyroid hormone on TRH biosynthesis in the paraventricular nucleus. Studies in two laboratories have now demonstrated that there is at least a two-fold increase in pro-TRH mRNA in hypothyroid animals which can be eliminated by thyroid hormone treatment (5,6). _In situ_ hybridization experiments showed that the increase in the TRH mRNA occurred exclusively in this region of the hypothalamus. If one compares euthyroid and hypothyroid animals with specific attention to the cell bodies in these nuclei, there may be as much as a ten-fold increase per cell body (5). More recently it has been demonstrated that stereotaxic implants of crystalline 3,5,3'triiodothyronine (T_3), but not the hormonally inactive 3,5,diiodo L-thyronine, led to a unilateral reduction in the immunostaining of these neurons as well as a marked unilateral decrease in the pro-TRH mRNA staining (7). There was no change in the serum TSH or T_3 in these hypothyroid rats with unilateral T_3 implants. Thus it is now possible to extend the thyroid hormone loop feedback to the regulation of hypothalamic TRH production.

Additionally, there has been considerable evidence of the physiological relevance of somatostatin in TSH regulation. Passive immunization to somatostatin leads to increases in serum TSH and hypothyroidism causes a reduction in somatostatin production by hypothalamic fragments (8,9). Somatostatin production can be increased by exposure of hypothalamic fragments to T_3 (9). Thus at least two arms of the hypothalamic TSH regulatory system are under the influence of thyroid hormone and respond in an opposite and appropriate fashion to thyroid hormone deprivation. The noradrenergic, dopaminergic and other peptidergic neurons also influence TSH release but TRH and somatostatin appear to be the most important with respect to thyroid hormone feedback regulation.

THYROID PITUITARY INTERRELATIONSHIPS

The effects of thyroid hormone on pituitary TSH synthesis and secretion have been studied for decades. Considering first the qualitative aspects of this system, it is well recognized that as thyroid hormone levels fall TSH rises and vice versa. In chronically hypo- or hyperthyroid rats these changes are due to alterations in the rate of TSH synthesis. However, more acute studies demonstrate that the effects of thyroid hormone on the thyrotroph are even more complex. Table 2 shows that when thyroid hormone is administered intravenously to hypothyroid rats there is a decrease in serum TSH within 30 minutes (10). Also shown is the increase in pituitary TSH concentration which accompanies this decrease indicating that it is accounted for by an inhibition of

Table 2

The acute decrease of serum TSH in hypothyroid rats after T_4or T_3 is due to blockade of pituitary TSH release, not synthesis*

	Plasma TSH (μU/ml)		Pituitary TSH concentrations (mU/mg)
	0	1 hr	1 hr
control	2300	2100	30
T_4	2000	1342	46
T_3	2100	1510	37

T_4 dose: 1.5 μg/100 g BW, T_3 dose: 0.15 μg/100 g BW

*Silva and Larsen, Endocrinology, 102:1783, 1978 (10).

pituitary TSH release. An equally rapid effect can be seen after T_4 infusion. An effect of T_3 to inhibit TRH induced TSH release can also be demonstrated _in vivo_ and _in vitro_ and is therefore independent of alterations in TRH secretion (11-13). The acute effect of T_3 is completely blocked by actinomycin D or inhibitors of protein synthesis (11-13). Thus this effect is extremely rapid but requires mRNA and protein synthesis. The data in Figure 2 demonstate that such an effect of T_3 can also be demonstrated with other TSH secretagogues besides TRH, in this case the phorbol ester, TPA (14). This is

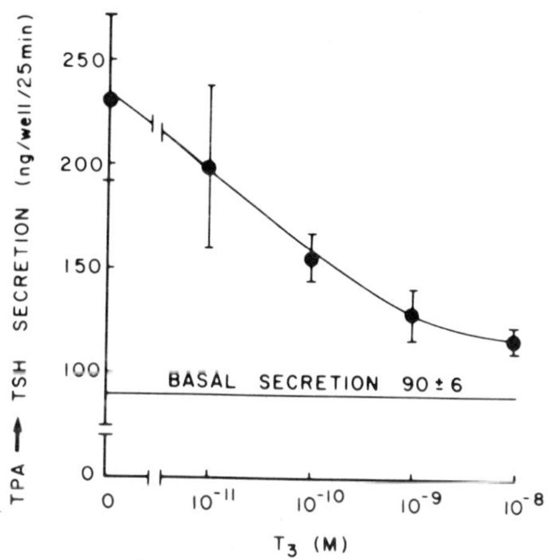

Figure 2. Triiodothyronine inhibits phorbol ester (TPA) induced TSH release (reprinted from Koenig et al, Biochem and Biophysical Research Communications 125:357, 1984 (14) with permission from Academic Press, Inc.).

important since it has been demonstrated that thyroid hormone can reduce the number of TRH receptors on pituitary tumor cells (15) and thus could influence the TRH message transduction system in a TRH-induced TSH release experiment. However, not only is the effect of T_3 on phorbol ester induced TSH release blocked blocked by cycloheximide (14) but also the release induced by increased Ca^{2+}, K^+ depolarization, or Ba^{2+} (13). Thus the effect of T_3 to inhibit secretagogue-induced TSH release is a general one and not specific to the stimulus used.

TSH is composed of two subunits, termed α and β, which are non-covalently but tightly associated. The α glycoprotein chain is common to FSH, LH and CG and the β subunit provides the receptor specificity for these glycoprotein hormones. When cDNAs became available for rat and mouse α and TSH β, it was possible to examine the effects of thyroid hormone on mRNA synthesis and mRNA content in the anterior pituitary. One extremely useful tool in this area is the mouse thyrotroph tumor. This has been employed with great success to study the effects of thyroid hormone on TSH synthesis. This tumor is maintained in hypothyroid mice and responds to thyroid hormone administration with a rapid decrease in the rate of transcription of both α and TSH β subunits (16,17). This decrease is significant by 30 minutes after T_3 administration and transcriptional activity continues to fall over the next four hours until it is virtually undetectable. As might be predicted, the effects on TSH β transcription occur sooner than those on the α subunit with a reduction of about 50% in the transcription rate within 30 minutes. It is of considerable interest that this effect of T_3 is not blocked by the protein synthesis inhibitor, cycloheximide (17). If one examines the TSH subunit mRNA content of pituitary tumors from mice treated in this fashion, one notes that the levels of mRNA for α and TSH β fall much more slowly than does the transcription rate. Assuming that the translation rate of these mRNA's is not affected by thyroid hormone, this can account for the persistence or even increase in TSH in the pituitary at a time when circulating TSH levels are falling. It is of note that T_3 does not inhibit TSH release in the mouse thyrotroph tumor as it does in normal rat pituitary.

Similar studies of TSH mRNA levels have been carried out in hypothyroid rats given acute treatment with thyroid hormone (18,19). One of these demonstrated a paradoxical increase in TSH β mRNA during the first six hours after intraperitoneal thyroid hormone administration though by 3 days the TSH β message had fallen to less than controls (19). At this point it is not certain whether the apparent differences in response between the mouse thyrotroph tumor and the hypothyroid rat pituitary are technological or physiological. Nonetheless, the persistence or slight increase of TSH β mRNA in the rat pituitary after T_3 is consistent with the previously mentioned increases in pituitary TSH during this time period (Table 2).

The cloning of the promoter region of the genes coding for TSH β and α subunit have permitted an evaluation of how the transcription of this gene might be regulated by thyroid hormone. An intriguing finding is the demonstration of two transcriptional start sites for the rat and mouse TSH β but apparently only a single site for human TSH β (20-22). These two sites are differentially regulated by thyroid hormone with transcription from the 3' site influenced by thyroid status to a much greater extent than is that from the upstream start site. There is considerable interest in the mechanism by which such regulation occurs. Studies of rat growth hormone (rGH) have identified a sequence between -189 and -165 which appears to be critically important in conferring the positive effects of T_3 on this promoter (23-25). This site, termed the T_3RE, was first identified by methylation interference footprinting using purified rat nuclear T_3 receptor (24). These and other studies have led to the search for similar sequences in the genes coding for α and β TSH as well as in TRH. It had been speculated that one such sequence might be found in the 5'untranslated region at +13 to +23 (20) although a similar sequence in the rGH promoter has subsequently been shown not to confer a T_3 response to a herterologous promoter (26). No sequences clearly analogous to the T_3RE of rat growth hormone in the TRH 5'flanking region have been identified although as a more certain consensus sequence is developed such sequences may be more readily apparent. Even if they are, it will have to be determined why for one promoter (e.g. rGH), transcriptional activity is enhanced by a T_3RE while in another (β TSH) it is suppressed by the presence of thyroid hormone.

THE THYROXINE ACTIVATION PROCESS IN HYPOTHALAMIC PITUITARY TSH REGULATION

Figure 3 demonstrates what was one of the most intriguing and puzzling aspects of the pituitary thyroid hormone axis subsequent to the discovery of T_3 and the development of techniques for its ready measurement. When rats are acutely deprived of iodine, serum T_4 falls serum T_3 remains constant but serum TSH rises (27). Since T_3 provides virtually all of the thyromimetic effect of T_4, it was not clear how such an apparent inverse relationship between serum T_4 and serum TSH could occur. A similar pattern of relationships between T_3, T_4, and TSH is also found in iodine deficient man as well

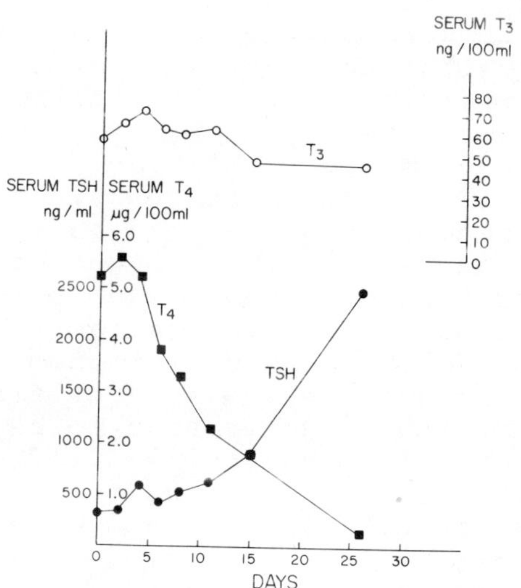

Figure 3. Early effects of iodine deficiency on serum T_3, T_4 and TSH in rats (data of Riesco et al, Endocrinology 100:303, 1977 (27).

as in early hypothyroidism (28). Another example of this phenomenon is found in constant T_3 infusion studies in thyroidectomized rats (29). When serum T_3 concentrations are maintained at pre-thyroidectomy levels by an implanted minipump, TSH rises demonstrating the importance of T_4 in the TSH feedback process. In order to maintain TSH at normal concentrations, the T_3 infusion rate had to be increased from 350 to 566 ng T_3/100 gm per day. Under these circumstances, serum T_3 rose to almost double the initial value and serum TSH remained normal. Thus one could conclude that in order to replace the feedback regulation of TSH due to the presence of serum T_4, an increase of 65% in the serum T_3 concentration was required.

Some years ago we performed more acute studies to examine this paradoxical effect of T_4 (10,30-32). When small doses of T_3 were given intravenously to hypothyroid rats, there was a transient suppression of TSH release as shown in Table 2. This was inversely proportional to the peak occupancy of the nuclear T_3 receptor binding sites (31). As the serum and nuclear T_3 concentrations fell over the next few hours, the serum TSH increased. Thus, there is a quantitative and chronological relationship between the degree of saturation of the pituitary nuclear receptors and the suppression of TSH release even though only a small fraction of hypothyroid male rat pituitary cells are thyrotrophs. If one administers an approximately 10 fold higher dose of T_4 (0.8 μg/100 gram body weight), we observed a rapid suppression of TSH release to a similar degree as occurred in the case of T_3. This was accompanied by an identical degree of nuclear T_3 receptor saturation. However because the half life of serum T_4 is so much longer than that of T_3, serum TSH remained suppressed. Isotopic studies demonstrated that the nuclear T_3 present after T_4 injection was derived from intracellular T_4 to T_3 conversion, presumably within the pituitary gland, by a process which was not susceptible to inhibition by propylthiouracil (PTU,32). A similar phenomenon of non-PTU supressible conversion could be demonstrated *in vitro* in hypothyroid pituitary fragments (33). However, if one employed the competitive deiodinase inhibitor, iopanoic acid, to block T_4 to T_3 conversion, then the effect of T_4 to inhibit TSH release was lost (34). In addition, T_3 did not appear in the pituitary nuclei supporting a cause and effect relationship between those two processes. These studies formed the basis for the identification of the so-called Type II T_4 deiodination process which is critically important in providing T_3 to the central nervous system and pituitary gland (reviewed in 35).

One of the characteristics of the Type II deiodinase activity is that it increases during hypothyroidism (36). It is not known whether such changes occur transcriptionally or post-translationally or both. For example, Type II deiodinase activity in pituitary homogenates increases about 10 fold as hypothyroidism progresses (36). This would seem to be counter-productive to the appropriate increase in TSH which should follow the fall in serum T_4. A potential explanation of this phenomenon is that there might be differential regulation of the deiodinase in pituitary cell subtypes. Koenig and Watson observed that thyrotrophs comprised only 3% of euthyroid pituitaries and about 12% of hypothyroid male rat pituitary cells (37). If dispersed cells are separated into different subtypes by a metrizamide density gradient, four fractions of pituitary cells each consisting predominantly of thyrotrophs, somatatrophs, mammotrophs, and gonadatrophs respectively can be prepared (37). This separation requires that the rats be hypothyroid so that the hyperplastic endoplasmic reticulum of the hypothyroid

Table 3

Distribution of cell types by electron microscopy in unfractionated anterior pituitary cells from chronically hypothyroid rats and four pools separated by density gradient centrifugation

	% of total identifiable cells				
	Unfractionated	Pool no.			
		1	2	3	4
Thyrotroph	13	42	14	6	12
Somatotroph	18	5	35	10	13
Mammotroph	32	0	14	62	27
Gonadotroph	18	10	11	13	30
Corticotroph	4	8	7	1	1
Agranular	15	34	20	8	17

Koenig and Watson, Endocrinology, 115:317, 1984 (37).

thyrotroph reduces the density of the cells. The distribution of the various cell types among four such pools is shown in Table 3. If these pools are placed into primary culture and exposed to T_3 for 24 hours and conversion of T_4 and T_3 is then measured, one can obtain an estimate of the responsivity of the deiodinase in each cell population to thyroid hormone (38). By inference, this also allows an estimate of the degree to which the deiodinase activity has increased during hypothyroidism. The data in Figure 4 demonstrate that the somatatroph and mammotroph pools show the greatest T_3 induced decrement in deiodinase activity of the four, with the thyrotroph and gonadotroph pools much less affected. Since none of the cell preparations is pure it is conceiveable that the differences are even more substantial. Thus, it is possible to explain the requirement for pituitary T_4 to T_3 conversion in the TSH suppression process on the presence of the deiodinase in thyrotrophs but the absence of an attentuation of the response of the thyrotroph to hypothyroidism by the fact that deiodinase activity in thyrotrophs does not increase in hypothyroidism. How such differential regulation occurs is unknown.

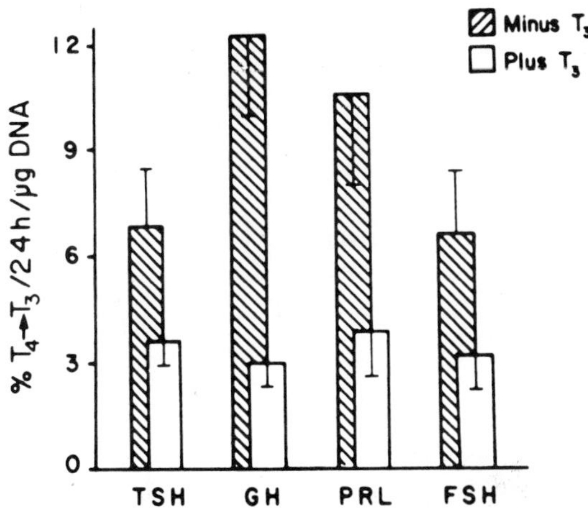

Figure 4. The influence of medium T3 concentrations on 5'-deiodinase activity was determined in cultured enriched populations of thyrotrophs, somatotrophs, mammotrophs, and gonadotrophs from chronically hypothyroid rats. The cells were maintained overnight in medium with 15% hypothyroid rat serum with or without 10^{-7} M T3. The following day, conversion of $[^{125}I]T_4$ to $[^{125}I]T_3$ was determined in serum-free medium with or without 10^{-8} M T3. The results of five experiments (mean ± SEM) are shown. (Reprinted from Koenig et al, Endocrinology 115:324, 1984 with permission from the Endocrine Society).

In Figure 5 are shown the sources of nuclear T3 in various euthyroid rat tissues. Most striking is the significant contribution of local T4 to T3 conversion via Type II deiodinase to the nuclear T3 in the cerebral cortex. For this reason we were quite surprised that the paraventricular nuclei of the hypothalamus had virtually no type II deiodinase activity (39). Also striking in this study was the high type II deiodinase activity in the arcuate nucleus median eminence area. In this critical area of the hypothalamus preservation of T3 production must be especially critical although its physiological role is unknown at the present time. The implication of the studies showing an inverse

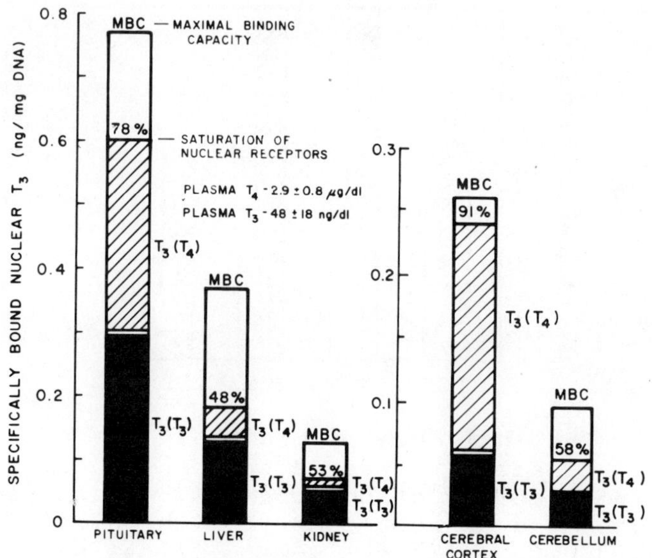

Figure 5. Sources of specifically bound nuclear T3 in various tissues of the euthyroid rat. $T_3(T_3)$ is the T_3 derived directly from the plasma. $T_3(T_4)$ is T_3 derived from intracellular monodeiodination of T_4.

relationship between TRH mRNA synthesis and T_3 together with the absence of Type II deiodinase activity in the paraventricular nuclei is that serum T_3 could be the physiological regulator of TRH synthesis. It is conceivable that this area of the hypothalamus receives a supply of T_3 from neighboring cells as opposed to its generation within those nuclei but this seems unlikely. This unexpected paradox serves to underline the complexity of the hypothalamic pituitary regulatory system and indicates the need for further experimentation before the precise interrelationships between circulating thyroid hormones and TRH and TSH synthesis can be understood. Nonetheless, in the context of the present conference, namely, the control of the thyroid gland, it is clear that the thyroid-pituitary axis has the capacity to respond not only to the active thyroid hormone, T_3, but to the prohormone thyroxine which is the principal secretory product of this gland.

REFERENCES

1. M. Szabo, N. Kovathana, K. Gordon, and L. A. Frohman, Effect of passive immunization with an antiserum to thyrotropin (TSH)-releasing hormone on plasma TSH levels in thyroidectomized rats, Endocrinology 102:799 (1978).
2. A. R. C. Harris, D. Christianson, M. S. Smith, S. L. Fang, L. E. Braverman, and A. G. Vagenakis, The physiological role of thyrotropin-releasing hormone in the regulation of thyroid-stimulating hormone and prolactin secretion in the rat, J Clin Invest 61:441 (1978).
3. M. Mori, I. Kobayashi, and K Wakabayashi, Suppression of serum thyrotropin (TSH) concentrations following thyroidectomy and cold exposure by passive immunization with antiserum to thyrotropin-releasing hormone (TRH) in rats, Metab 27:1485 (1978).
4. S. L. Lee, K. Stewart, and R. H. Goodman, J Biol Chem 263:16604 (1988).
5. T. P. Segerson, J. Kauer, H. C. Wolfe, H. Mobtaker, P. Wu, I. M. D. Jackson, and R. M. Lechan, Thyroid hormone regulates TRH biosynthesis in the paraventricular nucleus of the rat hypothalamus, Science 238:78 (1987).
6. R. T. Zoeller, R. S. Wolff, and K. J. Koller, Thyroid hormone regulation of messenger ribonucleic acid encoding thyrotropin (TSH)-releasing hormone is independent of the pituitary gland and TSH, Molecular Endocrinol 2:248 (1988).
7. E. M. Dyess, T. P. Segerson, Z. Liposits, W. K. Paull, M. M. Kaplan, P. Wu, I. M. D. Jackson, and R. M. Lechan, Triiodothyronine exerts direct cell-specific regulation of thyrotropin-releasing hormone gene expression in the hypothalamic paraventricular nucleus, Endocrinology 123:2291 (1988).
8. A. Arimura and A. V. Schally, Increase in basal and thyrotropin-releasing hormone (TRH)-stimulated secretion of thyrotropin (TSH) by passive immunization with antiserum to somatostatin in rats, Endocrinology 98:1069 (1976).
9. M. Berelowitz, K. Maeda, S. Harris, and L. A. Frohman, The effect of alterations in the pituitary-thyroid axis on hypothalamic content and in vitro release of somatostatin-like

immunoreactivity, Endocrinology 107:24 (1980).
10. J. E. Silva and P. R. Larsen, Peripheral metabolism of homologous thyrotropin in euthyroid and hypothyroid rats: acute effects of thyrotropin-releasing hormone, triiodothyronine, and thyroxine, Endocrinology 102:1783 (1978).
11. C. Y. bowers, K. L. Lee, and A. V. Schally, A study on the interaction of the thyrotropin-releasing factor and L-triiodothyronine: effects of puromycin and cycloheximide, Endocrinology 82:75 (1968).
12. W. Vale, R. Burgus, and R. Guillemin, On the mechanism of action of TRF: effects of cycloheximide and actinomycin on the release of TSH stimulated in vitro by TRF and its inhibition by thyroxine, Neuroendocrinology 3:34 (1968).
13. T. G. Gard, B. Bernstein, and P. R. Larsen, Studies on the mechanism of 3,5,3'-triiodothyronine-induced thyrotropin release in vitro, Endocrinology 108:2046 (1981).
14. R. J. Koenig, D. Senator, and P. R. Larsen, Phorbol esters as probes of the regulation of thyrotropin secretion, Biochem and Biophysical Res Com 125:353 (1984).
15. M. H. Perrone and P. M. Hinkle, Regulation of pituitary receptors for thyrotropin-releasing hormone by thyroid hormones, J Biol Chem 253:5168 (1978).
16. J. A. Gurr and I. A. Kourides, Regulation of thyrotropin biosynthesis, J Biol Chem 258:10208 (1983).
17. M. A. Shupnik and E. C. Ridgway, Triiodothyronine rapidly decreases transcription of the thyrotropin subunit genes in thyrotropic tumor explants, Endocrinology 117:1940, 1985.
18. F. E. Carr, E. C. Ridgway, and W. W. Chin, Rapid simultaneous measurement of rat α- and thyrotropin (TSH) β-subunit messenger ribonucleid acids (mRNAs) by solution hybridization: regulation of TSH subunit mRNAs by thyroid hormones, Endocrinology 117:1272 (1985).
19. J. A. Franklyn, D. F. Wood, N. J. Balfour, D. B. Ramsden, K. Docherty, W. W. Chin, and M. C. Sheppard, Effect of hypothyroidism and thyroid hormone replacement in vivo on pituitary cytoplasmic concentrations of thyrotropin-β and α-subunit messenger ribonucleic acids, Endocrinology 120:2279 (1987).

20. F. E. Carr, L. R. Need, and W. W. Chin, Isolation and characterization of the rat thyrotropin β-subunit gene, J Biol Chem 262:981 (1987).
21. O. Wolf, I. A. Kourides, and J. A. Gurr, Expression of the gene for the β subunit of mouse thyrotropin results in multiple mRNAs differing in their 5'-untranslated regions, J Biol Chem 262:16596 (1987).
22. F. E. Wondisford, S. Radovick, J. M. Moates, S. J. Usala, and B. D. Weintraub, Isolation and characterization of the human thyrotropin β-subunit gene, J Biol Chem 263:12538 (1988).
23. P. R. Larsen, J. W. Harney, and D. D. Moore, Sequences required for cell-type specific thyroid hormone regulation of rat growth hormone promoter activity, J Biol Chem 261:14373 (1986).
24. C. K. Glass, R. Franco, C. Weinberger, V. R. Albert, R. M. Evans, and M. G. Rosenfeld, A c-erb-A binding site in rat growth hormone gene mediates trans-activation by thyroid hormone, Nature 329:738 (1987).
25. R. J. Koenig, G. A. Brent, R. L. Warne, P. R. Larsen, and D. D. Moore, Thyroid hormone receptor binds to a site in the rat growth hormone promoter required for induction by thyroid hormone, Proc Natl Acad Sci USA 84:5670 (1987).
26. G. A. Brent, P. R. Larsen, J. W. Harney, R. J. Koenig, and D. D. Moore, Functional characterization of the rat growth hormone promoter elements required for induction by thyroid hormone with and without a cotransfected β type thyroid hormone receptor, J Biol Chem 264:178 (1989).
27. G. Riesco, A. Taurog, P. R. Larsen, and L. Krulich, Acute and chronic response to iodine deficiency in rats, Endocrinology 100:303 (1977).
28. P. R. Larsen, Feedback regulation of thyrotropin secretion by thyroid hormones. Thyroid-pituitary interaction. N Engl J Med 306:23 (1982).
29. J. M. Connors and G. A. Hedge, Feedback effectiveness of periodic versus constant triiodothyronine replacement, Endocrinology 106:911 (1980).
30. P. R. Larsen and R. D. Frumess, Comparison of the biological effects of thyroxine and triiodothyronine in the rat, Endocrinology 100:980 (1977).
31. J. E. Silva and P. R. Larsen, Pituitary nuclear 3,5,3'-triiodothyronine and thyrotropin secretion:

an explanation for the effect of thyroxine, Science 198:617 (1977).

32. J. E. Silva and P. R. Larsen, Contributions of plasma triiodothyronine and local thyroxine monodeiodination to triiodothyronine and nuclear triiodothyronine receptor saturation in pituitary, liver and kidney of hypothyroid rats. Further evidence relating saturation of pituitary nuclear triiodothyronine receptors and the acute inhibition of thyroid-stimulating hormone release, J Clin Invest 61:1247 (1978).
33. R. G. Cheron, M. M. Kaplan, and P. R. Larsen, Physiological and pharmacological influences on thyroxine to 3,5,3'-triiodothyronine conversion and nuclear 3,5,3'-triiodothyronine binding in rat anterior pituitary, J Clin Invest 64:1402 (1979).
34. P. R. Larsen, T. E. Dick, M. M. Markovitz, M. M. Kaplan, and T. G. Gard, Inhibition of intrapituitary thyroxine to 3,5,3'-triiodothyronine conversion prevents the acute suppression of thyrotropin release by thyroxine in hypothyroid rats, J Clin Invest 64:117 (1979).
35. P. R. Larsen, J. E. Silva, and M. M. Kaplan, Relationships between circulating and intracellular thyroid hormones: physiological and clinical implications, Endocrine Rev 2:87 (1981).
36. T. J. Visser, M. M. Kaplan, J. L. Leonard, and P. R. Larsen, Evidence for two pathways of iodothyronine 5'-deiodination in rat pituitary that differ in kinetics, propylthiouracil sensitivity, and response to hypothyroidism, J Clin Invest 71:992 (1983).
37. R. J. Koenig and A. Y. Watson, Enrichment of rat anterior pituitary cell types by metrizamide density gradient centrifugation, Endocrinology 115:317 (1984).
38. R. J. Koenig, J. L. Leonard, D. Senator, N. Rappaport, A. Y. Watson, and P. R. Larsen, Regulation of thyroxine 5'-deiodinase activity by 3,5,3'-triiodothyronine in cultured rat anterior pituitary cells, Endocrinology 115:324 (1984).
39. R. N. Riskind, J. M. Kolodny, and P. R. Larsen, The regional hypothalamic distribution of type II 5'-monodeiodinase in euthyroid and hypothyroid rats, Brain Res 420:194 (1987).

THYROID-STIMULATING HORMONE:

STRUCTURE AND FUNCTION

James A. Magner

Michael Reese Hospital

University of Chicago, Chicago, IL 60616

INTRODUCTION

Thyroid-stimulating hormone (TSH) is a pituitary-derived glycoprotein of molecular weight 28,000 that is composed of two noncovalently linked subunits, α and β. TSH is chemically related to the pituitary gonadotropins, luteinizing hormone (LH) and follicle-stimulating hormone (FSH), as well as to placental chorionic gonadotropin (CG). TSH is synthesized by thyrotropes of the anterior pituitary and stored in secretory granules. TSH is released into the circulation in a regulated manner, binds to thyroid cells and activates them to release thyroid hormones.

Since Smith[1], Allen[2] and others performed experiments in the early 20th century suggesting that the pituitary contained a thyrotrophic substance, the subunit structure of the glycoprotein hormones has been determined, and the amino acid sequences of TSH subunits from several species have been learned. In recent years great progress has been made in determining the structures of TSH α- and β-subunit genes and the chromosomal localizations and regulation of those genes. These techniques of molecular biology have also provided insights into the evolution of the glycoprotein hormones. The posttranslational processing events of TSH subunits have been elucidated in some detail, and the kinetics of the oligosaccharide processing and subcellular sites of subunit combination and processing have been studied. Studies of the secretion, metabolic clearance and bioactivity of TSH have demonstrated important biological roles for the TSH oligosaccharides. Although no glycoprotein hormone has been crystallized successfully, advanced computer techniques have allowed tertiary structures to be postulated, and use of monoclonal antibodies and other specialized techniques have allowed the function of domains of the subunits to be postulated.

Very sensitive radioimmunometric assays for TSH have come into wide use, and the physiology of TSH in man and several species has been well described. In addition to the more classic states of hyperthyroidism and primary hypothyroidism, the status of TSH in other states such as nonthyroidal illness, the syndrome of the inappropriate secretion of TSH, and central hypothyroidism has been investigated. Studies of the mechanism of action of TSH have explored the binding of TSH to thyroid plasma membranes and the activation of the adenylate cyclase-cyclic AMP system. TSH has dramatic effects on thyroid morphology, as well as on the metabolism of iodine, nucleic acids, proteins, carbohydrates and phospholipids.

EARLY STUDIES OF TSH

Several excellent reviews are available that recount the early attempts to define a pituitary thyrotrophic factor.[3-12] Many accounts of the discovery of such a factor begin by quoting Niépce or Rogowitsch.[13] Niépce performed autopsies on patients with cretinism, and in 1851 noted that seven had enlarged pituitary glands. In 1888, N. Rogowitsch performed thyroidectomies on rabbits and noted hyperplasia of the pituitaries. Although both studies demonstrated that there was some relationship between the thyroid and the pituitary gland, neither worker properly understood the phenomena. Niépce did not elaborate on his result, whereas Rogowitsch thought that the pituitary might be changed to take over the thyroid's function - the "vicarious function" hypothesis. It was not until the mid-20th century that the concept of the pituitary-thyroid axis was well formulated by Hoskins[14] and others.[15,16]

In 1912, a young anatomist at Berkeley, Philip E. Smith, chose to study amphibians (as a matter of economy) and attempted to learn the effect of pituitary removal in frogs. By 1916 he had noted that tadpoles without pituitaries grew slowly, had atrophied thyroid glands, and did not metamorphose. Smith correctly attributed this failure of metamorphosis to the atrophy of the thyroid, and not to the direct action of the hypophysis. Working independently at the University of Kansas, Bennet M. Allen performed hypophysectomies on tadpoles and noted similar results. By chance, Smith and Allen met in 1916 and discovered that each had been doing the same sort of work. Both presented data at the same meeting of the Western Society of Naturalists in August 1916[13], and their papers were published in the same volume of _Science_.[1,2] Smith went on to show that the pituitary secreted a substance that maintained thyroid size and metamorphosis in frogs, and that injection of a crude bovine pituitary extract could preserve the thyroid in hypophysectomized tadpoles.[17] He later demonstrated that injections of rat or bovine pituitary partially repaired the thyroid in hypophysectomized rats.[18]

In spite of the pioneering studies by Smith and Allen, credit for the discovery of a pituitary thyrotrophic factor is often given to Leo Loeb of St. Louis, or Max Aron of Strasbourg. Both reported independently in 1929 that crude extracts of bovine anterior pituitaries caused the thyroid glands of guinea pigs to enlarge and show histologic signs of cell growth and secretion.[19,20] Both referred to Smith's work and recognized that they were extending it to mammals; neither claimed proof of a specific thyrotrophic substance distinct from the growth- and gonad-stimulating activities that had been described by others.

During the 1930's a number of workers used biochemical means to prepare enriched samples of the thyrotrophic substance, an era when bioassays were difficult and imprecise. The Junkmann-Schöeller assay[21], for example, was based on histologic changes in the guinea pig thyroid, and these were widely interpretable and difficult to quantify. Roy O. Greep and colleagues[22] noted in 1935 that by changing the precipitant conditions, the thyrotrophic activity shifted from the LH-containing fractions to the FSH-containing fractions. Although this demonstrated that TSH was a separate pituitary hormone, the actual purification of TSH had to await the application of ion-exchange column chromatography.

In 1957 Peter Condliffe and Robert Bates at the NIH used diethylaminoethyl cellulose to generate enriched preparations of TSH.[23] John Pierce and colleagues, working independently at UCLA, used ion-exchange chromatography to enrich TSH activity. Both laboratories benefited by using the better McKenzie bioassay.[24] Finally, in 1969, Liao, working in Pierce's laboratory, prepared highly purified TSH.[25] Earlier attempts to determine the amino acid sequences of the glycoprotein hormones had failed because the subunit structure of these hormones had not been recognized; amino-terminal valine as well as phenylalanine was reported.[26] In 1967, Papkoff and Samy[27] achieved a major advance when they recognized that ovine LH consists of two nonidentical subunits, and that subunit combination is required for hormonal activity. In 1969 Condiffe[28] performed gel-filtration studies on reduced S-carboxymethyl TSH in which the presence of more than one peptide chain was suspected. Unequivocal recognition of the subunit nature of TSH by Pierce and colleagues resulted from an unusual combination of dissociation under one set of conditions and fractionation under another.[29] By 1971, Pierce and colleagues had defined the α- and β-subunits of TSH and their amino acid sequences, and had demonstrated that the β-subunit determined the biological specificity of the heterodimer.[29,30]

MOLECULAR BIOLOGY OF THE TSH SUBUNITS

Although it is true that the information required to produce a

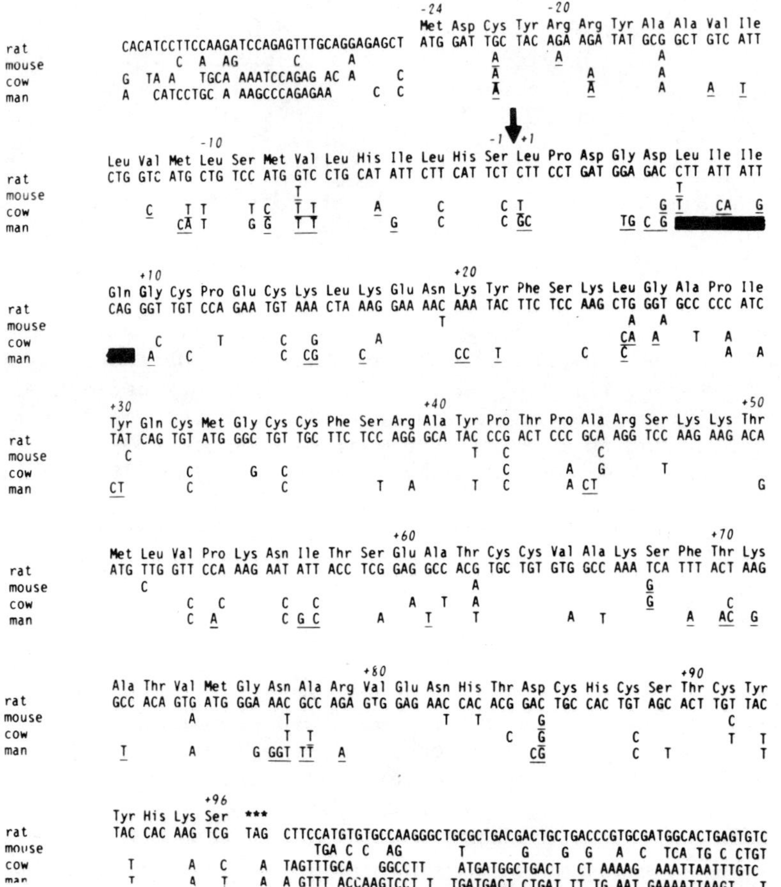

Fig. 1. Nucleotide sequences of cDNAs encoding the α-subunit of rat, mouse, bovine, and human glycoprotein hormones. The top nucleotide sequence represents the cDNA encoding rat pre-α-subunit, and the deduced amino acid sequence is shown directly above the nucleotide sequence. Numbers above the protein sequence indicate amino acid residues (-24 to -1, leader peptide; +1 to +96, α-subunit apoprotein). For comparison of the other sequences with that of the rat, different bases are indicated, and a blank space is present if a given nucleotide is identical with the corresponding one in the rat. Underlined nucleotides in the latter three sequences denote nucleotide substitutions that also result in amino acid substitutions. Solid arrow, site of leader peptide cleavage; ***, signal for termination of translation. The solid bar spanning 12 nucleotides in the human α-subunit cDNA represents a deleted segment of DNA occurring late in mammalian evolution. Reproduced with permission from Chin.[41]

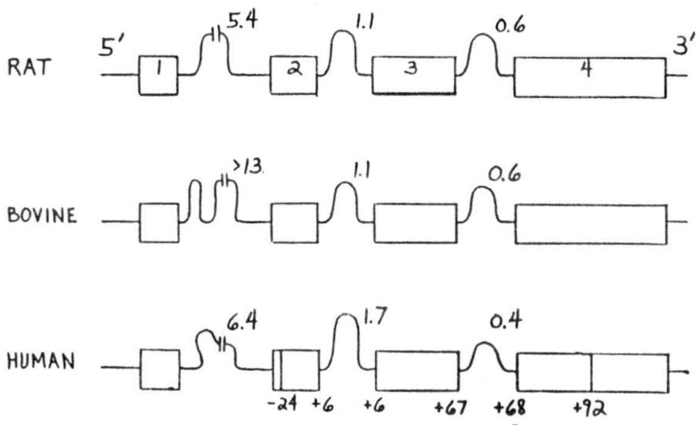

FIG. 2. Structure of the genes that encode the α-subunits of rat, bovine, and human glycoprotein hormones.

particular protein is encoded in the DNA in one or more genes, recent advances have disclosed that there may be regions of excess DNA interspersed between the DNA regions that actually code for amino acids in the final product.[31 32] These regions of excess DNA are called introns, while the coding sections of a gene are called exons. Both coding and noncoding regions are transcribed to produce a large precursor RNA. This large mRNA must then have the introns cut out, and the remaining segments spliced together. Additional required modifications include polyadenylation at the 3' end of the mRNA, and alteration of the 5' end of the mRNA, called "capping," that allows efficient translation.[33] The mature mRNA then is released into the cytoplasm and binds to ribosomes. Nascent secretory or membrane proteins generally contain a sequence of 20 to 30 hydrophobic amino acids termed the leader or signal sequence. This sequence may bind to a signal recognition particle to enable the nascent protein to move from the cytoplasmic space into the lumen of the rough endoplasmic reticulum.[34-39] All of these early biosynthetic events have been described for both the α- and β-subunits of TSH in several species. Several excellent reviews concerning the structure and expression of the thyrotropin subunit genes have appeared recently.[40-44]

THE α-SUBUNIT GENE

Fiddes and Goodman[45] first cloned and sequenced the complementary DNA (cDNA) of the human α-subunit in 1979, and two years later reported the gene structure.[46] The structures of α-subunit genes and mRNAs, and of the precursor proteins that they encode, have now been determined in several species. The mRNAs for the α-subunits are approximately 800 base pairs in size and each encodes a translation product of about 14,000 molecular weight that contains 116 to 120 amino acid residues.[45,47-49] Each product contains a 24-amino-acid residue amino-terminal signal peptide, and a 92 to 96 amino acid residue apoprotein. Each species possesses a single gene for the

α-subunit, which is generally expressed as a single form of mRNA in the pituitary gland or the placenta. Godine et al.[50], however, found evidence for two types of mRNAs encoding the α-subunit in the human placenta, perhaps due to the use of different promoters or alternative RNA processing.

A comparison of the cDNA sequences of rat, mouse, cow, and human α-subunits is shown in Fig. 1. The homology varies from 76% (human-rat) to 96% (rat-mouse).[45,47-49] Several regions are highly conserved, especially the region that codes for amino acid residues 10 to 50, a domain of the α-subunit believed to be in contact with the β-subunit. The human α-subunit is 4 amino acid residues smaller than the others due to a 12-nucleotide-long deleted segment of DNA that apparently occurred late in mammalian evolution. Chin et al.[51] showed that this gene segment deletion occurs at the site of one of the introns in the human α-subunit gene.

The genes encoding the α-subunits in the cow, human and rat have been isolated and characterized.[46,52-54] the genes are large: cow 13.7 kilobases (kb), human 9.4 kb, rat 7.7 kb. The organization of these genes is shown in Fig. 2. Non-coding sequences make up the bulk of each gene. The placement of the introns is identical in the α-subunit genes, although the sizes of the introns differ. One of the introns interrupts the codon for the sixth amino acid. Examination of the 5′ flanking region of the bovine α-subunit gene revealed characteristic promoter elements as well as an AT-rich area that may be important in control of the gene.[53] A cyclic AMP responsive element, containing the core 8-bp motif T (G or T) ACGTCA required for the induction of gene transcription by cAMP, is present in the region of the a-subunit gene between residues -146 and -128. Recently Bokar et al.[55] studied a mechanism for cAMP-regulated transcription common to a number of genes having the above core motif. Regulation of these genes appears to involve a nuclear factor or factors that have been conserved across tissue and species lines. The 3′ untranslated region of the α-subunit contains regions that differ substantially between mouse and rat, yet are nearly identical in human and cow.[49] The α-subunit gene has been localized to the long arm of chromosome 6 in man[56], and chromosome 4 in the mouse.[56,57]

THE MOUSE AND RAT TSH β-SUBUNIT GENES

The TSH β-subunits in several species are initially synthesized as precursors of approximately 17,000 molecular weight.[58,59] Maurer et al.[60] cloned the cDNA for the β-subunit of bovine thyrotropin. Gurr et al.[61] cloned the cDNA of mouse TSH β-subunit, and Chin et al.[62] and Croyle et al.[63] cloned the cDNA of rat TSH β-subunit. Fig. 3 shows the cDNA and deduced protein sequences of mouse and rat TSH β-subunit mRNAs. Each mRNA is 700 bases in size and encodes a precursor protein of 138 amino acids with 20 residues constituting a

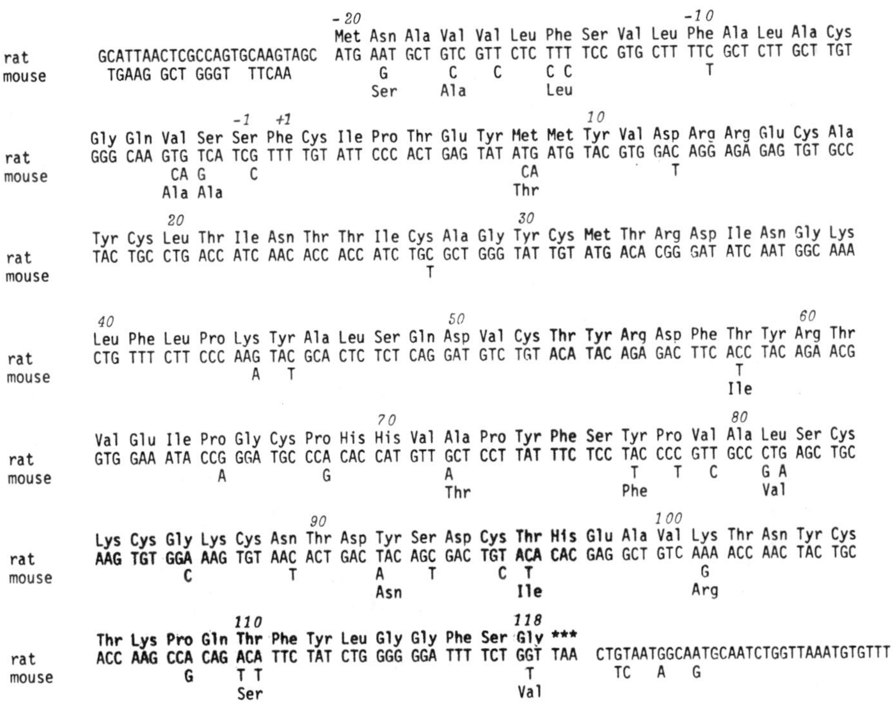

Fig. 3. Nucleotide sequences of cDNAs encoding the β-subunit of rat and mouse TSH. For notation, see legend to Fig. 1. Reproduced with permission from Chin.[41]

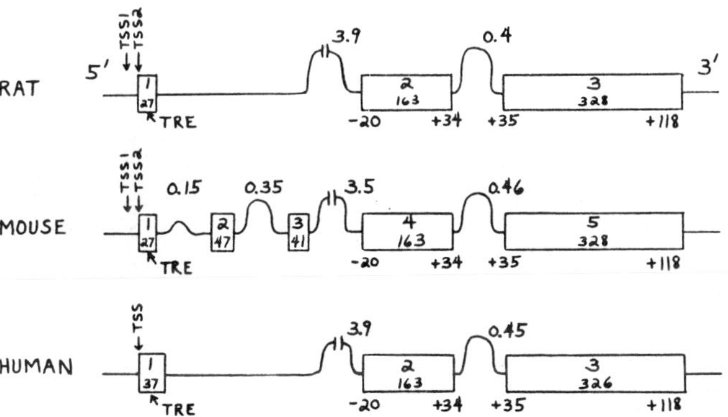

Fig. 4. Structures of the genes that encode the β-subunits of rat, mouse, and human TSH. See text for details.

signal peptide and 118 residues forming the β-subunit apoprotein. Thus, the predicted β-subunit apoproteins are slightly larger than those previously reported in other species (cow, pig and human). The mouse and rat TSH β-subunit cDNAs show 91% homology. There is a long sequence from residue +9 to residue +57 that is identical, and most of the few amino acid substitutions elsewhere are conservative in nature.

The rat TSH β-subunit gene (Fig. 4) is approximately 5 kb in size, and contains 3 exons and 2 introns.[63,64] There are two tandem promoters and two corresponding transcriptional start sites for the rat β-subunit gene in contrast to a single one in the rat α-subunit gene.[64] The TATA elements representing the promoter sites are present in two tandem copies located 43 base pairs apart in the 5′ flanking region. Carr et al.[64,65] have provided a variety of evidence that these promoters are differentially regulated by thyroid hormones; the transcript resulting from use of the downstream start site (mRNA 2) was more readily altered by thyroid hormones than was the transcript derived from the first start site (mRNA 1). The mouse TSH β-subunit gene also has dual transcriptional start sites and promoters, but it is unclear whether or not there is differential thyroid-hormone regulation of the transcripts in the mouse.[66,67]

Carr et al.[68] used several fragments of the 5′ flanking and coding regions of the rat TSH β-subunit gene to perform a deletion-mutation analysis. They identified a putative thyroid-hormone-responsive element (TRE) located near the downstream transcriptional start site in exon 1. The region is similar to the TRE recently identified in the rat growth hormone gene.[69-72] Additional experiments using thyroid-hormone receptor binding studies are in progress to establish this sequence as an authentic element crucial for the inhibition of transcription by thyroid hormone.[73] The thyroid hormone-receptor family encoded by the c-erbAs, however, has multiple members with varying affinities for thyroid hormone.[74-77] Recently Lazar et al.[78] isolated a novel rat c-erbA cDNA, r-erbA α-2, and its <u>in vitro</u> protein product. This 55,000 dalton protein binds a putative T_3-responsive sequence from the rat growth hormone gene, but the protein does not bind T_3. There appeared to be tissue-specific production of this product, and it was particularly abundant in brain. In future studies, Chin[44] proposes to examine the interactions of various specific thyroid hormone receptors or related proteins with the TRE in the rat TSH β-subunit gene.

In 1988, Gordon et al.[79] reported the structure and nucleotide sequence of the gene encoding the β-subunit of mouse thyrotropin. The mouse TSH β-subunit gene has been localized to chromosome 3.[57] The gene is 5 kb in size and consists of five exons and four introns.[79] The 5′ untranslated region of the mRNA is encoded (except for a single nucleotide) by exons 1, 2 and 3. The protein coding regions are encoded by exons 4 and 5 while the 3′ untranslated region is entirely contained in exon 5. Two transcriptional start sites, near two TATAAA sequences, were detected, but 99% of transcripts initiate at the downstream site. Transcription from both start sites was regulated by thyroidal status. Sequences homologous with putative thyroidresponse elements and cyclic AMP-responsive elements are present in the 5′ flanking region.

The organization of the mouse TSH β-subunit gene, with five exons and four introns, differs from that of other species, which have three exons and two introns (Fig. 4). A comparison between the nucleotide sequences of the mouse and rat TSH β-subunit genes reveals a high degree of homology, especially in the 5′ flanking region, in which 227 of 237 nucleotides, 95.8%, are identical in the two genes. In each rodent gene there are two sequences at positions -29 and -69 which resemble the consensus TATA box and which occur 29 bp upstream from each of the two RNA start sites at positions +1 and -40. A putative thyroid inhibitory element is present in the mouse TSH β-subunit at position -64 to -55 and consists of a 10 bp region with 80% homology with an inhibitory element found in the rat growth hormone gene.[80] This nucleotide sequence has been conserved in the rat TSH β-subunit gene,[63,64] but it has not yet been proven that its function has been conserved. A putative thyroid response element is present in the mouse TSH β-subunit gene within the first exon, positions +15 to +23. Finally, sequences in this gene at positions -191 to -183 and -593 to -584 are similar to a cyclic AMP responsive element in the rat somatostatin gene[81] and the rat phosphoenolpyruvate carboxykinase gene.[82]

THE HUMAN TSH β-SUBUNIT GENE

In 1985 Hayashizaki et al.[83] reported the cloning and sequence of a large portion of the human TSH β-subunit gene; Whitfield et al.[84] also reported a small part of the sequence. The Japanese group reported that the deduced precursor protein consists of 138 amino acids; a 20 amino acid signal peptide is followed by 112 amino acids expected from previous chemical studies of human TSH β-subunit, followed by an additional 6 hydrophobic amino acids that presumably are eliminated posttranslationally. One intron of 460 bp was detected, but an additional intron could not be ruled out because the 5′ and 3′ flanking regions were not well characterized.[83] Watanabe et al.[355] recently expressed the cDNAs for TSH α- and β-subunits in Chinese hamster ovary cells, and demonstrated that the hTSH secreted into the medium was bioactive in an _in vitro_ adenylate cyclase assay.

In 1988 Wondisford et al.[85] more completely characterized the gene (Fig. 4). They found three exons separated by two introns of 3.9 and 0.45 kb. Exons 2 and 3 in the mouse TSH β-subunit gene are not found in the human gene due to a lack of consensus sequences important in exon splicing. Moreover, exon 1 in the human gene contains only one transcriptional start site, unlike both the rat and mouse genes which each contain two sites. The genomic structure of the more 5' TATA box has been altered in humans, and the first exon in the human gene is longer than the corresponding exon in the mouse due to a 9 bp insertion. The human gene appears to have a thyroid response element at position +23 to +37 in the first exon. Wondisford et al.[85] speculate that the location of this putative control sequence downstream from the start of transcription may explain the down-regulation of this gene by thyroid hormone.

Miyai et al.[86,87] have recently reported an interesting clinical application of molecular biology approaches. In 1971 Miyai et al.[88] had been the first to report a case of congenital isolated TSH deficiency. The proposita were two sisters with congenital nongoitrous hypothyroidism, and were products of a consanguineous marriage. Serum TSH, assessed by bioassay and radioimmunoassay, was undetectable in the patients but was normal in their parents, suggesting a defect with autosomal recessive inheritance. Analysis of chromosome 1, the location of the human TSH β-subunit gene,[89,90] using a high-resolution chromosome banding technique failed to show any major alterations.[86] Genomic DNA Southern blot hybridization was performed using peripheral leukocyte DNA, but no gross abnormalities were noted, suggesting that any mutation in the TSH β-subunit gene must involve a very small region. Pituitary thyrotrophs were believed to be present in these patients because serum free TSH α-subunits were elevated in serum in the hypothyroid state, and increased after TRH administration.

It was not until 1988, when these patients' TSH β-subunit gene was cloned, that the nature of the gene defect was learned.[87] A single point mutation in the gene caused GGA to become AGA, and an amino acid was altered from Gly to Arg at position 129. This substitution is in the so-called "CAGY" region, which is conserved in all glycoprotein hormones and may play a role in TSH biosynthesis. When normal α and mutant β mRNA were injected into _Xenopus_ oocytes, intact TSH was not produced, unlike control experiments[91] using normal α and normal β mRNAs. Thus, these Japanese workers have described a type of familial congenital hypothyroidism due to isolated TSH deficiency which is an autosomal recessive disease due to a point mutation of the human TSH β-subunit gene.

REGULATION OF TSH SUBUNIT GENE EXPRESSION

Studies of the regulation of the TSH subunit genes have been summarized in several recent reviews.[41-44,92,93] Because the genes for the α- and β- subunits of TSH are located on different chromosomes, it is clear that there must be some degree of coordinated regulation of these genes so that intact hormone may be produced, yet substantial evidence suggests that there is differential control of gene expression. The effect of thyroid status on serum TSH levels was first studied in whole animals, but has more recently been studied in pituitary tissue, as well as in a useful model system, the mouse transplantable thyrotropic tumor, originally developed by Furth, et al.[94]

Early studies in several laboratories suggested that thyrotropin biosynthesis, as well as secretion, is augmented during hypothyroidism and inhibited by excess thyroid hormone.[95-100] Unbalanced production of α- and β- subunits of TSH (as well as of other glycoprotein hormones) occurred in certain circumstances both in vivo and in vitro.[101-108] Treatment of hypothyroid mice with T_4 caused a divergent inhibition of α- and TSH β-subunits.[109]

With the availability of specific cDNA probes encoding the α- and β-subunits of mouse and rat TSH, the influence of thyroid hormones on levels of subunit mRNAs was examined. Mice bearing thyrotropic tumors were treated with supraphysiologic doses of T_3 subcutaneously, and serum TSH levels declined rapidly within hours.[110-112] TSH α- and β-subunit mRNAs declined to 40% and 20% of their basal levels by 4 hours. Thus, T_3 given to these mice appeared to rapidly lower the steady-state levels of the subunit mRNAs in the thyrotrophs, and the effect was apparently greater on TSH β- than α-subunits. Negative regulation of TSH subunit mRNAs has also been reported in the pituitary tissues of euthyroid and hypothyroid mice and rats.[111-116]

Levels of mRNAs of TSH subunits have also been evaluated during withdrawal of thyroid hormones. In the rat in vivo there was a tenfold increase in pituitary TSH β-subunit mRNA, but only a threefold increase in α-subunit mRNA, 14 days after thyroidectomy, and these changes were reversed by T_3 treatment.[116] Similar results were also observed after treating rats with propylthiouracil for 10 weeks.[117] A paradoxical rise in serum TSH and TSH response to TRH has been reported in profoundly hypothyroid rats and man during the initial treatment period with thyroid hormone.[117-119] A biphasic dose-response relationship for inhibition by thyroid hormones has also been shown for TSH-producing cells in vitro[99], but this effect has not been observed in some other studies.[111,113,116]

Because steady-state levels of mRNAs are determined by both rates of gene transcription and mRNA turnover, nuclear "run-on" assays were performed to determine the contribution of the former. Shupnik et al.[112] reported that T_3 treatment rapidly decreased the transcription of both α- and TSH β-subunit genes. Supraphysiologic doses of T_3 reduced α- and TSH β-subunit gene transcription rates to 70% and 40% of basal levels after 30 minutes, and to 15% and 5% of basal levels after 4h. This inhibition of transcription occurred even in the presence of the protein synthesis inhibitor, cycloheximide, and was proportional to the degree of occupancy of nuclear thyroid hormone receptors, suggesting that the negative effect of T_3 on TSH subunit gene transcriptional is direct.[120] Earlier studies[100 121 122] suggested that the suppressive effects of thyroid hormone on TSH secretion were mediated by an inhibitory protein or a transferable factor that accumulated in the medium of T_3-treated cells. Thus, a clear distinction must be made between T_3 effects on gene transcription and T_3 effects on TSH secretion.

In 1986 Shupnik et al.[123] reported that TRH stimulated and dopamine inhibited the transcription of TSH subunit genes. TRH treatment of pituitary cells in vitro increased transcription of the α- and β-subunit genes of TSH three- to five-fold, and cytoplasmic levels of the mRNAs were increased. Franklyn et al.[124] also demonstrated a stimulatory effect of TRH on rat TSH β-subunit mRNA levels, and also noted a stimulatory effect of forskolin, an agent that stimulates adenylate cyclase activity. In contrast, Lippman et al.[125] were unable to demonstrate any effect of TRH on TSH subunit mRNA levels, and suggested that the regulatory effects of TRH are confined to the posttranslational processing and the release of TSH from thyrotropes.

Regulation of TSH subunit gene expression by estrogen, testosterone and glucocorticoids has been investigated in only a preliminary fashion. Estrogen appears to augment the inhibitory action of thyroid hormones[126], and testosterone appears to blunt the influence of hypothyroidism on TSH α- and β-subunit mRNA levels.[127] The physiological relevance of such observations remains uncertain.

POSTTRANSLATIONAL PROCESSING OF TSH

The outstanding feature of the glycoprotein hormones is their relatively high carbohydrate content; the α- and β-subunits of TSH are approximately 21% and 12% carbohydrate by weight, respectively. In addition to the novel information gleaned by techniques of molecular biology, as reviewed in prior sections, any serious discussion of TSH must review how the oligosaccharides are added to the subunit precursors and how they are processed posttranslationally. In fact, various lines of evidence indicate that the oligosaccharides of the glycoprotein hormones modulate their biologic activity, and play other important roles as well. In the following sections I will review early studies of immunoactive TSH subunits, including cell-free translation studies of subunit mRNAs as well as studies of the biosynthesis of TSH in intact cells. Over the years a more clear picture of the posttranslational processing of TSH has emerged, including insights into the subcellular compartmentalization of various processng steps, and the regulation of processing. Finally, investigations into the roles played by TSH oligosaccharides will be reviewed.

LARGE-MOLECULAR WEIGHT FORMS OF TSH

Early observations of large-molecular weight immunoreactive forms of TSH and gonadotropins raised the possibility that these hormones were synthesized from a common prohormone containing both the α- and β-subunits, analogous to proinsulin. It now seems clear that these large forms represent molecules of uncertain physiologic significance. Several workers had noted a variable amount of immunoreactive highmolecular weight forms of pituitary glycoprotein hormones in both pituitary extracts and serum. Klug and Adelman[128] described an age-related accumulation of unusually large forms of TSH in the rat. Kourides et al.[129] described two patients with a high-molecular weight TSH-β immunoreactive material that was the predominant form of TSH-β in the serum. Spitz et al.[127] described a clinically euthyroid man with only a high-molecular weight form of TSH in his serum; this TSH bound normally to receptors _in vitro_, but had low bioactivity (4% of normal) documented by decreased stimulation of the adenylate cyclase of human thyroid membranes. It is now believed that these large forms of TSH represent aberrant forms that have aggregated[131,132], or possibly storage forms of the hormone not normally seen in serum.

Instances of highly unbalanced or even isolated production of α- or β-subunits, both _in vivo_ and _in vitro_, suggested that the subunits were derived from different genes rather than from a prohormone form of TSH analogous to proinsulin. This became even more clear when separate mRNAs for α- and β-subunits of TSH were detected and studied in cell-free systems.

In early studies, mRNAs were extracted from mouse thyrotropic tumors and translated in wheat germ or reticulocyte lysate cell-free systems that were devoid of enzymes necessary for the proteolytic cleavage of polypeptide precursors or glycosylation.[133-138] The major cell-free translation product, representing up to half of the total ^{35}S-methionine-labeled proteins synthesized, had an apparent molecular weight of 14,000 to 17,000, depending on the conditions of the gel electrophoresis. This protein was shown to be closely related to standard TSH α-subunit on the basis of immunoprecipitation and tryptic peptide analysis. Although it did not contain carbohydrate, its molecular weight was about 3,000 daltons greater than the apoprotein portion of standard α-subunit, consistent with the presence of a signal peptide. This precursor form of α-subunit could be cleaved of the signal peptide and glycosylated when mRNA was translated in frog oocytes, or by the addition of microsomal membranes during translation in cell-free systems. By using a variety of labeled amino acid precursors, Giudice et al.[134] established a partial amino terminal sequence of this precursor form of α-subunit. There were substantial homologies noted among the signal sequences of mouse, human and bovine α-subunits, although the signal peptidase apparently cleaved between different amino acids in the different species.

The identification of the TSH β-subunit precursor in cell-free translation mixtures of mouse tumor mRNA proved more difficult. This difficulty arose in part because of the lesser amounts of the β-precursor synthesized as compared with α-precursor. Also, the β-precursor was poorly reactive with antisera raised against standard glycosylated β-subunits. Direct immunologic identification of the β-precursor required use of an antiserum directed at determinants in the primary structure of denatured, reduced, carboxymethyl-TSH β-subunit.[135] Gel electrophoresis of the β-precursor disclosed an apparent molecular weight of 15,500, or 2,500 daltons greater than the apoprotein portion of standard TSH β-subunit, consistent with the presence of a signal peptide. Kourides et al.[136] and Chin et al.[133] also successfully detected the precursor form of TSH β-subunit. Discrepancies in the molecular size of the β-precursor initially reported by different laboratories have now been resolved by modern molecular biology techniques, as discussed in a prior section.

BIOSYNTHESIS OF TSH IN INTACT CELL SYSTEMS

The cell-free mRNA translation studies just described were important to define the initial precursor forms of TSH subunits, since these forms are rapidly processed in vivo. Studies of TSH biosynthesis in intact cells, however, were necessary to elucidate the steps of posttranslational processing of TSH, including the glycosylation and combination of TSH subunits, and the sequential processing of the oligosaccharides.

Initial studies of TSH biosynthesis in primary cultures of dispersed mouse thyrotropic tumor cells used gel chromatography under nondenaturing conditions to distinguish the intact hormone from free subunits.[139] In labeling studies using ^{35}S-methionine, the earliest α-subunit form identified intracellularly during a 10-minute pulse was smaller than standard α but was converted to higher molecular weight α forms during a 60-minute chase period with excess unlabeled methionine; only this higher molecular weight form of α-subunit was found in intact TSH. Excess free α-subunits and TSH, but not free β-subunits, appeared in the media between 60 and 120 minutes of the chase period and were slightly larger than the respective intracellular forms.

TSH biosynthesis was studied subsequently using improved techniques including immunoprecipitation of TSH subunits, and analysis using sodium dodecyl sulfate (SDS) polyacrylamide gradient gel electrophoresis under reducing conditions.[140-143] After incubation of mouse thyrotrophic tumor tissue with ^{35}S-methionine for 10-minutes, most α-subunits were of molecular weight 18,000, while only a few were 21,000 daltons. When the pulse incubation was followed by chase incubations of variable length, the 18,000 form of α-subunit was progressively converted to the 21,000 form. After treatment with endoglycosidase H, both the 18,000 and 21,000 molecular weight forms of α-subunit were converted to an 11,000 form[141,143], consistent with the weight of the apoprotein portion of standard α-subunit. These data suggested that the 11,000 dalton, 18,000 dalton, and 21,000 dalton forms of the α-subunit have zero, one, and two asparagine-linked oligosaccharides, respectively.[143]

These experiments also demonstrated that ^{35}S-methionine-labeled β-subunits accumulated as an 18,000 dalton form that was converted to an 11,000 dalton form after endoglycosidase H treatment. Thus, it was concluded that the 11,000 and 18,000 dalton forms had zero and one asparagine-linked oligosaccharide units, respectively.[143] About 20% of the β-subunits had combined with excess α-subunits after a 20-minute pulse incubation. Use of subcellular fractionation techniques disclosed that combination of α- and β-subunits began in the rough endoplasmic reticulum (RER), and combining subunits had high-mannose, endoglycosidase H-sensitive oligosaccharides.[143] Interestingly, combination of LH α- and β-subunits at very early times of pulse labeling has been reported also, but subcellular fractionation techniques were not used to isolate RER-associated heterodimers.[144] TSH subunit precursors were processed slowly to forms with "mature" complex oligosaccharides that were resistant to endoglycosidase H.[141,143] TSH and excess free α-subunits, but no free β-subunits, were released into the medium after 60 to 240-minutes chase. The secreted species mostly had endoglycosidase H-resistant oligosaccharides.

Various lines of evidence had suggested that secreted free α-subunits had a slighly higher molecular weight than the form of α-subunit that combined with β-subunits[132,139-143], and this had been noted in studies of glycoprotein hormones other than TSH as well. In 1983 Parsons et al.[145] reported that the free α-subunit derived from bovine pituitaries is glycosylated at an additional site, the threonine at position 43. This threonine is located in a domain of the α-subunit believed to contact the β-subunit during heterodimer formation.[40] Thus, free α-subunits bearing this O-linked oligosaccharide are no longer able to bind β-subunits. It remains unclear whether the O-linked oligosaccharide is added to a subpoplation of α-subunits to keep them from binding β-subunits during biosynthesis, implying a regulatory role, or whether the O-linked oligosaccharide is merely added to excess α-subunits that have this domain exposed because limiting quantities of β-subunits have been exhausted.

Studies of hCG biosynthesis similar to those described above for TSH have been performed using choriocarcinoma cells or human placental extracts.[146-150] Biosynthesis of the α-subunit occurs in a similar manner, including O-glycosylation. The choriogonadotropin β-subunit is synthesized in a somewhat different manner because it contains two (rather than one) asparagine-linked oligosaccharides as well as carboxy-terminal O-linked oligosaccharides. Another major difference is that excess choriogonadotropin β-subunits as well as excess α-subunits are released by cells.

HIGH-MANNOSE OLIGOSACCHARIDES OF TSH SUBUNIT PRECURSORS

A number of studies in recent years have shown that nascent TSH subunit pepetides are cotranslationally glycosylated with precursor oligosaccharides rich in mannose; these are subsequently trimmed and other sugar residues are then added to make complex-type asparagine-linked oligosaccharides. A generalized scheme for this type of post-translational processing is illustrated in Fig. 5. In 1970 Behrens and Leloir[151] demonstrated that hepatocytes contain lipid-linked oligosaccharides that serve as intermediates in glycoprotein biosynthesis. The oliosaccharide $(glucose)_3$ $(mannose)_9$ (N-acetylglucosamine)$_2$, abbreviated Glc_3 Man_9 $GlcNAc_2$, is preassembled in the RER linked by phosphates at the reducing terminus to a long organic molecule containing approximately 20 polyprene units, the dolichol phosphate carrier. Asparagine residues in nascent peptides destined to become glycosylated in an N-linked fashion are present in the sequence (asparagine)-(X)-(serine or threonine). There is a cotranslational *en bloc* transfer of the oligosaccharide from the dolichol carrier to the asparagine in the nascent chain.[152] The first two glucose residues are then rapidly trimmed, followed by cleavage of the third glucose. Mannose residues are then progressively cleaved until a "core" unit remains, followed by addition of GlcNAc and other residues to build complex forms.

Tunicamycin is a drug that inhibits the formation of the oligosaccharide-dolichol carrier precursors, and thereby prevents glycosylation of asparagine residues in nascent proteins.[153] Tunicamycin in doses of 1 to 5 ug/ml caused the appearance of new forms of TSH α- and β-subunits of about 11,000 to 12,000 daltons[140]; these forms incorporated ^{35}S-methionine but not ^{3}H-glucosamine, confirming that they were not glycosylated. These nonglycosylated TSH subunits were subject to intracellular aggregation and proteolytic degradation, presumably because the nascent peptides had not folded properly, and correct internal disulfide bonding had not been achieved.[132,154] Thus, nascent TSH subunits that had never been glycosylated due to the actions of tunicamycin failed to fold properly, and α- and β-subunit combination did not occur. This contrasts with the finding that deglycosylation by enzymes or chemical means of mature secreted TSH does not prevent subunit combination. The explanation for this apparent paradox is that the mature subunits have already folded and have had internal disulfide bonds stabilize their conformations to a degree necessary for subunit binding.

In contrast to the rapid (less than 30 min) processing of many different glycoproteins thus far studied, the high-mannose oligosacc-

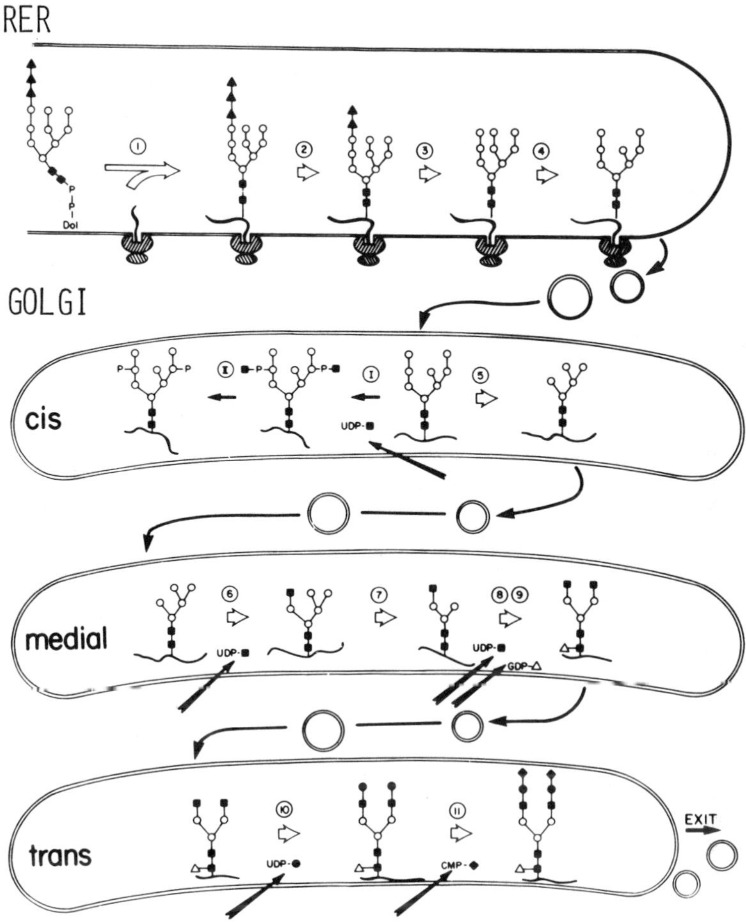

Fig. 5. Schematic pathway of oligosaccharide processing on newly synthesized glycoproteins. The reactions are catalyzed by the following enzymes: (1) oligosaccharyltransferase, (2) α-glucosidase I, (3) α-glucosidase II, (4) ER α1,2-mannosidase, (I) N-acetylglucosaminylphosphotransferase, (II) N-acetylglucosamine-I-phosphodiester α-N-acetylglucosaminidase, (5) Golgi α-mannosidase I, (6) N-acetylglucosaminyltransferase I, (7) Golgi α-mannosidase II, (8) N-acetylglucosaminyltransferase II, (9) fucosyltransferase, (10) galactosyltransferase, (11) sialyltransferase. The symbols represent: ■, N-acetylglucosamine; ○, mannose; ▲, glucose; △, fucose; ●, galactose; ◆, sialic acid. Reproduced with permission from Kornfeld and Kornfeld.[156]

harides of the TSH subunits are much more slowly processed.[132,141,155,156] Using mouse thyrotrophic tumor cells, Weintraub et al.[132] found that after an 11-minute pulse nearly all of the intracellular α- and TSH β-subunits were of the high-mannose type. After 30 minutes of chase only a few α-subunits in cells developed complex, endoglycosidase H-resistant oligosaccharides. The proportion of intracellular α-subunits of complex type increased progressively with time, but even after 18h chase reached only 76%. There was also a time-dependent increase in intracellular β-subunits of complex type. Secretion of TSH and α-subunits did not begin until about 60 minutes, and media species were predominantly of complex type.

Metabolic pulse-chase labeling studies employing ^{3}H-mannose, rather than radiolabeled amino acids, have provided substantial new information about TSH high-mannose oligosaccharide biosynthesis and processing.[155-157] After incubation of thyrotrophic tumor cells with ^{3}H-mannose for 60-minutes, the lipid-linked oligosaccharides were extracted from the cells; these precursor oligosaccharides bound to the dolichol carrier were found to be predominantly $Glc_{3-2}Man_9GlcNAc_2$, $Man_{9-8}GlcNAc_2$ and $Man_5GlcNAc_2$.[156] These species are generally similar to lipid-linked oligosaccharides extracted from hepatocytes and other cell types.[152,153] After short 10-minute incubations of thyrotrophs with ^{3}H-mannose, $Glc_3Man_9GlcNAc_2$ oligosaccharides were detected bound to some cellular glycoproteins, but this very early glucose-containing precursor was not found linked to nascent TSH subunits[155-157], suggesting either that TSH subunits were initially glycosylated with a non-glucosylated precursor, or that the glucose residues were very rapidly trimmed from the TSH subunits. It was only in 1988, when Stannard et al.[158] employed the glucosidase inhibitor 1-deoxynojirimycin that it became clear that very rapid glucose trimming was the more likely explanation. In the earlier studies[155-157] it was also apparent that there was differential processing of the high-mannose units of TSH as compared to free α-subunits, which also differed from that of the bulk of glycoproteins in these cells. For instance, the rate of trimming of a mannose residue from $Man_9GlcNAc_2$ to produce $Man_8GlcNAc_2$ units appeared to be much faster for free α-subunits; after a 60-minute incubation with ^{3}H-mannose, $Man_8GlcNAc_2$ units predominated in free α-subunits, whereas $Man_9GlcNAc_2$ units still predominated in TSH heterodimers and in other cellular glycoproteins. This transient intermediate, $Man_8GlcNAc_2$, also seemed to accumulate to a greater degree in free α-subunits as compared to TSH or other cellular glycoproteins. Trimming the three glucose and the first mannose residues of the high-mannose oligosaccharides clearly occurred in the rough endoplasmic reticulum, as documented by subcellular fractionation techniques.[155] Accumulation of the transient intermediate $Man_5GlcNAc_2$ was also particularly marked for free α-subunits as compared with TSH or other cellular glycoproteins, and was best recognized in subcellular fractions enriched in Golgi elements.[155]

It had been reported in an earlier subcellular fractionation study by Magner et al.[143] that combination of α- and TSH β-subunits began in the rough endoplasmic reticulum at early times, and that these combining subunits had endoglycosidase H-sensitive, high-mannose oligosaccharides. In light of the ^{3}H-mannose experiments in 1984, it was clear that the oligosaccharides on these combining subunits were most likely $Man_9GlcNAc_2$ and $Man_8GlcNAc_2$ but it was not until 1987 that this was more rigorously demonstrated.[159] Also, differential processing of α- versus β-subunit of the TSH heterodimer was noted; after a 60-minute incubation with ^{3}H-mannose, the α-subunits of heterodimers had both $Man_9GlcNAc_2$ and $Man_8GlcNAc_2$ oligosaccharides present, whereas the β-subunits of heterodimers had predominantly $Man_9GlcNAc_2$ units.[159] $Man_8GlcNAc_2$ oligosaccharides became particularly prominent on α-subunits of heterodimers after chase incubations, or after prolonged pulse incubations, and this phenomenon was observed in pituitaries from euthyroid and hypothyroid mice as well as in mouse thyrotrophic tumor tissue. Although the processing of high-mannose oligosaccharides of α-subunits of heterodimes resembled that of free α-subunits more closely than that of β-subunits of heterodimers, the differences between the oligosaccharides detected on the two varieties of α-subunits remained substantial enough to suggest that heterodimer formation did affect α-subunit oligosaccharide processing.[159]

Of note, the kinetics of the high-mannose oligosaccharide processing of the α- and β-subunits of chorionic gonadotropin has also been described. [160] Analogous to the situtation for TSH, it appears that the tendency of the heterodimer to become enriched in $Man_9GlcNAc_2$ intemediates is explained in part by the accumulation of that species on β-subunits. Moreover, processing of α-subunit oligosaccharides was found to be affected if α-subunits combined with β-subunits.[161] A single report[162] has described hCG subunit processing in subcellular fractions of choriocarcinoma cells. Very recently, experiments employing site-specific mutagenesis to prevent glycosylation at particular Asn residues have explored the roles of specific hCG α-subunit[163] and hCG β-subunit[164] oligosaccharides, but the kinetics of processing at individual glycosylation sites has not yet been defined for hCG.

Miura et al.[165] determined the structures of high mannose oligosaccharides at the individual glycosylation sites of mouse TSH. Mouse thyrotropic tumor tissue was incubated with ^{3}H-mannose with or without ^{14}C-tyrosine for 2, 3, or 6 hours, and for a 3 hour pulse followed by a 2 hour chase. TSH heterodimers or free α-subunits were obtained from tissue homogenates using specific antisera. After reduction and alkylation, subunits were treated with trypsin. Tryptic fragments bearing labeled oligosaccharides were then separated using reverse phase HPLC. Knowledge of the theoretical tryptic glycopeptides of mouse α-subunits and TSH β-subunits (Fig. 6) facilitated the interpretation of the HPLC profiles (Fig. 7). For example, HPLC

A. Tryptic glycopeptides of mouse α-subunits

Asn*Ile Thr Ser Glu Ala Thr Cys Cys Val Ala Lys
56 67
Val Glu Asn*His Thr Glu Cys His Cys Ser Thr Cys Tyr Tyr His Lys
80 82 95

B. Tryptic glycopeptide of mouse TSH β-subunit

Glu Cys Ala Tyr Cys Leu Thr Ile Asn*Thr Thr Ile Cys Ala Gly-
15 23 29
Tyr Cys Met Thr Arg
34

Fig. 6. Theoretical tryptic glycopeptides of mouse TSH α-subunits (A) and TSH β-subunits (B). The asterisks mark the positions of the oligosaccharides. Reproduced with permission from Miura et al.[165]

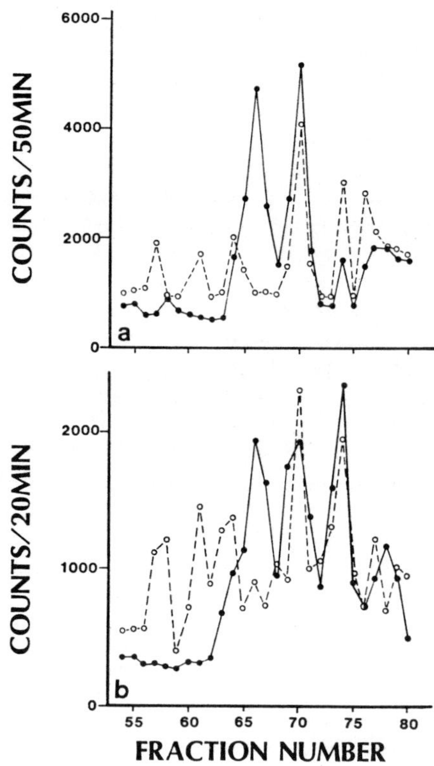

Fig. 7. Reverse phase HPLC of ^{3}H-mannose and ^{14}C-tyrosine double labeled tryptic fragments of free α-subunits (a) and TSH heterodimers (b). Closed circles, ^{3}H-mannose; open circles, ^{14}C-tyrosine. Reproduced with permission from Miura et al.[165]

analysis of tryptic fragments of free α-subunits showed two main ^{3}H-mannose-labeled peaks at fractions 66 and 70 (Fig. 7a). Both of these tryptic peptides contained ^{3}H-mannose-labeled N-linked oligosaccharides, but only the second peptide contained ^{14}C-tyrosine. This allowed the identification of these two tryptic fragments as the peptides bearing the oligosaccharide units linked to Asn^{56} and Asn^{82}, respectively. Analogously, HPLC analysis of the tryptic peptides of TSH revealed three main ^{3}H-mannose-labeled peaks (Fig. 7b). The first and second peaks had retention times and patterns of ^{3}H and ^{14}C radioactivity exactly the same as those of free α-subunits and, therefore, must have been derived from the α-subunits of the TSH heterodimers. The third ^{3}H-mannose-labeled peak also comigrated with a ^{14}C-tyrosine peak, so that this species likely represented the tryptic fragment from the TSH β-subunit that contained both the Asn-linked oligosaccharide unit and tyrosine.

Having unambiguously identified the peaks of radioactivity in the HPLC profiles in this manner, the ^{3}H-mannose-labeled oligosaccharides of each tryptic fragment were released using endoglycosidase H and were analyzed by paper chromatography. The chromatographic profiles of the high mannose oligosaccharides at individual glycosylation sites of mouse free α-subunits are shown in Fig. 8, and oligosaccharides at individual glycosylation sites of mouse TSH are shown in Fig. 9. $Man_9GlcNAc_2$ and $Man_8GlcNAc_2$ units predominated at each time point and at each specific glycosylation site, but the processing of high mannose oligosaccharides differed at each glycosylation site. The processing at Asn^{23} of TSH β-subunits was slower than that at Asn^{56} or Asn^{82} of α-subunits. The processing at Asn^{82} was slightly faster than that at Asn^{56} for both α-subunits of TSH heterodimers and free α-subunits. These differences were attributed to local conformational differences that affected the interaction of the TSH subunits with the cellular processing enzymes.[165]

This HPLC technique was employed by Miura et al.[166] to study the differential susceptibility to N-glycanase (peptide-N4-[N-acetyl-β-glucosaminyl] asparagine amidase) of oligosaccharides at the individual glycosylation sites of mouse TSH and free α-subunits. N-glycanase treatment of native molecules did not cleave oligosaccharides efficiently at Asn^{56} of α-subunits and Asn^{23} of TSH β-subunits, whereas oligosaccharides at Asn^{82} of α-subunits were more susceptible regardless of whether or not the α-subunits were combined with β-subunits. Heat denaturation, reduction, and the presence of detergents did not substantially increase the cleavage by N-glycanase of the protected oligosaccharides, suggesting that the primary structures of the TSH subunits influenced the efficiency of enzyme action at the specific sites. In contrast, Ronin et al.[167] reported that denaturation of human TSH increased its sensitivity to deglycosylation, and that native combined and free subunits were differentially susceptible to a mixture of N-glycanase and endoglycosidase F. Lee et al.[168], in a study of bovine TSH, found that under nondenaturing

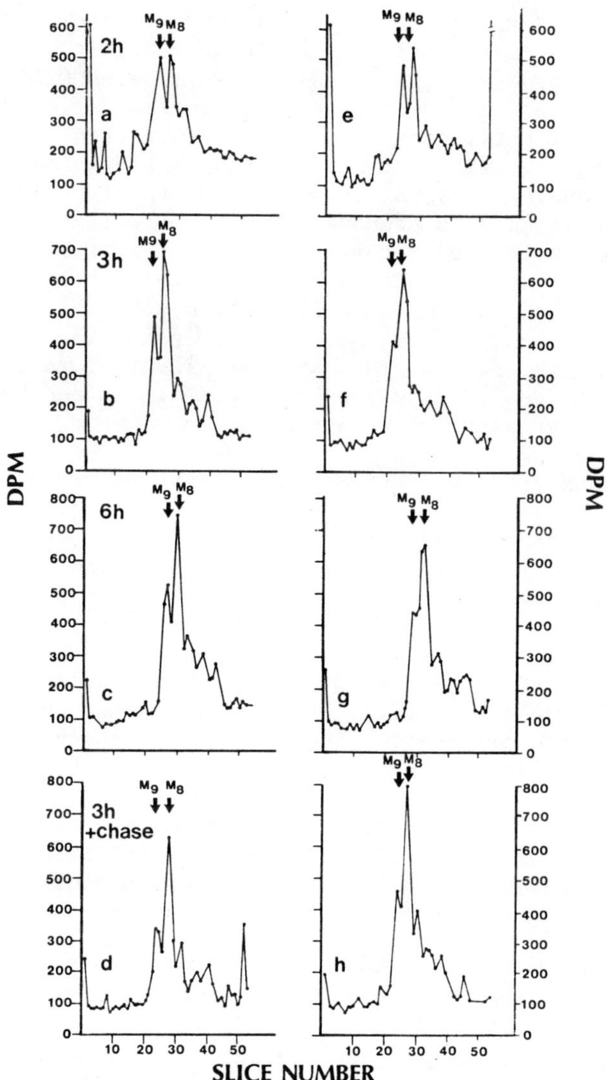

Fig. 8. High mannose (M) oligosaccharides from individual glycosylation sites of free α-subunits. Mouse thyrotropic tumor tissue was incubated with ^{3}H-mannose for 2h (a and e), 3h (b and f), or 6h (c and g) and for a 3h pulse, 2h chase (d and h). Tryptic fragments of free α-subunits were treated with endoglycosidase H, and the released oligosaccharides were analyzed by paper chromatography. Left panels (a-d) show oligosaccharides from Asn^{56}, and right panels (e-h) show oligosaccharides from Asn^{82} of the free α-subunit. The arrows mark the position of migration of the standards $Man_9GlcNAc$ and $Man_8GlcNAc$. Reproduced with permission from Miura et al.[165]

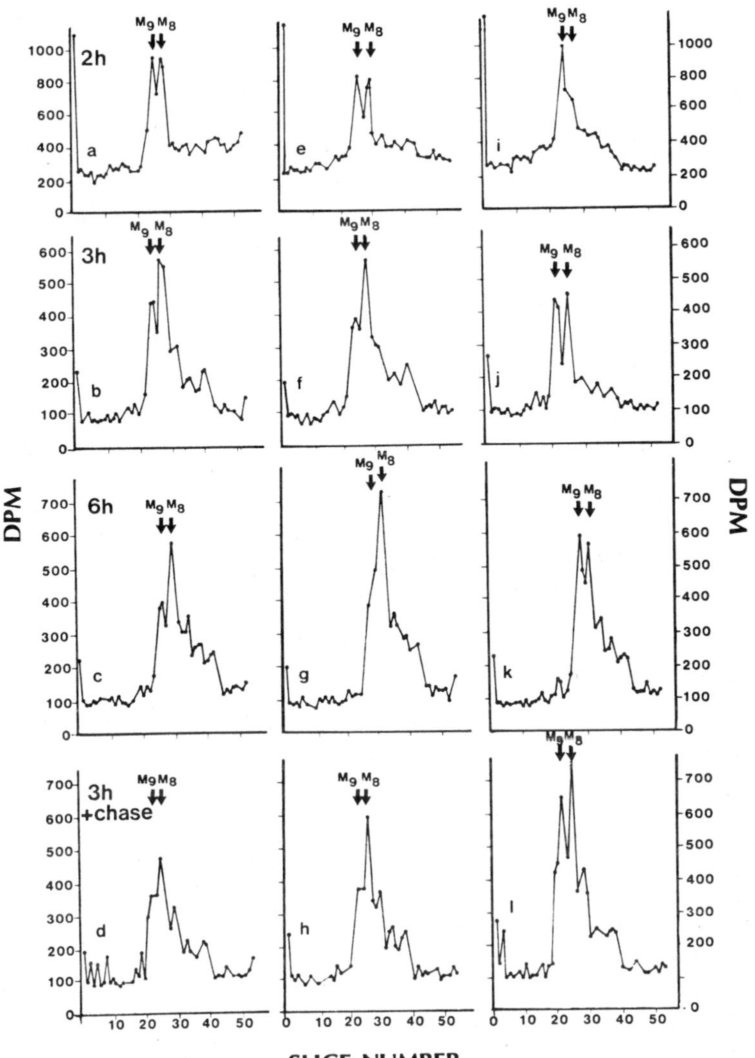

Fig. 9. Paper chromatographic profiles of high mannose (M) oligosaccharides from individual glycosylation sites of TSH heterodimers. Mouse thyrotropic tumor tissue was prepared as described in the legend to Fig. 8. Left panels (a-d) show oligosaccharides from Asn^{56} of α-subunits, middle panels (e-h) show oligosaccharides from Asn^{82} of α-subunits, and right panels (i-l) show oligosaccharides from Asn^{23} of β-subunits. The arrows mark the positions of migration of the standards $Man_9GlcNAc$ and $Man_8GlcNAc$. Reproduced with permission from Miura et al.[165]

conditions N-glycanase did not readily cleave one of the oligosaccharides of α-subunits, and that cleavage was not substantially improved after denaturation and reduction of the subunits. The reason for these differences in N-glycanase susceptibility remain unclear, but may reflect differences in the primary sequences of the subunits from different species.

Swedlow et al.[169] studied the susceptibility of equine gonadotropins to N-glycanase. They reported that one of two oligosaccharides of α-subunits were cleaved (although which Asn-linked unit could not be determined), and this resulted in a gonadotropin with only 22% of the potency of native LH in a testicular membrane assay. If the ovine LH α-subunits behaved similarly to the mouse α-subunits in our digestions[166], then this leads to the prediction that the more carboxylterminal Asn-linked oligosaccharide is the more important for the bioactivity of the hormones.

Interestingly, our studies[165,166,170] of the individual glycosylation sites of mouse TSH suggest that there is a correlation between Asn sites that are rapidly processed posttranslationally and that are relatively more susceptible to N-glycanase.

Matzuk and Boime[163] employed site-specific mutagenesis of the two Asn-linked glycosylation sites of hCG α-subunits to study the function of the individual high mannose chains as regards α-β-subunit assembly and hormone secretion. Absence of the oligosaccharide at Asn^{78} (analogous to Asn^{82} of mouse α-subunit) caused hCG α-subunits to be degraded quickly in the cell, although this mutant subunit was partially stabilized if bound to hCG β-subunits. Absence of the oligosaccharide at Asn^{52} (analogous to Asn^{56} of mouse α-subunit) did not perturb the stability or transport of hCG α-subunit, but did decrease hCG heterodimer secretion. They concluded that there were site-spectific functions of the α-subunit oligosaccharides. Recently these workers reported an analogous mutagenesis study of hCG β-subunits, and concluded that the oligosaccharides of the β-subunit are vital for proper folding of the nascent peptides.[164] Absence of the oligosaccharide at position 30, which is analogous to the Asn^{23} oligosaccharide in TSH β-subunits, had a more profound effect than did absence of the oligosaccharide at position 13.

Thus, these studies of the high mannose oligosaccharides of TSH and other glycoprotein hormones suggest that the chief intracellular roles of these carbohydrate units are to affect the folding of the nascent peptides to facilitate proper disulfide bond formation, and to avert proteolysis and aggregation of subunits. These high mannose oligosaccharides are also the substrates upon which the final complex oligosaccharides are built, and these mature structures may influence the metabolic clearance rate and intrinsic bioactivity of the secreted hormone, as will be discussed in forthcoming sections of this chapter.

PROCESSING OF TSH OLIGOSACCHARIDES TO COMPLEX FORMS

Much less information is available concerning the late steps as compared to the early steps of TSH posttranslational processing. As shown in the generalized scheme depicted in Fig. 5, the conversion of high mannose oligosaccharides to complex oligosaccharides containing fucose, N-acetylglucosamine, galactose, N-acetylgalactosamine, sulfate and sialic acid residues is believed to occur principally in the Golgi apparatus. Techniques used to explore late processing steps have included metabolic labeling studies employing various radioactive sugars, use of subcellular fractionation and/or of drugs that block intracellular transport, determination of enzymatic activities, and analyses of TSH by lectins and a variety of other analytical techniques.

Early studies of the carbohydrate compositions of the various glycoprotein hormones reported significant differences in the structures of their complex oligosaccharides.[171-193] Moreover, classical biochemical techniques, such as isoelectric focusing, had suggested for many years that TSH was extremely heterogeneous, and that the oligosaccharide moieties contributed significantly to this heterogeneity.[26,194-204] It was suspected that this biochemical heterogeneity was related to heterogeneity in hormone binding affinity, cyclase generation, metabolic clearance and bioactivity, as will be discussed in a later section.

SIALYLATION AND SULFATION OF TSH SUBUNITS

During the 1970's it was noted that some but not all of the TSH heterogeneity was removed by use of neuraminidase to cleave sialic acid residues. In 1980 a key observation was made by Parsons and Pierce[205], who found that some of the oligosaccharides of bovine TSH α-subunits, bovine LH α-subunits, and human LH, but not hCG, are sulfated. They speculated that the negatively charged sulfate may play some functional role comparable to that of the negatively charged sialic acid. Shortly thereafter Hortin et al.[206] demonstrated the metabolic incorporation of ^{35}S-sulfate into the oligosaccharides of the α- and β-subunits of bovine lutropin. Anumula and Bahl[207] obtained similar results using ovine lutropin. Gesundheit et al.[208] showed that mouse TSH subunits could also be metabolically labeled with sulfate and sialic acid. Moreover, TSH secreted in the presence of thyrotropin-releasing hormone (TRH) had a lower sulfate to mannose ratio, and a lower sialic acid to mannose ratio, than did spontaneously secreted TSH, suggesting that differential sulfation and sialylation may represent a point of regulation by TRH. Gesundheit et al.[208] speculated that such biochemical modulation of TSH by TRH might explain in part the previously observed[199,209,210] variability in the isoelectric point, bioactivity and metabolic clearance rate of

TSH in different physiological states. Prior studies of pituitary gonadotropins had demonstrated that changes in carbohydrate structure occurred during the ovulatory cycle[211], and that intracellular sialylation increased with castration and decreased when gonadal steroids were replaced.[212] More recently, altered sialylation of rat lutropin has been evaluated.[213] Sardanons et al.[214] have reported that gonadotropin-releasing hormone increases the sulfation and the bioactivity of rat LH.

Because sulfate is linked to GalNAc residues whereas sialic acid is linked to Gal residues in the oligosaccharides of the glycoprotein hormones [215-218] Smith and Baenziger[219] have postulated that a key posttranslational step in pituitary tissue is the addition of GalNAc rather than Gal to GlcNAc residues of precursor oligosaccharides (Fig. 10). GalNAc rarely is present in the N-linked oligosaccharides of glycoproteins other than some of the glycoprotein hormones. These authors identified a GalNAc-transferase in bovine pituitary membranes that specifically recognizes glycoprotein hormones.[219] Although these workers have focused on explaining different patterns of glycosylation of LH and FSH, it is likely that this enzyme also exists in thyrotropes. Although there is presently no evidence that this GalNAc transferase is under hormonal control, it is possible that regulation of this enzyme could partially explain how TSH oligosaccharide structures are modulated. A pituitary sulfotransferase (not present in placenta) is specific for the oligosaccharide sequence GalNAc-GlcNAc-Man and does not require the peptide for recognition. A subcellular fractionation study has directly confirmed that the subcellular site of the sulfation of mouse TSH and free α-subunits is the Golgi apparatus[220], and sulfotransferase activity has been observed in Golgi-derived membranes from bovine[221] and mouse[222] pituitary tissue.

Baenziger and Green[218] have determined the structures and the distributions of sulfated and sialylated oligosaccharides on several pituitary glycoprotein hormones (Figs. 11,12,13). For bovine TSH, 48% of the oligosaccharides contain two sulfates, 32% have one sulfate, 18% are neutral, and 2% have one sulfate and one sialic acid; no oligosaccharides contain sialic acid residues exclusively. The oligosaccharides of human TSH are somewhat different: 25% have one sulfate, 21% have one sulfate and one sialic acid, 18% are neutral, 12% have two sialic acid residues and 5% have one sialic acid residue. The distributions of sulfated and sialylated oligosaccharides of bovine LH and FSH, ovine LH and FSH, and human LH and FSH were also reported, and each hormone had a unique spectrum of oligosaccharide moieties. Of note, these data refer to hormones derived from pituitary tissues, not secreted hormones. Moreover, there may not be a "correct" distribution of structures present on a given hormone, as the proportions may vary in different physiologic states. Yet the identical structures are found on these hormones regardless of the type of hormone or animal species.

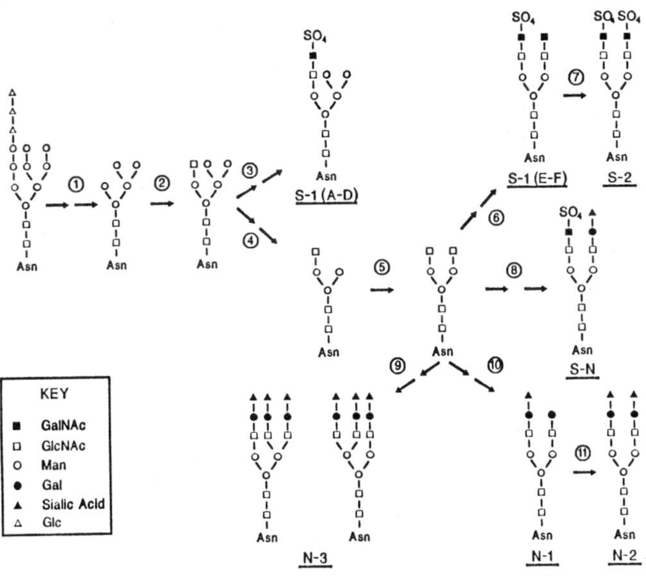

Fig. 10. Proposed pathway for synthesis of sulfated and sialylated Asn-linked oligosaccharides on the pituitary glycoprotein hormones. A key branchpoint in the pathway is the addition of GalNAc (step 6) vs. Gal (steps 9 and 10) to peripheral GlcNAc residues. Reproduced with permission from Baenziger and Green.[218]

KEY

- ■ GalNAc
- □ GlcNAc
- ○ Man
- ● Gal
- ▲ Sialic Acid

Designation:	S-1(A)	S-1(B)	S-1(C)	S-1(D)	S-1(E)	S-1(F) n=1	S-2 n=2	S-N
Hormone								
bLH	15	8	2	2	2	16	22	
bFSH	3	2	1	1	1	3	1	1
bTSH	12	5	1	2	1	11	48	2
oLH	27	9	9	5		6	13	4
oFSH	1	1	2	2		8	16	10
hLH	3	3	4	8	1		7	23
hFSH	1			1				5
hTSH	5	10		10			18	21

[% OF TOTAL OLIGOSACCHARIDES]

Fig. 11. Structures and distributions of the sulfated oligosaccharides on the pituitary glycoprotein hormones. Reproduced with permission from Green and Baenziger.[216,217]

KEY: ■ GalNAc, □ GlcNAc, ○ Man, ● Gal, ▲ Sialic Acid

Designation:	N-1(A)	N-1(B) n=1	N-2(B) n=2	N-1(C) n=1	N-2(C) n=2	N-2(D) n=1	N-3(D) n=2	N-1(E) n=1	N-2(E) n=2	N-3(E) n=3	N-1(F) n=1	N-2(F) n=2	N-2(G) n=2	N-3(G) n=3	N-2(H) n=2	N-3(H) n=3
Hormone																
bLH																
bFSH	2	3	33			6	11									
bTSH																
oLH		1														
oFSH	1	2	5					5	4	4	2	2		3		
hLH	10	6	10	3	6											
hFSH	3	3	12	9	7						4	7	7	13	6	12
hTSH	5		12													

[% OF TOTAL OLIGOSACCHARIDES]

Fig. 12. Structures and distribuitons of the sialylated oligosaccharides on the pituitary glycoprotein hormones. Reproduced with permission from Green and Baenziger.[216,217]

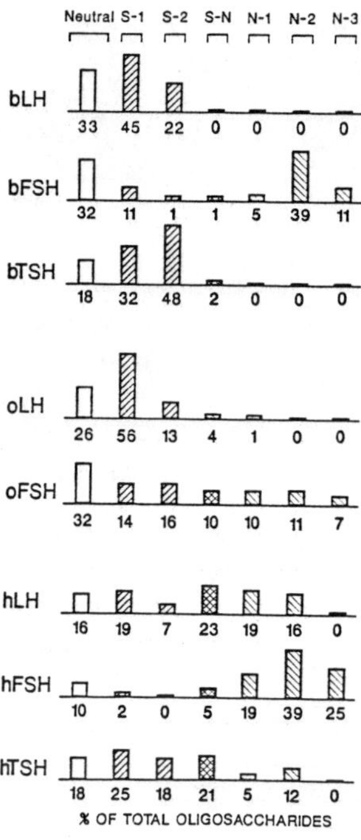

Fig. 13. Relative distributions of neutral, sulfated, and sialylated oligosaccharides on the pituitary glycoprotein hormones. Reproduced with permission from Baenziger and Green.[218]

Concerning secreted hTSH, Miura et al.[223] have recently studied sera from euthyroid subjects and patients with primary and central hypothyroidism. To assess the degree of sialylation, they analyzed the binding of hTSH to a Gal-specific lectin, ricin (RCA_{120}), after preincubation of the hormone with or without neuraminidase. TSH in the the sera of patients with primary hypothyroidism was more sialylated than that from euthyroid or central hypothyroid patients, and the amount of sialylation appeared to increase with the duration of primary hypothyroidism over several months. An analogous increase in sialylation and decrease in sulfation of secreted mouse TSH with time over several months has also been reported by DeCherney et al.[224] Pituitaries from euthyroid mice, or mice made hypothyroid for 3 or 12 months, were incubated with ^{3}H-glucosamine. Labeled secreted TSH was immunoprecipitated, α- and β- subunits were separated, and the endoglycosidase F-released oligosaccharides were analyzed by anion-exhange HPLC. Chromatograms of the α-subunit-derived oligosaccharides showed seven distinct species corresponding to differently sialylated or sulfated carbohydrates. Oligosaccharides with one or two sialic acids increased, while species with one or two sulfates decreased, as the duration of hypothyroidism became prolonged. Moreover, hypothyroidism of 12 months duration caused the appearance of a new tri-sialylated species.

Recently Murray et al.[356] used periodate to oxidize the side chains of the sialic acid residues of hFSH and hCG, and then derivatized those residues with alanine or other small molecules. The chemically altered hormones were resistant to neuraminidase; when injected into rats the circulating halftime was increased 7- to 10-fold. When tested in vitro for steroid production by Leydig cells, the derivatized hFSH and hCG were less potent than the standard hormones, although a maximum biological response could be attained by using larger doses of the derivatives. These data suggest that the sialic acid residues of glycoprotein hormones may play some role in modulating their biological properties.

FUCOSYLATION OF TSH SUBUNITS

Studies of a wide variety of glycoproteins suggested that complex-type N-linked oligosaccharides may contain fucose linked α 1,6 to the innermost GlcNAc residue; a peripheral GlcNAc may contain fucose in an α 1,3 or α 1,4 linkage or Gal may be substituted with a fucose residue in an α 1,2 or α 1,6 linkage.[152] Some of the transferases catalyzing the incorporation of L-fucose from GDP-β-fucose into oligosaccharide chains have been purified, and their substrate specificities have been characterized.[225-228] Fucosidases that cleave peripheral but not core fucose residues also have been used as probes of complex oligosaccharide structure. Almond α-L-fucosidase I will cleave only fucose linked α 1,3 or α 1,4 to GlcNAc.[229] An α-L-fucosidase from *Aspergillus niger*[230], and an α-L-fucosidase from human serum[231], preferentially cleave fucose linked α 1,2 to Gal.

Studies of hepatic subcellular fractions suggested that fucosyltransferoses are localized in the cis or proximal Golgi apparatus.[232] This is consistent with the observation that 6-α-L-fucosyltransferase ("core fucosyltransferase") may use GlcNAc-terminated oligosaccharides as acceptor substrates.[225,228] Thus, addition of fucose to the core GlcNAc occurs following the action of Golgi GlcNAc-transferase I and prior to the addition of peripheral Gal or GalNAc. Molecules having a bisecting GlcNAc residue, or peripheral addition of Gal β1,4 or sialic acid-Gal β 1,4, are no longer substrates for the 6-α-fucosyltransferase.[227,228] The purpose of fucose addition to glycoproteins during their biosynthesis, and the roles of fucose in the mature product, are not known for any glycoprotein.

Over the years, compositional studies of the glycoprotein hormones reported a small and variable amount of fucose, often less than one residue per hormone molecule.[26,185,195,196,198,205] In 1980 Weintraub et al.[140] demonstrated the metabolic incorporation of ^{3}H-fucose into mouse TSH subunits, but this study design could provide little quantitative information. Then, in 1984, Chapman et al.[233] used a lectin affinity technique to demonstrate that choriogonadotropin α-subunits synthesized by tumor cells were more highly fucosylated than α-subunits made by nonmalignant cells. Recently, Kobata[234] more definitively established the oligosaccharide structures of hCG, and reported increased core fucose in hCG synthesized by malignant cells as compared to nonmalignant cells. These studies suggest that the fucose content of a glycoprotein hormone may be modulated under certain circumstances, presumably because of an increase in cellular fucosyltransferase activity. Earlier autoradiographic studies from Canada had suggested the peculiar finding that fucosylation of TSH[235] or gonadotropins[236] generally occurred in the Golgi apparatus of resting pituicytes, but occurred in both the RER and Golgi of stimulated pituicytes. Cytologists had long noted that after thyroidectomy, thyrotropes enlarged and developed hypertrophied RER. The autoradiographic studies suggested that the distribution of fucosylating enzymes was being altered in stimulated thyrotropes. More critical study of this phenomenon would prove difficult, as will be discussed below.

Early light microscopic studies of thyrotropes suggested that TSH was being stored not only in secretory granules, but also in granules within hypertrophied cisternae.[237-239] In an early electron microscopic study, Farquhar and Rinehart[240] demonstrated that the cisternae were RER and that the aldehyde fuchsin-positive granules were dense intracisternal inclusions. The intracisternal granules became more numerous with increasing time after thyroidectomy, and their existence was confirmed by other investigators.[241-245]

To attempt to confirm that RER-associated fucosylation occurred in stimulated mouse thyrotropes, in 1986 Magner et al.[246] incubated pituitaries from hypothyroid mice with ^{3}H-fucose and performed a subcellular fractionation study using sucrose gradients. Most fucosylation occurred in Golgi elements. Although RER-enriched cell fractions contained ^{3}H-fucose-labeled TSH subunits in amounts believed to exceed the degree of contamination with Golgi or secretory granule elements, it was difficult to conclude definitively that RER-associated fucosylation had occurred. Granules that may have represented the poorly understood intracisternal granules were seen in some electron micrographs of RER-enriched gradient fractions, but these may also have represented classical secretory granules that were contaminating the RER-enriched fractions. Moreover, use of the drugs monensin and CCCP in this study could provide only suggestive evidence that atypical compartmentalization of oligosaccharide processing enzymes were present in stimulated thyrotropes. Thus, this novel study perhaps raised more questions than it answered. For example, perhaps the controversial RER-associated intracisternal granules of stimulated thyrotropes, and their possible content of fucosylated molecules, are related to RER-associated degradation of TSH during biosynthesis, a phenomenon reported in other cell types.

One further attempt was made to clarify the concept of RER-associated fucosylation in thyrotropes. Miura et al.[247] incubated mouse thyrotropic tumor tissue with ^{35}S-methionine for 2 to 30 min, then tested the affinity of labeled TSH subunits for lentil lectin, which requires the presence of a core fucose residue for glycoprotein binding.[248] Although small amounts of TSH subunits bound to the lectin at early times, further studies will be needed to determine whether or not fucosylation may occur in the RER as well as the Golgi of hypertrophied thyrotropes.

In 1986 Magner and Papagiannes[249] employed a double-label technique to estimate the relative fucose content of mouse TSH and free α-subunits. Thyrotropic tumor minces were incubated simultaneously with ^{35}S-methionine and ^{3}H-fucose, and TSH subunits were immunoprecipitated and analyzed by gel electrophoresis. Secreted free α-subunits were approximately five-fold richer in fucose than was TSH. Within the TSH heterodimer the β-subunit contained about twice as much fucose as the α-subunit, in agreement with the results of Gesundheit et al.[250,251] Magner and Papagiannes[249] reported that a brief incubation of the tumor tissue with 0.1 uM TRH before and during metabolic labeling aparently did not modulate the fucose/methionine ratio, a result also confirmed by Gesundheit et al.[251] in a study of hypothyroid mouse hemipituitaries.

STUDIES OF TSH BIOSYNTHESIS EMPLOYING INHIBITORS OF INTRACELLULAR TRANSLOCATION

To determine the subcellular sites of TSH subunit posttranslational processing, Magner and coworkers analyzed subunit precursors in subcellular fractions of thyrotropic tumor or pituitary tissue.[143,155,220,246] This approach is subject to several sources of error, however, most notably the cross-contamination of subcellular fractions. An alternative approach was to study unfractionated thyrotropes that putatively had become enriched in subunit precursors within certain subcellular compartments while being incubated with drugs that inhibited the intracellular translocation of newly synthesized proteins. Use of such drugs, however, raises other methodological questions, such as the accuracy of the known site(s) of action of the drugs. In spite of these questions, drugs such as monensin, which blocks intracellular transport in middle Golgi elements[252], and carboxyl cyanide m-chlorophenylhydrazone (CCCP), which blocks transport from RER to proximal Golgi elements[253], have been used in dozens of recent studies of a wide variety of tissues.[254-258]

Ponsin and Mornex[259] were the first to study the effects of monensin on the biosynthesis of TSH. Enzymatically dispersed pituitary cells from euthyroid rats were incubated with ^{3}H-proline or ^{3}H-glucosamine in the absence or presence of TRH and/or monensin. It was concluded that TRH stimulated the terminal glycosylation of TSH, and this was inhibited by 25 uM monensin. Some of these data are difficult to interpret, however, because the chosen sugar, ^{3}H-glucosamine, may be present in TSH oligosaccarides in either the core or the periphery.

Magner et al.[246] used monensin and CCCP to try to localize the subcellular compartment responsible for fucosylation of TSH subunits. They incubated pituitaries from thyroidectomized mice with ^{35}S-methionine or ^{3}H-fucose for 2 hours, and then chase incubated the tissue in the absence of radioactivity for 3 hours in the presence of monensin, CCCP or no drug. TSH and free α-subunits were immunoprecipitated from cell lysates and chase media and analyzed by gel electrophoresis. Monensin and CCCP partially inhibited the appearance of the ^{3}H-fucose-labeled subunits in the media; the distribution of the ^{3}H-fucose-labeled subunits between lysates and media was similar to that of the ^{35}S-methionine-labeled subunits. These results suggested that although some fucosylation occurred in the Golgi apparatus, at least some of the ^{3}H-fucose was being incorporated into TSH subunits relatively early in the secretory pathway, proximal to the site(s) of action of monensin and CCCP. Thus, at least some fucosylation of subunits was occurring in the RER or very proximal Golgi apparatus. Monensin and CCCP were employed in a similar fashion by Magner et al.[220] in a study of TSH sulfation, and it was concluded that most sulfation occurred relatively late in the secretory pathway, distal to the sites of action of the translocation inhibitors.

Because the drug CCCP might have diverse actions within cells due to reductions in ATP levels, it was desirable to test an alternative drug that blocked intracellular transport between RER and proximal Golgi. The drug brefeldin A, a fungal metabolite of a 13-member macrocyclic lactone ring, appeared to be a potential candidate.[260-263] This drug caused dilatation of the RER in hepatocytes without lowering cellular ATP levels. Takatsuki and Tamura[261] observed that brefeldin A caused the intracellular accumulation of vesicular stomatitis virus G-protein containing endoglycosidase H-sensitive oligosaccharides lacking capping sugars such as N-acetylglucosamine or galactose. Misumi et al.[262] found in rat hepatocytes that the drug inhibited the proteolytic conversion of proalbumin to albumin and blocked terminal glycosylation of α^1-protease inhibitor and haptoglobin, yet the drug blocked neither proteolytic processing of haptoglobin proform (an RER event), nor cellular uptake of ^{125}I-asialofetuin (endocytosis). Oda et al.[263] found that brefeldin A caused a precursor form of complement C3 to accumulate within rat hepatocytes. Thus, the results of all of these workers suggested that a major action of brefeldin A is to block intracellular transport between the RER and the Golgi apparatus.

Using brefeldin A kindly provided by Dr. A. Takatsuki, Magner and Papagiannes[264] first tested this drug in an endocrine system. When pituitary tissue from hypothyroid mice was incubated with 5 or 10 ug of brefeldin A/ml for 3.5 hours, marked dilatation of the RER and mild swelling of the Golgi apparatus occurred in all pituitary cell types. At 5 ug/ml the drug did not inhibit protein synthesis, but markedly reduced protein secretion. After a 2 hour pulse with ^{35}S-methionine, followed by a 4 hour chase, brefeldin A at 5 ug/ml reduced the release of TSH and free α-subunits into the medium by 94% and 99%, respectively; subunits that accumulated within cells were forms with molecular weights of 2000-4000 less than normal. Brefeldin A also partially inhibited the release into the medium of TSH or free α-subunits labeled with ^{3}H-fucose or ^{35}S-sulfate.

Subsequently, Perkel et al.[265] studied the effects of brefeldin A on the processing of the high mannose oligosaccharides of TSH, free α-subunits, and cellular glycoproteins. Mouse pituitary thyrotropic tumor tissue was incubated with ^{3}H-mannose in pulse-chase fashion in the presence or absence of 5 ug of brefeldin A/ml. TSH and free α-subunits were obtained from cell lysates using specific antisera. Endoglycosidase H-released ^{3}H-oligosaccharides were analyzed by paper chromatography. Brefeldin A inhibited the posttranslational processing of TSH, free α-subunits, and cellular glycoproteins, resulting in the accumulation of the oligosaccharides $Man_8GlcNAc_2$, $Man_7GlcNAc_2$, $Man_6GlcNAc_2$, and $Man_5GlcNAc_2$. Use of subcellular fractionation disclosed that these brefeldin A-induced changes occurred as early as the RER compartment. The species retained within the RER under those conditions may have been subject to ongoing processing by endoplasmic reticulum (α,1-2) mannosidase, resulting in the accumulation of $Man_{8-5}GlcNAc_2$ oligosaccharides within the RER.

Incidental to the brefeldin A data, the study by Perkel et

al.[265] also reported the subcellular distribution of fucosyltransferase activity, a marker enzyme rarely reported. The mean fucosyltransferase activities were highest in the Golgi-derived subcellular fractions, suggesting that most fucosylation of TSH and free α-subunits in this tumor tissue occurred in the Golgi apparatus.

In another study Perkel et al.[266] explored whether or not brefeldin A affected oligosaccharide processing at multiple subcellular sites even though its chief action was to inhibit RER to Golgi transport. Pituitaries from hypothyroid mice were incubated with ^{35}S-methionine, ^{3}H-mannose, ^{3}H-galactose, ^{3}H-fucose, ^{3}H-N-acetylmannosamine, or ^{35}S-sulfate for 2 hours in the absence or presence of 5 ug of brefeldin A/ml or 2 uM monensin. TSH and free α-subunits were immunoprecipitated from tissue lysates and analyzed by gel electrophoresis, or tryptic glycopeptides of TSH were separated by HPLC. Labeled oligosaccharides were analyzed by paper chromatography. Brefeldin A did not prevent the initial glycosylation at any specific asparagine site of TSH. Glucose-trimming from the very early oligosaccharides of glycoproteins was slowed by brefeldin A, presumably because the distortion of the RER morphology by the drug interfered with the efficient interaction of glucosidases with substrates. Both monensin and brefeldin A inhibited fucosylation, sulfation,and sialylation more markedly than mannose incorporation, suggesting a direct effect on the Golgi apparatus, in agreement with a recent study by Fujiwara et al.[267]

In summary, use of monensin and CCCP have provided some insights into the subcellular localization of TSH processing, particularly concerning fucosylation and sulfation. In turn, thyrotropic model systems have proved useful in testing the relatively little-used inhibitor, brefeldin A, which potentially may be a useful drug in the study of many endocrine and nonendocrine tissues.

ENDOCRINE REGULATION OF TSH BIOSYNTHESIS AND GLYCOSYLATION

The hormonal regulation of the TSH subunit genes has been addressed in an earlier section of this chapter. The huge literature concerning the regulation of TSH secretion is beyond the scope of this chapter; only the few studies dealing directly with the regulation of TSH biosynthesis and glycosylation will be reviewed here.

During the late 1960's Wilber and Utiger[268,269] performed immunoassay studies of TSH in rat pituitaries, as well as metabolic incorporation experiments using ^{14}C-glucosamine. In 1971 Wilber[270] observed a curious effect of TRH on the metabolic incorporation of a labeled sugar and a labeled amino acid into TSH. TRH appeared to stimulate the incorporation of glucosamine into TSH by a factor of 11.4, but only stimulated the incorporation of alanine by a factor of 1.5. A provocative implication of these data was that the processes of glycosylation and translation of TSH are differentially regulated by TRH. Subsequently, Cacicedo et al.[271] and Marshall et al.[272] employed labeled amino acids and found small effects of TRH on the de novo biosynthesis of TSH. Some of these studies have been summarized recently.[273] Twelve years were to pass, however, before Wilber's intriguing glucosamine/alanine phenomenon would be further explored.

In 1983 Ponsin and Mornex[259] reported that TRH caused a selective stimulation of TSH glycosylation. Using dispersed rat pituitary cells they documented that TRH increased the relative incorporation of ^{3}H-glucosamine into TSH. In 1985 Taylor and Weintraub[274] incubated pituitaries from euthyroid or hypothyroid rats with ^{14}C-alanine and ^{3}H-glucosamine, and demonstrated that the hypothyroid state caused increased relative glycosylation of α-subunits of TSH heterodimers. There was little or no altered glycosylation of β-subunits of TSH heterodimer, or of free α-subunits, that was detectable by the methods employed. In another study[275] these workers incubated pituitaries from euthyroid rats with TRH for 24 hours in vitro and demonstrated that glucosamine incorporation into secreted TSH increased 3-fold while alanine incorporation remained level. In this case, the increased glucosamine incorporation was present in both the α- and β-subunits of TSH heterodimers, but was not present in secreted free α-subunits. Such alterations in TSH oligosaccharides might explain the altered isoforms of rat TSH detected in different physiological states.[276-278]

Taylor et al.[279] also studied the effects of in vivo bolus versus continuous TRH administration on TSH secretion, biosynthesis, and glycosylation in normal and hypothyroid rats. The animals were treated with TRH intermittently or continuously for 5 days, then pituitaries were removed and incubated in vitro with ^{35}S-methionine and ^{3}H-glucosamine, with or without TRH, for 6 or 24 hours. TSH was immunoprecipitated and analyzed by gel electrophoresis. The relative incorporation of ^{3}H-glucosamine and ^{35}S-methionine in TSH was significantly altered in the normal but not in the hypothyroid rats after continuous in vivo TRH; for α-subunit of the TSH heterodimer the glucosamine: methionine ratio increased from 0.31 ± 0.03 to 0.53 ± 0.04 after 4 days of TRH treatment. This change presumably reflected altered TSH oligosaccharide structures induced by the TRH treatment.

Evidence has also been presented that TRH might influence early posttranslational steps of TSH oligosaccharide processing. In vivo administration of TRH to recently thyroidectomized rats caused the high mannose species $Glc_1Man_9GlcNAc_2$ and $Glc_1Man_8GlcNAc_2$ to become more predominant on intracellular TSH heterodimers and free β-subunits.[157] It was not clear whether this effect was due to a TRH-related alteration in the kinetics of oligosaccharide processing, or to actual addition of glucose residues posttranslationally as has rarely been reported.[280] Increased predominance of glucose-containing high mannose units induced by TRH was not detected, however, in another study performed under somewhat different conditions.[159]

Because of the difficulty of applying classical biochemical techniques to determine precisely the TSH oligosaccharide structural changes induced by TRH, a more general approach using various lectins has been used. A lectin is a substance that binds only one or a few sugars with relative specificity and allows inferences to be made about whether or not certain sugar residues or structures are present in an oligosaccharide. As has been reviewed recently[281,282], glycopeptides applied to the lectin concanavalin A (con A) are eluted in three general classes: 1.) unbound glycopeptides that have bisecting, triantennary and multiantennary complex structures, 2.) weakly bound glycopeptides that elute with 10mM α-methylglucoside that have biantennary complex or truncated hybrid oligosaccharides, and 3.) strongly bound glycopeptides that elute with 500mM α-methylmannoside that have high mannose or hybrid oligosaccharides (Fig.14). Gesundheit et al.[250] incubated pituitaries from hypothyroid mice with ^{3}H-mannose with or without 0.1 uM TRH for 18 hours. TSH heterodimers were immunoprecipitated by anti-TSH β serum, digested with pronase, and the resultant TSH glycopeptides were applied to con A-Sepharose. In the absence of TRH, the percentages of ^{3}H-mannose-labeled secreted TSH glycopepetides that were unbound, weakly bound and strongly bound to con A were 37%, 55%, and 8%, respectively; TRH caused these percentages to change to 26%, 68%, and 6%, respectively. Thus, TRH <u>in vitro</u> promoted the secretion of TSH molecules slightly enriched in biantennary complex or truncated hybrid oligosaccharides. TRH did not alter the pattern of con A binding of glycopeptides from intrapituitary TSH. Con A-Sepharose chromatography of ^{3}H-glucosamine- and ^{3}H-fucose-labeled secreted TSH glycopeptides showed similar increases in weakly bound species induced by TRH. Analyses of ^{3}H-mannose-labeled TSH glycopeptides using erythroagglutinating phytohemagglutinin-Sepharose and leukoagglutinating phytohemagglutinin-Sepharose disclosed no significant differences in TRH-treated vs. control samples. Presumably TRH affected the final structure of secreted TSH oligosaccharides by activating or inhibiting specific glycosyltransferases, or by altering the intracellular secretory pathway. Moreover, this TRH-induced alteration of TSH oligosaccharides is believed to have enhanced the hormone's intrinsic bioactivity.[283]

Modulation of TSH oligosaccharide structure has also been observed <u>in vivo</u> as well as <u>in vitro</u>. Taylor et al.[284] studied rats with hypothalamic hypothyroidism and found altered forms of TSH. Bilateral paraventricular nuclear lesions were created in adult male rats. Two weeks later the pituitaries were incubated with ^{3}H-glucosamine for 24 hours. Secreted and intrapituitary TSH was immunoprecipitated, digested with pronase, and the glycopeptides were analyzed by con A chromatography. Compared to sham controls, the lesioned animals contained a greater proportion of secreted TSH glycopeptides that bound weakly to con A, indicating a shift from multiantennary oligosaccharides in control rats to biantennary or truncated hybrid oligosaccharides in lesioned rats. In contrast, thyroidectomized animals, compared to normal and hypothalamus-lesioned animals, had more secreted TSH glycopeptides that did not bind con A. Thus, the characteristics of the oligosaccharides of secreted TSH differed in hypothalamic vs. primary hypothyroidism despite equally low serum thyroid hormone levels in vivo. Another example of modulation of TSH oligosaccharides in vivo was reported by Gyves et al.[285], who characterized secreted TSH synthesized during maturation of the pituitary-thyroid axis in the rat. Secreted TSH at the time of parturition showed predominantly biantennary oligosaccharides that contained less sialic acid by anion exchange HPLC analysis compared to adult rats. Conversely, neonatal or adult hypothyroidism in rodents increased sialylation and decreased sulfation of secreted TSH. Interestingly,

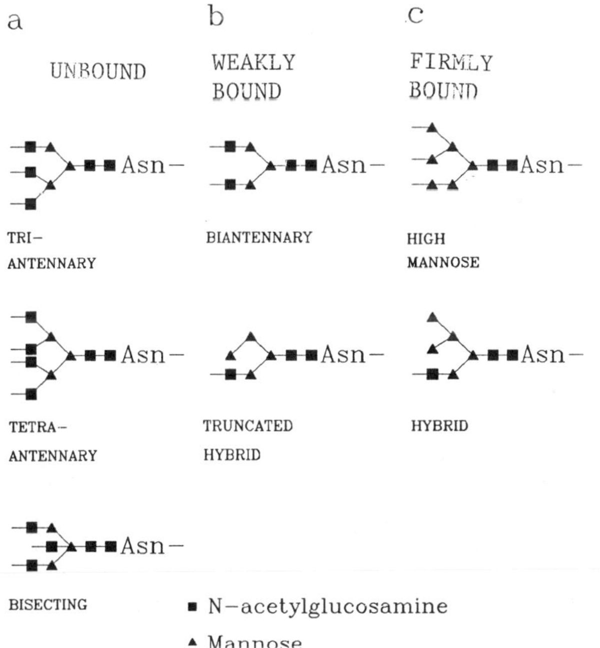

Fig. 14. Representative types of Asn-linked oligosaccharides that are unbound, weakly bound, or strongly bound to concanavalin A. See text for details. Adapted with permission from a figure by Taylor et al.[284]

in the latter study[285], incubation of rat pituitaries with TRH *in vitro* caused increases in the amount of secreted TSH glycopeptides that bound weakly to con A, a finding apparently in conflict with the study of the presumed TRH-deficient, hypothalamus-lesioned rats by Taylor et al.[284]

The lectin binding characteristics of TSH oligosaccharides have been investigated in a few other instances. Gesundheit et al.[286] reported that TSH and α-subunits secreted by an aggressive human pituitary adenoma had more bisecting and multiantennary oligosaccharide units than did TSH and α-subunits from a less aggressive tumor. Joshi and Weintraub [204]studied bovine and mouse TSH from a variety of sources; fractionation by gel chromatography revealed multiple isoforms of TSH with widely different ratios of biological to immunological activity. To determine whether these forms of TSH differed in their oligosaccharide structures, affinity chromatography using con A, wheat germ agglutinin and soybean agglutinin was performed. A less bioactive form of TSH had decreased amounts of exposed N-acetylgalactosamine and/or β-linked galactose than did the forms with higher bioactivity. Lee et al.[287] have reported that patients with severe nonthyroidal illness secrete forms of TSH with reduced con A binding. Miura et al.[223] used ricin to delineate different degrees of sialylation of TSH in sera of euthyroid, primary and central hypothyroid subjects. TSH from hypothyroid sera was the most sialylated, and the degree of sialylation increased with the duration of hypothyroidism. Perkel et al.[288] used serial lectin affinity chromatography to separate human TSH into subclasses. Serum from 29 primary hypothyroid patients and 10 euthyroid subjects was evaluated. TSH from these diverse patients behaved similarly when applied to con A and lentil lectin. For the hypothyroid patients, the percentages of TSH heterodimers that were unbound, weakly bound or strongly bound to con A were $10.8 \pm 0.6\%$ (mean $\pm$SEM), $37.3 \pm 1\%$ and $52 \pm 1.2\%$, respectively; for the euthyroid subjects these percentages were $13.1 \pm 1.7\%$, $26.7 \pm 2.6\%$ and $60.1 \pm 3.2\%$. The percentages of TSH heterodimers that bound to lentil lectin for the hypothyroid and euthyroid patients were $52 \pm 1.6\%$ and $62 \pm 2.7\%$, respectively. Serial use of the con A and lentil lectins allowed five major subclasses of TSH to be defined based on the branching of the oligosaccharides, and the presence or absence of a core fucose residue. The subclasses of TSH present in sera of hypothyroid and euthyroid patients were similar. Manasco et al.[289] reported similar data concerning the con A binding of TSH from sera of hypothyroid patients, and analyses of TSH from sera of patients with central hypothyroidism revealed a slight increase in forms of TSH that failed to bind con A.

BIOACTIVITY OF TSH

Although the carbohydrate moiety is not required for the biological activity of some glycoproteins, the oligosaccharides of the glycoprotein hormones appear to be important for hormone activity. As discussed in prior sections of this chapter, the high mannose precursor oligosaccharides protect nascent TSH subunits from intracellular proteolysis and aggregation and allow proper nascent chain folding to occur so that correct internal disulfide bonding is facilitated, proper subunit conformation is attained, and α-β-subunit combination may proceed. The final complex oligosaccharides determine properties of metabolic clearance *in vivo* and intrinsic biological activity *in vitro*.

The relationship between glycosylation and bioactivity was first addressed in glycoprotein hormones other than TSH. Removal of terminal sialic acid residues from the glycoprotein hormone hCG caused its plasma half-life in the rat to fall from 53 to 1 minute[290-292] with concomitant loss of *in vivo* hormone effect, but desialylated hCG retained about 50% of its steroidogenic potency *in vitro*.[293,294] Removal from intact hCG of galactose[292] or other residues in addition to sialic acid by enzymatic [292,295-299] or chemical[300-305] means had little effect on hormone binding to receptors in target tissues *in vitro*[292,295,296,298-305], but markedly diminished cAMP generation [295,296,298-305], and variably but generally reduced steroidogenesis. [295,297,299,302,303,305] Deglycosylation of purified α- and β-subunits of hCG followed by recombination with native subunits suggested that intact carbohydrate of both subunits is necessary for normal cAMP generation [303,304], but that α-subunit oligosaccharides are particularly important for bioactivity in gonadal tissues[299,300] and thyroid membranes.[306] Lutropin oligosaccharides were also thought to influence steroidogenic activity, particularly those of the α-subunit.[307]

In recent years the notion of gonadotropin oligosaccharide participation in hormone bioactivity has become more complicated as it has been recognized that the specific features of deglycosylating agents and of hormone assay systems must be carefully considered.[308] For example, forms of hCG that have little cAMP-generating ability *in vitro*, may still cause substantial steroidogenesis *in vitro*[302,309] suggesting that minimal amounts of the second messenger, cAMP, are sufficient to evoke a maximal end organ response. Forms of hCG that act as competitive antagonists *in vitro* may not inhibit the effects of native hCG *in vivo* as assessed by changes in uterine weight.[302] Cole et al.[310] used endoglycosidase F to remove the oligosaccharides of human and ovine LH; when tested for ability to promote testosterone release by rat testicular interstitial cells *in vitro* the deglycosylated hormones were 2 to 3 times less potent than native LH, but could still induce maximal testosterone responses. Thus, workers who had used hydrogen fluoride to deglycosylate hormones and found almost no *in vitro* bioactivity may have inadvertantly damaged the peptides in addition to removing some of the carbohydrates.

Recently Patton et al.[311] demonstrated that deglycosylated hCG, and a recombinant molecule composed of deglycosylated hCG α-subunit and native hCG β-subunit, had residual agonist activity in women. Infusions of these modified hormones into women for 24 to 48 hours produced a significant rise of serum progesterone levels in the mid-luteal phase. Liu et al.[312] prepared deglycosylated and desialylated hCG and reported that although deglycosylated hCG had impaired ability to generate cAMP in vitro, the modified hormones caused a normal short-term rise of plasma testosterone in vivo. This occurred in spite of the fact that the desialylated and deglycosylated hCG molecules were rapidly cleared from the plasma. Thus, when assessing the contribution of oligosaccharides to the bioactivity of a glycoprotein hormone, details concerning the method of deglycosylation, techniques of in vitro or in vivo assay, appropriateness of biological end-points, species differences, and other factors must be carefully weighed.

Few studies of the relationship between TSH oligosaccharides and hormone bioactivity have been performed. Probably the first such study was by Webster et al.[200] Human pituitary TSH originally prepared by Dr. Anne Stockell Hartree was subjected to isoelectric focusing covering the pH range 3-10, and immunoreactive TSH of six subtypes was detected. The bioactivity of each of these subtypes was tested in the McKenzie mouse assay, and the immunologic to biologic potency ratio was determined for each. Subtypes I, II, III, IIIa, IV, and V had pI values of 7.25, 6.62, 6.08, 5.93, 5.45, and 5.18, respectively, and the immunologic to biologic ratio was greater than 70, 64.1, 5.1, 4.6, 5.7, and 5.8, respectively. Pretreatment of TSH with neuraminidase before isoelectric focusing caused two new forms of TSH to appear with pI values of 8.7 and 8.1, but did not eliminate the TSH heterogeneity, suggesting that the charge differences in the molecules were due to residues other than sialic acid.

In 1980 Takai et al.[313] analyzed radioiodinated bovine thyrotropin by HPLC, and assayed fractions for cAMP response in monolayers of cultured thyroid cells. Surprisingly, there was discordance between the eluted positions of radiolabeled TSH and bioactive TSH. The same authors confirmed this discordance using a technique other than HPLC, namely polyacrylamide gel electrophoresis.[314] Moreover, different preparations of TSH behaved somewhat differently. Bovine TSH partially purified in their laboratory was subjected to polyacrylamide disc gel electrophoresis and revealed five individual protein bands, confirming the presence of TSH isohormones. When tested in the in vitro cAMP-generating assay, four of the five bands had bioactivity, and their potencies differed substantially. These authors speculated that the biologically less active material present to various degrees in different TSH preparations represented degradation products, TSH components at different stages of biosynthesis, or non-TSH impurities.

Joshi and Weintraub[204] provided evidence that diverse forms of TSH exist naturally that have different biopotencies. They examined the interaction of mouse tumor and bovine pituitary TSH with standard bovine TSH on the activation of adenylate cyclase in human thyroid membranes. Tumor extract, serum from tumor-bearing mice, culture media from dispersed thyrotropic cell incubations, and two preparations of purified bovine TSH (Sigma and Pierce) were fractionated on Sephadex G-100 (1.2 X 200cm). For each column fraction, immunoactivity was determined by radioimmunoassay, and TSH bioactivity was assessed by stimulation of adenylate cyclase activity by human thyroid membranes. Pierce bovine TSH had multiple immunoactive components with ratios of biological: immunological activity (B/I) of 0.59 to 1.42. Sigma bovine TSH, mouse tumor extract, mouse serum, and culture media were even more heterogeneous with many immunoreactive components and a lower range of B/I of 0.04 to 1.01. When single doses of those fractions with the lowest B/I ratios were mixed with multiple doses of Armour TSH standard (B/I = 1), there was 30-56% inhibition of adenylate cylcase stimulation. Double reciprocal plots showed competitive inhibition for the low B/I forms in most cases; TSH forms in culture media had the highest inhibitory activity. To determine the chemical differences between the different forms of TSH, affinity chromatography using concanavalin A, wheat germ agglutinin, and soybean agglutinin was performed. Compared with the apparent higher molecular weight form with higher B/I, the apparent lower molecular weight form with lower B/I contained decreased amounts or availability of N-acetylgalactosamine or β-galactose.

Dahlberg et al.[315] reported the existence of naturally occurring forms of human TSH having varying B/I ratios. TSH from sera of hypothyroid patients and normal subjects was immunoaffinity purified up to 400-fold, and then tested for cAMP generating activity using cultured FRTL-5 rat thyroid cells. The TSH B/I ratios varied from less than 0.25 to 1.21 among four euthyroid persons and eight patients with primary hypothyroidism. An inverse correlation was found between B/I ratios of immunopurified basal TSH and the serum-free T_4, and T_3. B/I ratios of TSH from three hypothyroid patients before and after acute stimulation by TRH showed no significant change, despite major changes in serum TSH. Thus, there appeared to be an inverse relationship between the metabolic status of an individual and the intrinsic bioactivity of TSH. It was presumed that TSH oligosaccharide structure differed in different physiologic states, providing the basis for the differences in TSH bioactivity.

Several groups have directly tested the role of the oligosaccharide moieties in thyrotropin action. Berman et al.[316] studied human TSH treated with anhydrous hydrogen fluoride, and bovine TSH treated with trifluoromethane sulfonic acid. Deglycosylated human TSH was 6-fold more potent than native human TSH, but was much less potent than Pierce bovine TSH, in inhibiting ^{125}I-TSH binding to porcine thyroid membranes. In contrast, the deglycosylated bovine TSH had greatly impaired receptor binding activity, perhaps due to damage during deglycosylation. The ability of the several forms of TSH to stimulate adenylate cyclase activity in vitro was tested using thyroid membranes. Deglycosylated human TSH retained about 80% of its potency, whereas the chemically-treated bovine TSH had little activity. When added to increasing concentrations of native bovine TSH (Sigma), however, the deglycosylated human TSH antagonized the ability of bovine TSH to generate cAMP. These data suggested that although the effects of TSH deglycosylation are not as dramatic as for the gonadotropins, the oligosaccharides of TSH appear to be required for maximal activation of adenylate cyclase by the hormone. Amir et al.[317] deglycosylated highly purified bovine TSH with anhydrous hydrogen fluoride. Amino acid and carbohydrate analyses of the original and deglycosylated preparations indicated that 85% of the carbohydrate originally present had been removed, and that the protein moiety was unaltered. In a TSH radioreceptor assay, native and deglycosylated bovine TSH bound to human thyroid membranes with equal affinity, since both caused a half-maximal inhibition of ^{125}I-bovine TSH binding at approximately equal concentrations (Fig. 15). The deglycosylated hormone displayed only about one third the activity of native TSH, however, in stimulating adenylate cyclase activity in human thyroid membranes. The deglycosylated hormone also antagonized the adenylate cyclase-stimulating activity of native TSH in this system, but only weakly, since abolition of the native TSH effect required a 40-fold excess of the deglycosylated TSH (Fig. 16). In cultures of FRTL-5 rat thyroid cells the deglycosylated TSH was not as effective as native hormone in stimulating cell growth (as judged by ^{3}H-thymidine incorporation) or causing release of cAMP into the medium (Fig. 17). The deglycosylated TSH evoked a smaller response than did native TSH in an in vivo mouse assay (Fig. 18). These authors concluded that the oligosaccharides of TSH are not required for receptor recognition, but are essential for the full expression of biological activity. These results and conclusions are in general agreement with those of Amr et al.[318], who studied the activity of chemically deglycosylated TSH using human thyroid membranes.

Although they did not employ deglycosylation, Menezes-Ferreira et al.[283] studied the modulation of rat TSH bioactivity by thyroid hormone and TRH. These factors presumably altered the TSH oligosaccharides. Normal or thyroidectomized rats were injected with TRH in vivo for 24 hours, then rat pituitaries were incubated in vitro for 6 hours in the absence or presence of 10mM TRH. The biological activity of TSH in pituitary extracts and media was measured in terms of stimulation of adenylate cyclase in human thyroid membranes. The bioactivity of TSH from various experimental groups apparently increased or decreased by about a factor of 2 compared to control. Hypothyroidism caused TSH remaining within pituitaries to be less bioactive, and favored the effect of TRH to cause secretion of more bioactive hormone. TRH caused the synthesis of more bioactive forms of TSH, and enhanced their release into the medium.

In 1987 Nissim et al.[319] reported a new sensitive TSH bioassay

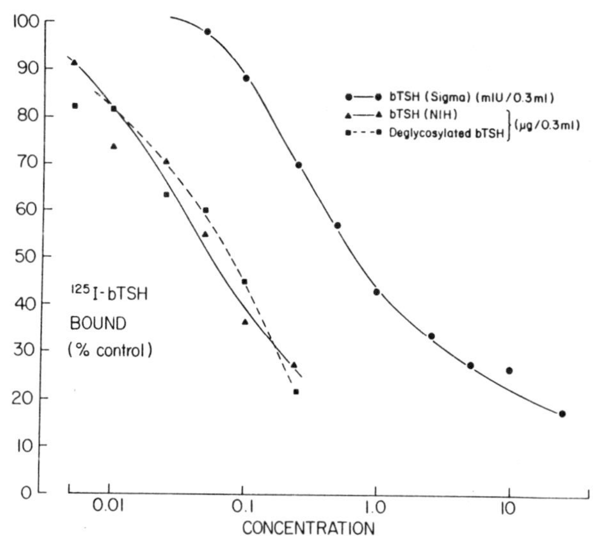

Fig. 15. Inhibition of binding of ^{125}I-bovine TSH to human thyroid membranes by bovine TSH or deglycosylated TSH. Reproduced with permission from Amir et al.[317]

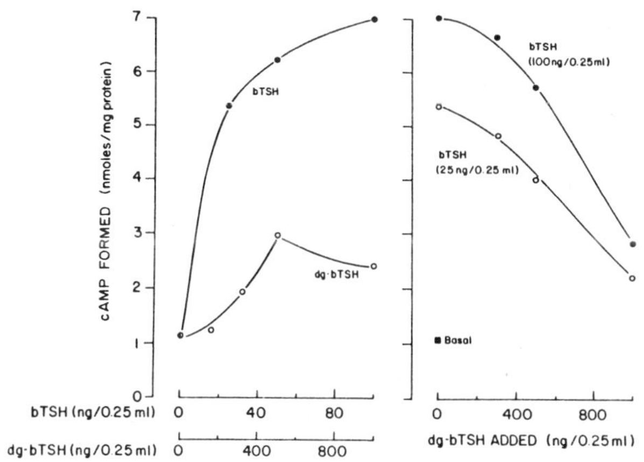

Fig. 16. Antagonistic effect of deglycosylated bovine TSH on adenylate cyclase activity induced by bTSH. Intact bTSH and dg-bTSH were either tested alone (left) or in combination (right). In the latter experiments, bTSH and dg-bTSH were mixed together before the addition of human thyroid membranes. Reproduced with permission from Amir et al.[317]

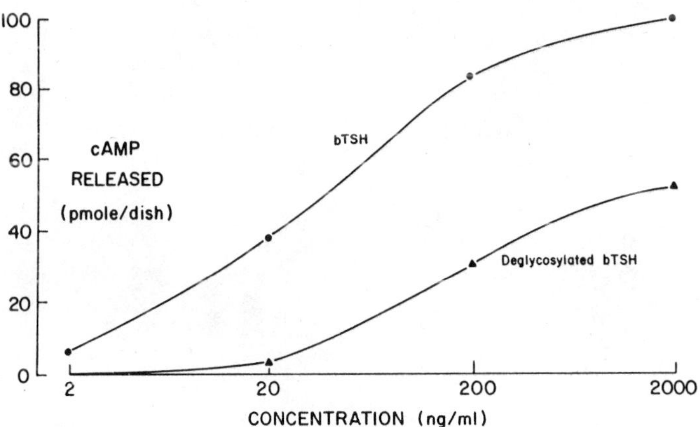

Fig. 17. Stimulation of cAMP release by bTSH and dg-bTSH in FRTL5 cells. Reproduced with permission from Amir et al.[317]

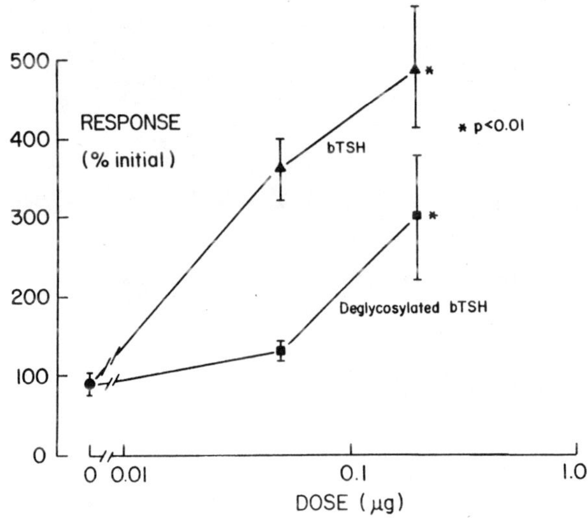

Fig. 18. Bioactivity of bTSH and dg-bTSH in an in vivo mouse assay. The response was the release of ^{125}I from the thyroid at 2h after test samples were injected into the tail vein. Reproduced with permission from Amir et al.[317]

based on iodide uptake in rat FRTL-5 thyroid cells. They measured the bioactivity of TSH from various sources in the new assay, as well as in an adenylate cyclase assay. They also enzymatically deglycosylated bovine and human TSH and compared the bioactivities of these reagents to that of native hormones in both assays. In the iodide uptake assay, pituitary-derived TSH from different species had substantially different biopotencies; human TSH was 29- and 10-fold less potent than bovine and rat TSH, respectively. Immunoaffinity-purified human serum TSH was tested in both bioassays. In the adenylate cyclase bioassay, serum TSH showed increased bioactivity in patients with primary hypothyroidism or TSH-secreting pituitary tumor compared to that in normal subjects, but in the iodide uptake bioassay minimal differences were detected among the different groups. Concerning studies of deglycosylated human and bovine TSH, peptide-N-glycosidase and endo-β-N-acetylglucosaminidase F were used to remove one oligosaccharide chain from TSH α-subunit, and all three chains from TSH, respectively. The removal of one oligosaccharide chain from both human and bovine TSH significantly decreased their biologic activity about 2-fold in both the adenylate cyclase assay and the iodide uptake assay. Paradoxically, removal of all three oligosaccharide chains decreased their bioactivity only in the iodide uptake assay; these disparate results suggested that second messengers other than cAMP may play a role in TSH action. One lesson of this study is that the assessment of the bioactivity of hormones is a complex business, and is clearly assay-dependent.

Another approach to the investigation of the biological function of the oligosaccharides of the glycoprotein hormones is to use techniques of molecular biology to create mutant hormone subunits that lack asparagine glycosylation sites, as has been discussed earlier for the case of hCG.[163,164] However, deglycosylation of mature hormone might theoretically be a more suitable technique because a mutant hormone that is never glycosylated during biosynthesis likely would have aberrant folding and incorrect internal disulfide bond formation, and therefore might be a poor candidate molecule for assessing the role of the oligosaccharides in bioactivity. Nevertheless, in a recent elegant study Matzuk et al.[354] used site-directed mutagenesis to create hCG molecules lacking oligosaccharides at certain sites, and reported that the carbohydrate at Asn^{52} of the α-subunit was particularly important for bioactivity in an *in vitro* assay measuring progesterone production by MA-10 cells. An alternative approach would be to use monoclonal antibodies to study the relationship between the immunologic structure and the bioactivity of TSH. In a recent interesting study, Costagliola et al.[320] employed monoclonal antibodies to the peptide portions of TSH, but did not test antibodies to the oligosaccharides. Twenty-four monoclonal antibodies to 11 different antigenic regions of human TSH were tested for both binding to TSH and inhibition of TSH stimulation of adenylate cyclase in human thyroid membranes. Using various antibodies, biopotency was inhibited 3-92%. This technique extends prior studies of the effects of chemical modifications of TSH. Monoclonal antibodies directed to human and equine chorionic gonadotropins were prepared by Bidart et al.[321], and were used as probes for the topographic analysis of epitopes on the human α-subunit. Certain amino acid residues in separate regions of the primary sequence were postulated to be topographically adjacent.

Evaluation of TSH bioactivity in certain clinical settings has also been informative. In 1979 Faglia et al.[322] studied TSH levels in plasma of 89 patients with hypothyroidism due to various hypothalamicpituitary disorders. Basal TSH was slightly elevated in about 25% of the patients, suggesting that the hormone had inappropriately low bioactivity in these patients. The serum T_3 response to TRH was absent or low in 40 out of 53 patients in whom it was evaluated. Administration of T_3 (100ug/day for 3 days) reduced both basal and TRH-stimulated TSH levels. TSH was of normal size by gel chromatography. Plasma TSH values determined by cytochemical bioassay of both basal and TRH-stimulated samples from five patients were markedly lower than those obtained by radioimmunoassay. Thus, it was believed that some patients with central hypothyroidism secreted forms of TSH with low bioactivity. In a follow-up study in 1983[323] α-subunit and β-subunit of TSH were measured in the sera of five patients with idiopathic central hypothyroidism, in seven normal persons, and in five patients with primary hypothyroidism both before and after administration of TRH. Patients with central hypothyroidism had an excess of circulating TSH β-subunits. One patient with central hypothyroidism was given oral TRH (40 mg/day for 4 weeks). This patient's serum free T_4 level rose from 9 pmol/l at the start of the study to 27 pmol/l at 2 weeks, and was 18 pmol/l at 4 weeks; at the end of the trial the serum TSH was about 0.5 ng/ml, only slightly higher than at the start, suggesting that TRH caused a more bioactive form of TSH to be synthesized. Presumably a qualitatively different form of TSH was made after chronic exposure to TRH.

In a study of TSH from seven patients with hypothalamic hypothyroidism, Beck-Peccoz et al.[324] evaluated the adenylate cyclase-stimulting bioactivity and the receptor-binding activity of the immunoaffinity purified hormone. The TSH of each patient was defective in both activities as compared with TSH from normal persons. After long-term administration of TRH for 20 to 30 days, both activities of TSH returned to normal in six of the seven patients, and resulted clinically in enhanced serum thyroid hormone levels. Thus, in some cases of hypothalamic hypothyroidism, secreted TSH lacks biologic activity because of impaired binding to its receptor; TRH treatment can correct these defects. TRH regulates both the secretion of TSH and, presumably, specific structural features required for hormone action. Recently, Miura et al.[223] have reported qualitative differences in the structure of TSH from euthyroid, primary hypothyroid, and central hypothyroid patients.

In 1981 Spitz et al.[325] reported the case of a healthy 29 year-old man with a very high serum level of a qualitatively abnormal TSH. The serum levels of T_4, T_3 resin uptake and T_3 were normal, but the TSH was 75 uU/ml. Sephacryl G-200 gel chromatography of the patient's serum showed that the TSH immunoreactivity eluted near the void volume (mol. wt. greater than 200,000 daltons). The function of the TSH was studied in both a radioreceptor and adenylate cyclase assay. The thyroid membrane binding properties of this large TSH were relatively normal, but the potency in the adenylate cyclase assay was only 4% that of TSH from controls. Although the precise biochemical nature of this abnormal TSH remains unknown, it represents a clear example of a naturally occurring form of TSH with normal ability to bind to the receptor but decreased ability to stimulate second messenger. In contrast, a form of TSH with increased bioactivity was reported by Beck-Peccoz et al.[324] They described a 40 year-old man with acromegaly and hyperthyroidism who had elevated total and free thyroid hormone levels in the blood, but a TSH of 1.2-1.5 uU/ml. High levels of serum free α-subunit were present. Six months after pituitary adenomectomy, serum thyroid hormone levels and the patient's clinical status were normal, and the basal TSH was 0.4 uU/ml. Gel filtration of serum TSH prior to surgery revealed an appearent mol. wt. of about 29,000 daltons, slightly smaller than that of TSH from control sera. After surgery, TSH in the patient's serum appeared to be of normal mol. wt. When tested *in vitro* in an adenylate cyclase assay, the biological to immunological ratio of the patient's abnormal TSH was significantly higher than that of control TSH, with B/I of 6.9-0.2 vs. 4.4-1.1. When cultured *in vitro*, adenoma fragments actively secreted growth hormone and TSH. Immunostaining of the tumor showed that all cells were positive for growth hormone and α-subunits, but only a very few cells had TSH β-subunits. This case illustrates that a small amount of TSH with increased biological activity is capable of producing hyperthyroidism if the hormone is secreted autonomously. Although the biochemical nature of the abnormal TSH remains unknown, it is possible that differences in the oligosaccharide moieties may have been responsible for the altered bioactivity.

METABOLIC CLEARANCE STUDIES OF TSH

One of the potential roles of the oligosaccharides of TSH is the modulation of the hormone's metabolic clearance rate (MCR). One could postulate that, if it is true that these oligosaccharide structures are influenced by endocrine stimuli in various physiologic states, then qualitatively different forms of TSH might be secreted having intrinsic bioactivity (as might be measured *in vitro*), MCR, and *in vivo* bioactivity (that might reflect both *in vitro* bioactivity and MCR) appropriate for a particular physiologic state.

Early studies[326-339] investigating the MCR and distribution of

TSH in the rat and other species have used both radioactively labeled and unlabeled TSH, and have quantified the unlabeled hormone by various means, including _in vivo_ and _in vitro_ bioassays and RIA. In these cases the TSH preparations tested were derived from the pituitaries of euthyroid animals, and thus included heterogeneous forms of TSH, including precursor forms. In 1962 Bakke and Lawrence[330] studied the disappearance rate and distribution of bovine, rat and human TSH after intravenous injection into euthyroid rats. The rates of disappearance did not differ substantially for TSH of different species, and the half-life was about 12 minutes. In agreement with other workers of that era, they found that the kidney cleared a substantial portion of the TSH. In 1978 Silva and Larsen[335] carefully studied the peripheral metabolism of homologous radioiodinated TSH in euthyroid and hypothyroid rats. They carefully checked the validity of following TSH disappearance by using RIA by also evaluating trichloroacetic acid (TCA)-precipitable activity, and by immunoprecipitating TSH. The disappearance rate of TCA-precipitable ^{125}I (t1/2 = 28 min) was significantly longer than that of immunoprecipitable ^{125}I (t1/2=22 min), although other workers in the next decade who purified iodinated TSH more carefully using longer columns did not find this discrepancy. The disappearance rate of immunoprecipitable iodinated TSH was identical to that of noniodinated rat TSH and of the TRH-induced TSH increment in euthyroid rats. The disappearance rate of suppressible TSH (after T_3 treatment) in hypothyroid animals was only slightly longer than the rate of disappearance of immunoprecipitable iodinated TSH (40 vs. 36 min) in the same rats. The calculated MCR of TSH was slightly lower in hypothyroid rats (18.3±3.0 ml/h/100g BW, mean ±SD) than it was in euthyroid rats (22.6±2.1). Other studies have reported that the MCR of TSH is slightly reduced in hypothyroidism[334-336], but Connors et al.[340] reported that MCR decreased as a function of age but was not decreased by severe hypothyroidism.

In 1986 Constant and Weintraub[341] investigated whether TSH from different sources and from different physiological states might have different metabolic clearance characteristics. They also studied the effects of chemical deglycosylation of TSH on MCR, as well as the targeting and distribution of radiolabeled pituitary TSH. They compared purified pituitary rat TSH, TSH from crude pituitary extracts of normal and hypothyroid rats, TSH from hypothyroid rat sera, and TSH secreted by hypothyroid rat pituitaries incubated _in vitro_. After intravenous injection into euthyroid rats, ^{125}I-labeled rat TSH was determined by acid precipitation in serum and various organs, and unlabeled TSH was measured by RIA. The MCR of TSH from normal pituitary extracts (0.53±0.02 ml/min) was similar to that of unlabeled purified rat TSH (0.52±0.03), while those from hypothyroid pituitary extracts (0.32±0.03) and hypothyroid sera (0.33±0.01) were decreased. The reduced MCR of TSH from hypothyroid pituitaries was due to a decreased distribution volume (8.4±0.6 ml) compared to that from normal pituitaries (11.4±0.7). The decreased MCR of circulating TSH from hypothyroid sera reflected an increase in its t1/2 (12.6±0.5 min) vs. that from both normal (5.1±0.5) and hypothyroid (5.7±0.4) pituitaries. The t1/2 of *in vitro* secreted TSH was intermediate between those of circulating and pitutiary forms of TSH from hypothyroid rats. These investigators also compared the clearances of native and deglycosylated bovine TSH; the MCR were 0.59±0.02 ml/min and 0.71±0.02 ml/min, respectively, and the t1/2 were 4.7±0.02 min and 3.8±0.1 min, respectively. Thus, the metabolic clearance of TSH differed between pituitary and serum forms of TSH, and varied with the physiological state of the animal from which the TSH was derived. Because chemical deglycosylation increased the clearance of TSH, it was speculated that the basis for changes in TSH clearance was related to the oligosaccharide structures of the TSH. This conjecture is consistent with what is known about the clearance of glycoproteins in general[342-344], although Lefort et al.[345] have downplayed the role of the hepatic galactose receptor in the normal clearance of hCG, and Blithe and Nisula[346] have reported that free α-subunits and α-subunits from hCG heterodimers have similar clearance rates in spite of differences in sialic acid content, perhaps because exposed galactose residues in both types of subunits are actually present in similar amounts. Rosa et al.[347] clearly showed, however, that desialylated hCG had a markedly accelerated clearance rate in humans as compared to intact hCG. Only future invesigations will determine with certainty whether or not modulation of oligosaccharide structures of the glycoprotein hormones is a physiologic mechanism for adjusting the MCR of these hormones.

RECENT STRUCTURE-FUNCTION STUDIES EMPLOYING SYNTHETIC PEPTIDES

During the 1970's, chemical modifications were made to glycoprotein hormone subunits to gain insight into functional domains of the molecules; these studies have been reviewed elsewhere.[40,348,349] Most such studies have concerned the gonadotropins rather than TSH. For example, lysine-49 in the α-subunit must lie near the β-subunit of bovine lutropin because it can be cross-linked to Asp-111 in β by carbodiimide[350]; modification of lysine-49 in the α-subunit inhibits subunit combination. Interestingly, the Asp-111 present in LH β-subunit is replaced by threonine or serine in TSH and FSH, respectively. Tyrosine-41 in the α-subunit cannot be iodinated or nitrated in the heterodimer, but can be affected in the free α-subunit, suggesting that it lies in the contact domain. Crosslinking experiments using LH and its receptor suggest that both the α- and the β-subunit interact with the plasma membrane receptor.

Comparison of α-subunit sequence data from several species has permitted an analysis of conserved regions that may have functional importance. Ten half-cystine residues in the α-subunit have been conserved. The amino-terminal region up to the first half-cystine is heterogeneous and is probably less important for heterodimer formation or receptor binding. Residues 27 to 67 are highly conserved, as are residues 82 to 92 in the carboxyl-terminus. Chemical modification studies[40,348,349] have suggested that these two regions of the α-subunit are important for receptor binding. For example, derivatization of Arg-35 and Arg-42 in the native hormone using 1,2-cyclohexanedione causes loss of biological activity.[348] Nitration of the tyrosines in the carboxyl-terminus of hCG α-subunit, or enzymatic cleavage of two to five amino acids from this region, reduces the affinity of receptor binding.[40]

Chemical modification studies, however, may be misleading due to poor definition of the precise residue that was modified, the presence of unreacted hormone, and unanticipated effects on secondary and tertiary structure. To avoid these pitfalls, a synthetic peptide strategy has recently been employed by Ryan et al.[193,351-353] A series of short peptides replicating the entire amino acid sequence of human α-subunit was synthesized by Merrifield solid phase methods; the peptides were designed to be "overlapping" (replicating α-subunit residues 1-15, 11-25, 21-35, etc.). They also prepared a series of monoclonal antibodies from mice immunized with hCG α-subunit; some monoclonals inhibited the binding of hCG and hLH to rat ovarian membranes. Finally, certain of the synthetic peptides were found to inhibit binding of ^{125}I-hCG to these monoclonals, and some of the synthetic peptides could directly inhibit hCG or LH binding to ovarian receptors. Regions of the α-subunit between residues 26 and 46, and between 76 and 92 were found to be important for receptor binding, in agreement with prior chemical modification studies.

Peptides from these same two regions also inhibited ^{125}I-bovine TSH binding to human thyroid membranes and FRTL-5 rat thyroid cells and stimulation by TSH of adenylate cyclase activity in FRTL-5 cells.[35] Peptide 26-46 also inhibited this stimulation by serum from ten patients with Graves' disease. Analogous studies have been performed by these authors using synthetic peptides replicating sequences in the hCG and hLH β-subunits, but thus far not with TSH β-subunits.

A MODEL OF ALPHA-SUBUNIT STRUCTURE

Although there is no crystallographic information available for the glycoprotein hormones, Ryan et al.[351] have used computer techniques to model the structure of the α-subunit and of the hCG β-subunit. Regions of the α-subunit amino acid sequence were assumed to have particular secondary structures (α-helix, β-sheet, β-turn and random coil), and bond angle information and the amino acid sequence was entered into MAKEPOLYPEPTIDE, a computer program available on the PROPHET system. The resultant atomic coordinates were then downloaded to MOGLI, a molecular graphics program. The model was adjusted to bring together half-cystines forming well-established disulfide bonds (Cys-11-35, and 14-36), and then the remaining disulfides were accommodated (Cys-32-64, 63-91, and 86-88). Disulfides were placed at the surface of the molecule near the β-subunit interface surface. The models are constantly being updated and the final structures have not been solved. In a 1988 version, however, residues Tyr^{92}, Try^{93}, and Phe^{21} were placed on the surface away from the subunit interface, while Leu^{30} was placed in the interior. Oligosaccharide-linked residues, Asn^{56} and Asn^{82}, as well as all His and Arg residues, were located at the surface. Two regions thought to be receptor binding domains (residues 34-49 and residues 80-96) appear to be in separate loops in the molecule. Two residues thought to be in the subunit interface (Try^{41} and Lys^{49}) are located in an overlap region; it is possible that a receptor binding domain lies very near a β-subunit binding domain. Future studies will be required to further clarify α-subunit structure.

CONCLUDING COMMENTS

TSH is an extraordinarily complicated molecule, being about 200 times larger than thyroxine, the thyroid product whose secretion it controls. It would seem that a much smaller peptide could have acted as a unique signal to travel from the pituitary thyrotrope to the thyroid. Apparently, the emergence of the family of the glycoprotein hormones through the ages, by gene duplication or other mechanisms, resulted in a complicated thyrotrophic hormone that may have unusual control mechanisms. The hormone's qualitative structure as well as the amount of hormone secreted appear to be regulated. Unlike most glycoproteins, the oligosaccharides of TSH appear to play vital functional roles. Precursor forms of the oligosaccharides allow nascent subunits to fold properly during biosynthesis and prevent subunit degradation and aggregation. Mature oligosaccharides influence the hormone's metabolic clearance rate and biological activity. Some studies suggest that the structures of the oligosaccharides may be regulated by endocrine factors during TSH biosynthesis so that qualitatively different forms of TSH are secreted in different physiologic states. Aberrant clinical states exist in which TSH has inappropriately low or high biological activity. Thus, TSH may be a prototype of a new class of physiologically vital glycoproteins whose biological functions depend critically on proper oligosaccharide structures. Perhaps improper carbohydrate structures on such glycoproteins may explain some currently poorly understood endocrine and nonendocrine disease states.

ACKNOWLEDGEMENT

Expert secretarial assistance was provided by Margaret Nickless.

REFERENCES

1. P. E. Smith, Experimental ablation of the hypophysis in the frog embryo, <u>Science</u> 44:280 (1916).

2. B. M. Allen, The results of extirpation of the anterior lobe o the hypophysis and of the thyroid of Rana pipiens larvae, Science 44:755 (1916).
3. P. E. Smith, Relations of the activity of the pituitary and thyroid glands, Harvey Lectures Ser. 25:129 (1931).
4. A. White, The isolation and chemistry of anterior pituitary hormones influencing growth and metabolism, in: The Chemistry and Physiology of Hormones, ed., F.R. Moulton. Lancaster (1944).
5. A. White, Preparation and chemistry of anterior pituitary hormones, Physiol. Rev. 26:574 (1946).
6. A. Albert, The biochemistry of the thyrotropic hormone, Ann. N Acad. Sci. 50:466 (1949).
7. M. Sonenberg, Chemistry and physiology of the thyroid stimulating hormone, Vitamins Hormones 16:205 (1958).
8. R. W. Bates and P.G. Condliffe, Studies on the chemistry and bioassay of thyrotropins from bovine pituitaries, transplantable pituitary tumors of mice, and blood plasma, Recent Progr. Hormone Res. 16: 309 (1960).
9. J. G. Pierce, M.E. Carsten and L.K. Wynston. Purification and chemistry of the thyroid-stimulating hormone, Ann. NY Acad Sci. 86:612 (1960).
10. R. W. Bates and P.G. Condliffe, The physiology and chemistry o thyroid stimulating hormone, in: The Pituitary Gland, G.W. Harris and B.T. Donovan, eds., Berkeley: Univ. of Californi Press, (1966).
11. P. G. Condliffe and J. Robbins, Pituitary thyroid-stimulating hormone and other thyroid-stimulating substances, in: Hormones in Blood (2nd ed.), ed., C.H. Gray and A.L. Bacharach, New York, (1967).
12. J. G. Pierce, Chemistry of thyroid-stimulating hormone, in: Handbook of Physiology, The Pituitary Gland, American Physiological Society, Bethesda, (1974).
13. C. T. Sawin, Defining thyroid hormone: its nature and control, in: Endocrinology, People and Ideas, S.M. McCann, ed., American Physiological Society, Bethesda, (1988).
14. R. G. Hoskins, The thyroid-pituitary apparatus as a servo (feedback) mechanism, J. Clin. Endocr. 9:1429 (1949).
15. K. Brown-Grant, The "feedback" hypothesis of the control of thyroid function, Ciba Found. Colloq. Endocrinol. 10:97 (1957).
16. S. Reichlin, Functions of the median eminence gland, New End. J.Med. 275:600 (1966).
17. P. E. Smith and I.P. Smith, The repair and activation of the thyroid in the hypophysectomized tadpole by the parenteral administration of fresh anterior lobe of the bovine hypophysis, J.Med. Res. 43:267 (1922).
18. P. E. Smith, Ablation and transplantation of the hypophysis in the rat, Anat. Rec. 32:221 (1926).

19. M. Aron, Action de la prehypophyse sur le thyroide chez le cobaye, C.R. Seances Soc. Biol. Fil. 102:682 (1929).
20. L. Loeb and R.B. Bassett, Effect of hormones of anterior pituitary on thyroid gland in the guinea pig, Proc. Soc. Exp. Biol. Med. 26:860 (1929).
21. K. Junkmann and W. Schoeller, Uber das thyreotrope Hormon des Hypophysenvorderlappens, Klin. Wochenschr. 11:1176 (1932).
22. R. O. Greep, Separation of a thyrotropic from the gonadotropic substances of the pituitary, Am. J. Physiol. 110:692 (1935).
23. P. G. Condliffe and R.W. Bates, Chromatography of thyrotrophin on diethylaminoethyl cellulose, Arch. Biochem. Biophys. 68:229 (1957).
24. J. M. McKenzie, Bio-assay of thyrotrophin in man, Physiol. Rev. 40:398 (1960).
25. T.-H. Liao, G. Hennen, S.M. Howard, B. Shome, and J.G. Pierce, Bovine thyrotropin. Countercurrent distribution and a comparison with the isolated subunits of luteinizing hormone, J. Biol. Chem. 244:6458 (1969).
26. B. Shome, D.M. Brown, S.M. Howard, and J.G. Pierce, Bovine, human and porcine thyrotropins: molecular weights, amino- and carboxyl-terminal studies, Arch. Biochem. Biophys. 126:456 (1968).
27. H. Papkoff and T.S.A. Samy, Isolation and partial characterization of the polypeptide chains of ovine interstitial cell-stimulating hormone, Biochim. Biophys. Acta 147:175 (1967).
28. P. G. Condliffe, Biochemical specificity of thyrotropins, in: La Specificite Zoologique des Hormones Hypophysaires et de Leurs Acitivites, Paris: Centre Natl. Rech. Sci., (1969).
29. T.-H. Liao and J.G. Pierce, The presence of a common type of subunit in bovine thyroid stimulating and luteinizing hormones, J. Biol. Chem. 245:3275 (1970).
30. T.-H. Liao and J.G. Pierce, The primary structure of bovine thyrotropin. II. The amino acid sequences of the reduced, S-carboxymethyl α and β chains, J. Biol. Chem. 246:850 (1971).
31. W. Gilbert, Why genes in pieces? Nature 271:501 (1978).
32. F. Crick, Split genes and RNA splicing, Science 204:264 (1979).
33. J. Darnell, Variety in the level of gene control in eucaryotic cells, Nature 297:365 (1982).
34. G. Blobel and B. Dobberstein, Transfer of proteins across membranes, I. Presence of proteolytically processed and unprocessed nascent immunoglobulin light chains on membrane-bound ribosomes of murine myeloma, J. Cell Biol. 67: 835 (1975).
35. J. A. Magner, Information in the signal peptide? J. Theor. Biol. 99:831 (1982).
36. M. Hortsch and D.I. Meyer, Pushing the signal hypothesis: What are the limits? Biol. Cell 52:1 (1984).
37. Y. Fujimoto, Y. Watanabe, M. Uchida and M. Ozaki, Mammalian

signal peptidase: Partial purification and general characterization of the signal peptidase from microsomal membranes of porcine pancreas, J. Biochem. 96:1125 (1984).

38. C. A. Kaiser, D. Preuss, P. Grisafi and D. Botstein, Many random sequences functionally replace the secretion signal sequence of yeast invertase, Science 235:312 (1987).

39. M. Sjostrom, S. Wold, A. Wieslander, and L. Rilfors, Signal peptide amino acid sequences in *Escherichia coli* contain information related to final protein localization. A multivariate data analysis, EMBO J. 6:823 (1987).

40. J. G. Pierce, and T.F. Parsons, Glycoprotein hormones: structure and function, Annu. Rev. Biochem. 50:465 (1981).

41. W. W. Chin, Organization and expression of glycoprotein hormone genes, *in*: The Pituitary Gland, Imura, ed., Raven, New York (1985).

42. J. M. Hershman and A.E. Pekary, Regulation of thyrotropin secretion, *in*: The Pituitary Gland, Imura, ed., Raven, New York (1985).

43. W. W. Chin, Glycoprotein hormone genes, in: Habener ed: Molecular Cloning of Hormone Genes. Humana, Clifton (1987).

44. W. W. Chin, Hormonal regulation of thyrotropin and gonadotropin gene expression, Clinical Research 36(5):484 (1988).

45. J. C. Fiddes and H.M, Goodman, Isolation, cloning and sequence analysis of the cDNA for the α-subunit of human chorionic gonadotropin, Nature 281:351 (1979).

46. J. C. Fiddes and H.M. Goodman, The gene encoding the common alpha subunit of the four human glycoprotein hormones, J. Mol. Appl. Genet. 1:3 (1981).

47. W. W. Chin, H.M. Kronenberg, P.C. Dee, F. Maloof and J.F. Habener, Nucleotide sequence of the mRNA encoding the pre-α-subunit of mouse thyrotropin, Proc. Natl. Acad. Sci. U.S.A 78:5329 (1981).

48. J. E. Godine, W.W. Chin, and J.F. Habener, α-subunit of rat pituitary glycoprotein hormones: primary structure of the precursor determined from the nucleotide sequence of cloned cDNAs, J. Biol. Chem. 257:8368 (1982).

49. J. H. Nilson, A.R. Thomason, M.T. Cserbak, C.L. Moncman and R.P. Woychik, Nucleotide sequence of a cDNA for the common α-subunit of the bovine pituitary glycoprotein hormones, J Biol. Chem. 258:4679 (1983).

50. J. E. Godine, W.W. Chin, and J.F. Habener, Detection of two precursors to each of the subunits of human chorionic gonadotropin translated from placental mRNA in the wheat germ cell-free system, Biochem. Biophys. Res. Commun. 104:463 (1982).

51. W. W. Chin, J.V. Maizel, Jr., and J.F. Habener, Differences in sizes of human compared to murine alpha subunits of the glycoprotein hormones arises by a four-codon gene deletion or insertion, Endocrinology 112:482 (1983).

52. M. Boothby, R.W. Ruddon, C. Anderson, D. McWilliams, and I. Boime, A single gonadotropin α-subunit gene in normal tissue and tumor-derived cell-lines, J. Biol. Chem. 256:5121 (1981).

53. R. G. Goodwin, C.L. Moncman, F.M. Rottman, and J.H. Nilson, Characterization and nucleotide sequence of the gene for the common α-subunit of the bovine pituitary glycoprotein hormones, Nucleic Acid Res. 11:6873 (1983).

54. J. Burnside, P.R. Buckland and W.W. Chin, Isolation and characterization of the gene encoding the α-subunit of the rat pituitary glycoprotein hormone, Gene 70:67 (1988).

55. J. A. Bokar, W.J. Roesler, G.R. Vandenbark, D.M. Kaetzel, R.W. Hanson and J.H. Nilson, Characterization of the cAMP responsive elements from the genes for the α-subunit of glycoprotein hormones and phosphoenolpyruvate carboxykinase (GTP), J.Biol. Chem. 263:19740 (1988).

56. S. L. Naylor, W.W. Chin, H.M. Goodman, P.A. Lalley, K.H. Grzeschik and A.Y. Sakaguchi, Chromosomal assignment of genes encoding the α- and β-subunits of glycoprotein hormones in man and mouse, Somatic Cell Genet. 9:757 (1983).

57. I. A. Kourides, P.E. Barker, J.A. Gurr, D.D. Pravtcheva and F.H. Ruddle, Assignment of the genes for the α- and β-subunits of thyrotropin to different mouse chromosomes, Proc. Nat. Acad. Sci. U.S.A. 81:517 (1984).

58. W. W. Chin, J.F. Habener, J.D. Kieffer and F. Maloof, Cell-free translation of the messenger RNA coding for the α-subunit, J. Biol. Chem. 253:7985 (1978).

59. I. A. Kourides and B.D. Weintraub, mRNA-Directed biosynthesis of α-subunit of thyrotropin: Translation in cell-free and whole-cell systems, Proc. Nat. Acad. Sci. U.S.A. 76:298 (1979).

60. R. A. Maurer, M.L. Croyle and J.E. Donelson, Sequence of a cloned cDNA for the beta subunit of bovine thyrotropin predicts a protein containing both NH_2 and COOH terminal extensions, J. Biol. Chem. 259:5024 (1984).

61. J. A. Gurr, J.F. Catterall and I.A. Kourides, Cloning of cDNA encoding the pre- β subunit of mouse thyrotropin, Proc. Natl. Acad. Sci. U.S.A. 80:2122 (1983).

62. W. W. Chin, J.A. Muccini and L. Shin, Cloning and characterization on of cDNAs encoding the precursor of the β-subunit of rat thyrotropin, Biochemistry (submitted).

63. M. L. Croyle, A. Bhattacharya, D.F. Gordon, Analysis of the organization and nucleotide sequence of the chromosomal gene for the β-subunit of rat thyrotropin, DNA 5:299 (1986).

64. F. E. Carr, L.R. Need, W.W. Chin, Isolation and characterization of the rat thyrotropin β-subunit gene: Differential regulation of two transcriptional start sites by thyroid hormone, J. Biol. Chem. 62:981 (1987).

65. F. E. Carr, and W.W. Chin, Differential thyroid-hormone-regulated rat TSH β gene expression detected by blot hybridization, Mol. Endo. 2:667 (1988).
66. W. M. Wood, D.F. Gordon and E.C. Ridgway, Expression of the β-subunit gene of murine thyrotropin results in multiple messenger ribonucleic acid species which are generated by alternative exon splicing, Mol. Endo. 1:875 (1987).
67. O. Wolf, I.A. Kourides and J.A. Gurr, Expression of the gene for the β-subunit of mouse thyrotropin results in multiple mRNAs differing in their 5'-untranslated regions, J. Biol. Chem. 262:16596 (1987).
68. F. E. Carr, J. Burnside, and W.W. Chin, Thyroid hormones regulate rat TSH β gene promoter activity expressed in GH_3 cells, Ann. Mtg. American Thyroid Assn., Abstract T-66, (1987).
69. M. D. Crew and S.R. Spindler, Thyroid hormone regulation of the transfected rat growth hormone promoter, J. Biol. Chem. 261:5018 (1986).
70. F. Flug, R.P. Copp, J. Casanova, Cis-acting elements of the rat growth hormone gene which mediate basal and regulated expression by thyroid hormone, J. Biol. Chem. 262:6373 (1987).
71. C. K. Glass, R. Franco, C. Weinberger, A c-erb-A binding site in rat growth hormone gene mediates trans-activation by thyroid hormone, Nature 329:738 (1987).
72. R. J. Koenig, G.A. Brent, R.L. Warne, Thyroid hormone receptor binds to a site in the rat growth hormone promoter required for induction by thyroid hormone, Proc. Natl. Acad. Sci. U.S.A. 84:5670 (1987).
73. D. S. Darling, J. Burnside and W.W. Chin, Thyroid hormone receptor binds to a region of the rat TSH beta gene, Endocrine Society, Abstract #1135 (1988).
74. J. Sap, A. Munoz, K. Damm, Y. Goldberg, J. Ghysdael, A. Leutz, H. Beug and B. Vennstrom, The c-erb-A protein is a high-affinity receptor for thyroid hormone, Nature 324: 6350 (1986).
75. C. Weinberger, C.C. Thompson, E.S. Ong, R. Lebo, D. Gruol and R.M. Evans, The c-erb-A gene encodes a thyroid hormone receptor, Nature 324:641 (1986).
76. C. C. Thompson, C. Weinberger, R. Lebo, R.M. Evans, Identification of a novel thyroid hormone receptor expressed in the mammalian central nervous system, Science 237:1610 (1987).
77. M. A. Lazar, and W.W. Chin, Regulation of two c-erb-A messenger ribonucleic acids in rat GH_3 cells by thyroid hormone, Mol. Endo. 2:479 (1988).
78. M. A. Lazar, R.A. Hodin, D.S. Darling and W.W. Chin, Identification of a rat c-erbA α-related protein which binds deoxyribonucleic acid but does not bind thyroid hormone, Mol. Endo. 2:893 (1988).
79. D. F. Gordon, W.M. Wood and E.C. Ridgway, Organization and nu-

cleotide sequence of the gene encoding the β-subunit of murine thyrotropin, DNA 7:17 (1988).

80. P. A. Wight, M.D. Crew and S.R. Spindler, Discrete positive and negative thyroid hormone-responsive transcription regulatory elements of the rat growth hormone gene, J. Biol. Chem. 262:5659 (1987).

81. M. R. Montminy, K.A. Sevarino, J.A. Wagner, G. Mandel and R.H. Goodman, Identification of a cyclic-AMP-responsive element within the rat somatostatin gene, Proc. Nat. Acad. Sci. U.S.A. 83:6682 (1986).

82. M. J. Short, A. Wynshaw-Boris, H.P. Short and R.W. Hanson, Characterization of the phosphoenolpyruvate carboxykinase (GTP) promoter-regulatory region, J. Biol. Chem. 261:9721 (1986).

83. Y. Hayashizaki, K. Miyai, K. Kato and K. Matsubara, Molecular cloning of the human thyrotropin-β subunit gene, FEBS Lett. 188:394 (1985).

84. G. K. Whitfield, R.E. Powers, J.A. Gurr, O. Wolf and I.A. Kouride, Isolation of a gene encoding human thyrotropin beta subunit, in: Frontiers in Thyroidology, G. Medeiros-Neto and E. Gaitan, eds., Plenum Medical Book Co., NY (1986).

85. F. E. Wondisford, S. Radovick, J.M. Moates, S.J. Usala and B.D. Weintraub, Isolation and characterization of the human thyrotropin β-subunit gene: differences in gene structure and promoter function from murine species, J. Biol. Chem. 263:12538 (1988).

86. K. Miyai, Y. Endo, Y. Iijima, O. Kabutomori, and Y. Hayashizaki, Serum free thyrotropin subunit in congenital isolated thyrotropin deficiency, Endocrinol. Japon. 35(3):517 (1988).

87. K. Miyai, Y. Hayasizaki and K. Matsubara, Familial hypothyroidism due to thyrotropin gene abnormality, International Congress of Endocrinology, Kyoto, Symposium 76, (1988).

88. K. Miyai, M. Azukizawa and Y. Kumahara, Familial isolated thyrotropin deficiency, New Eng. J. Med. 285:1043 (1971).

89. S. Fukushige, T. Murostsu and K. Matsubara, Chromosomal assignment of human genes for gastrin, thyrotropin (TSH)-β subunit and c-erb B-2 by chromosome sorting combined with velocity sedimentation and Southern hybridization, Bioch. Biophy. Res. Commun. 134:477 (1986).

90. N. C. Dracopoli, W.J. Rettig, G.K. Whitfield, G.J. Darlington, B.A. Spengler, J.L. Biedler, L.J. Old and I.A. Kourides. Assignment of the gene for the β-subunit of thyroid-stimulating hormone to the short arm of human chromosome 1, Proc. Natl. Acad. Sci. U.S.A. 83:1822 (1986).

91. Y. Hayashizaki, Y. Endo, K. Miyai and K. Matsubara, The production of active human thyroid-stimulating hormone from α and β mRNAs in Xenopus laevis oocytes, Bioch. Biophys. Res. Commun. 152:703 (1988).

92. J. A. Franklyn and M.C. Sheppard, Regulation of TSH gene trans-

cription, European J. Clin. Invest. 16:452 (1986).

93. J. A. Franklyn and M.C. Sheppard, Thyrotrophin gene regulation, J. Endocr. 117:161 (1988).

94. J. P. Furth, J. Moy, J. Hershman and G. Ueda, Thyrotropic tumor syndrome, Arch. Pathol. 96:217 (1973).

95. J. L. Bakke and N. Lawrence, Influence of propylthiouracil and thyroxine on synthesis and secretion of thyroid stimulating hormone in the hypothyroid rat, Acta Endocrinol. (Copenh.) 46:111 (1964).

96. C. Y. Bowers, A.V. Schally, G.A. Reynolds, and W.D. Hawley, Interactions of L-thyroxine or L-triiodothyronine and thyrotropin-releasing factor on the release and synthesis of thyrotropin from the anterior pituitary gland of mice, Endocrinology 81:741 (1967).

97. G. P. Vanrees, The effect of triiodothyronine and thyroxine on thyrotropin levels in the anterior pituitary gland and blood serum of thyroidectomized rats, Acta Endocrinol. (Copenh.) 51:619 (1966).

98. A. G. Vagenakis, Regulation of TSH secretion, in: Clinical Neuroendocrinology: A Pathophysiological Approach, G. Tolis, ed., Raven Press, New York, (1979).

99. M. C. Gershengorn, Regulation of thyrotropin poduction by mouse pituitary thyrotrophic tumor cells in vitro by physiological levels of thyroid hormones, Endocrinology 102:1122 (1978).

100. G. T. Gard, B. Bernstein, and P.R. Larsen, Studies of the mechanism of 3,5,3'-triiodothyronine-induced suppression of secretagogue-induced thyrotropin release in vitro, Endocrinology 108:2046 (1981).

101. B. D. Weintraub and S.W. Rosen, Ectopic production of the isolated beta subunit of human chorionic gonadotropin, J. Clin. Invest. 52:3135 (1973).

102. A. H. Tashjian Jr., B.D. Weintraub, N.J. Barowsky, A.S. Rabson and S.W. Rosen, Subunits of human chorionic gonadotropin: unbalanced synthesis and secretion by clonal cell strains derived from a bronchogenic carcinoma, Proc. Natl. Acad. Sci. U.S.A. 70:1419 (1973).

103. S. W. Rosen and B.D. Weintraub, Ectopic production of the isolated alpha subunit of the glycoprotein hormones. A quantitative marker in certain cases of cancer, N. Engl. J. Med. 290:1441 (1974).

104. I. A. Kourides, B.D. Weintraub, E.D. Ridgway, and F. Maloof, Pituitary secretion of free alpha and beta subunit of human thyrotropin in patients with thyroid disorders, J. Clin. Endocrinol. Metab. 40:872 (1975).

105. C. Hagen, and A.S. McNeilly, Identification of human luteinizing hormone, follicle-stimulating hormone, luteinizing hormone β-subunit and gonadotropin α-subunit in foetal and adult pituitary glands, J. Endocrinol. 67:49 (1975).

106. M. R. Blackman, M.R. Gershengorn, and B.D. Weintraub, Excess production of free alpha subunits by mouse pituitary thyro-

trophic tumor cells in vitro, Endocrinology 102:499 (1978).

107. I. A. Kourides, M.B. Landon, B.J. Hoffman, and B.D. Weintraub, Excess free alpha relative to beta subunits of the glycoprotein hormones in normal and abnormal human pituitary glands, Clin. Endocrinol. 12:407 (1980).

108. E. C. Ridgway, J.D. Kieffer, D.S. Ross, M. Downing, H. Mover and W.W. Chin, Mouse pituitary tumor line secreting only the alpha subunit of the glycoprotein hormones: development from the thyrotropic tumor, Endocrinology 113:1587 (1983).

109. D. S. Ross, M.F. Downing, W.W. Chin, J.D. Kieffer, and E.C. Ridgway, Changes in tissue concentrations of thyrotropin, free thyrotropin β, and α-subunits after thyroxine administration: comparison of mouse hypothyroid pituitary and thyrotropic tumors, Endocrinology 112:2050 (1983).

110. J. A. Gurr, and I.A. Kourides, Regulation of thyrotropin biosynthesis. Discordant effect of thyroid hormones on α and β subunit mRNA levels, J. Biol. Chem. 258:10208 (1983).

111. W. W. Chin, M.A. Shupnik, D.S. Ross, J.F. Habener and E.C. Ridgway, Regulation of the alpha and thyrotropin beta-subunit messenger ribonucleic acids by thyroid hormones, Endocrinology 116:873 (1985).

112. M. A. Shupnik, W.W. Chin, J.F. Habener and E.C. Ridgway, Transcriptional regulation of the thyrotropin subunit genes by thyroid hormones, J. Biol. Chem. 260:2900 (1985).

113. M. L. Croyle, and R.A. Maurer, Thyroid hormone decreases thyrotropin β-subunit on mRNA levels in rat anterior pituitary, DNA 3:231 (1984).

114. J. A. Gurr, and I.A. Kourides, Ratios of α to TSHβ mRNA in normal and hypothyroid pituitaries and TSH-secreting tumors, Endocrinology 115:830 (1984).

115. J. A. Franklyn, D.F. Wood, N.J. Balfour and M.C. Sheppard, Effect of triiodothyronine treatment on thyrotrophin β- and α-messenger RNAs in the pituitary of the euthyroid rat, Mol. Cell. Endocr. 60:1 (1988).

116. F. E. Carr, E.C. Ridgway and W.W. Chin, Rapid simultaneous measurement of rat alpha- and thyrotropin (TSH) beta-subunit messenger ribonucleic acids (mRNAs) by solution hybridization: regulation of TSH subunit mRNAs by thyroid hormones, Endocrinology 117:1272 (1985).

117. J. A. Franklyn, D.F. Wood, N.J. Balfour, D.B. Ransden, K. Docherty, W.W. Chin, and M.C. Sheppard, Effect of hypothyroidism and thyroid hormone replacement in vivo on pituitary cytoplasmic concentrations of thyrotropin β and α subunit mRNAs, Endocrinology 120:2279 (1987).

118. S. A. D'Angelo, D.H. Paul, D.R. Wall and D.M. Lombardi, Pituitary thyrotropin rebound phenomenon and kinetics of secretion in the goitrous rat: differential effects on synthesis and release, Endocrinology 99:935 (1976).

119. E. C. Ridgway, I.A. Kourides, W.W. Chin, D.S. Cooper and F. Maloof, Augmentation of pituitary thyrotrophin response to

TRH during subphysiological tri-iodothyronine therapy in hypothyroidism, Clinical Endocrinology 10:343 (1979).

120. A. Shupnik, L.J. Ardisson, M.J. Meskell, J. Bornstein and E.C. Ridgway, Triiodothyronine (T_3) regulation of thyrotropin subunit gene transcription is proportional to T_3 nuclear receptor occupancy, Endocrinology 118:367 (1986).

121. C. Y. Bowers, K.L. Lee, and A.V. Schally, A study of the interaction of the thyrotropin-releasing factor and L-triiodothyronine: effects of puromycin and cycloheximide, Endocrinology 82:75 (1966).

122. S. Melmed, J. Park, and J.M. Hershman, Triiodothyronine induces a transferable factor which suppreses TSH secretions in cultured mouse thyrotropic tumor cells, Biochem. Biophys. Res. Comm. 98:1022 (1981).

123. M. A. Shupnik, S.L. Greenspan, and E.C. Ridgway, Transcriptional regulation of thyrotropin subunit genes by thyrotropinreleasing hormone and dopamine in pituitary cell culture. J. Biol. Chem. 261:12675 (1986).

124. J. A. Franklyn, M. Wilson, J.R. Davis, D.B. Ramsden, K. Docherty, and M.C. Sheppartd, Demonstration of thyrotrophin β-subunit messenger RNA in rat pituitary cells in primary culture: evidence for regulation by thyrotrophin-releasing hormone and forskolin, J. Endocrin. 111:R1 (1986).

125. S. S. Lippman, S. Amr, and B.D. Weintranb, Discordant effects of thyrotropin-releasing hormone on pre- and posttranslational regulation of TSH biosynthesis in rat pituitary, Endocrinology 119:343 (1986).

126. J. A. Franklyn, D.F. Wood, N.J. Balfour, D.B. Ransden, K.Docherty, and M.C. Sheppard, Modulation by oestrogen of thyroid hormone effects on thyrotrophin gene expression, J. Endocrin. 115:53 (1987).

127. J. Franklyn, J. Ahlquist, N. Balfour, S. King, and M.C. Sheppard, Testosterone and the effects of thyroid status on pituitary and hepatic mRNAs, Endocrinology 120:T69 (1987).

128. T. L. Klug and R.C. Adelman, Evidence for a large thyrotropin and its accumulation during aging in rats, Biochem. Biophys. Res. Commun. 77:1431 (1977).

129. I. A. Kourides, B.D. Weintraub, and F. Maloof, Large molecular weight TSH-β: The sole immunoactive form of TSH-β in certain human sera, J. Clin. Endocrinol. Metab. 47:24 (1978).

130. I. M. Spitz, D. LeRoith, H. Hirsch, P. Carayon, F. Pekonen, Y. Liel, R. Sobel, Z. Chorer and B.D. Weintraub, Increased high-molecular-weight thyrotropin with impaired biologic activity in a euthyroid man, N. Engl. J. Med. 304:278 (1981).

131. B. D. Weintraub, G. Krauth, S.W. Rosen, and A.S. Rabson, Differences between purified ectopic and normal alpha subunits of human glycoprotein hormones, J. Clin. Invest. 56:1043 (1976).

132. B. D. Weintraub, B.S. Stannard, and L. Meyers, Glycosylation of

thyroid-stimulating hormone in pituitary tumor cells. Influence of high-mannose oligosaccharide units on subunit aggregation, combination and intracellular degradation, Endocrinology 112:1331 (1983).

133. W. W. Chin, J.R. Habener, J.D. Kieffer, and F. Maloof, Cell-free translation of the messenger RNA coding for the α subunit of thyroid-stimulating hormone, J. Biol. Chem. 253:7985 (1978).

134. L. C. Giudice, M.J. Waxdal, and B.D. Weintraub, Comparison of bovine and mouse pituitary glycoprotein hormone pre-α subunits synthesized in vitro, Proc. Natl. Acad. Sci. U.S.A. 76:4798 (1979).

135. L. C. Guidice, and B.D. Weintraub, Evidence for conformational differences between precursor and processed forms of TSH-β subunit, J. Biol. Chem. 254:12679 (1979).

136. I. A. Kourides, N.C. Vamvakopoulos, and G.M. Maniatis, mRNA-directed biosynthesis of α- and β-subunits of thyrotropin, J. Biol. Chem. 254:11106 (1979).

137. I. A. Kourides and B.D. Weintraub, mRNA-directed biosynthesis of α-subunit of thyrotropin: Translation in cell-free and whole-cell systems, Proc. Natl. Acad. Sci. U.S.A. 76:298 (1979).

138. N. C. Vamvakopoulos and I.A. Kourides, Identification of separate mRNAs coding for the α- and β-subunits of thyrotropin, Proc. Natl. Acad. Sci. U.S.A. 76:3809 (1979).

139. B. D. Weintraub, and B.S. Stannard, Precursor-product relationships in the biosynthesis and secretion of thyrotropin and its subunits by mouse thyrotropic tumor cells, FEBS Lett. 92:303 (1978).

140. B. D. Weintraub, B.S. Stannard, D. Linnekin, and M. Marshall, Relationship of glycosylation to de novo thyroid-stimulating hormone biosynthesis and secretion by mouse pituitary tumor cells, J. Biol. Chem. 255:5715 (1980).

141. W. W. Chin and J.F. Habener, Thyroid-stimulating hormone subunits: Evidence from endoglycosidase-H cleavage for late presecretory glycosylation, Endocrinology 108:1628 (1981).

142. W. W. Chin, F. Maloof, and J.F. Habener, Thyroid-stimulating hormone biosynthesis, J. Biol. Chem. 256:3059 (1981).

143. J. A. Magner and B.D. Weintraub, Thyroid-stimulating hormone subunit processing and combination in microsomal subfractions of mouse pituitary tumor, J. Biol. Chem. 257:6709 (1982).

144. H. Hoshina and I. Boime, Combination of rat lutropin subunit occurs early in the secretory pathway, Proc. Natl. Acad. Sci. U.S.A. 79:7649 (1982).

145. T. F. Parsons, G.A. Bloomfield, and J.G. Pierce, Purification of an altenative form of the α-subunit of the glycoprotein hormones from bovine pituitaries and identification of its O-linked oligosaccharides, J. Biol. Chem. 258:240 (1983).

146. R. W. Ruddon, C.A. Hanson, and N.J. Addison, Synthesis and

processing of human chorionic gonadotropin subunits in cultured choriocarcinoma cells, Proc. Natl. Acad. Sci. U.S.A. 76:5143 (1979).

147. R. W. Ruddon, C.A. Hanson, A.H. Bryan, G.J. Putterman, E.L. White, F. Perini, K.S. Meade, and P.H. Aldenderfer, Synthesis and secretion of human chorionic gonadotropin subunits by cultured human malignant cells, J. Biol. Chem. 255:1000 (1980).

148. R. W. Ruddon, A.H. Bryan, C.A. Hanson, F. Perini, L.M. Cccorulli, and B.P. Peters, Characterization of the intracellular and secreted forms of the glycoprotein hormone chorionic gonadotropin produced by malignant cells, J. Biol. Chem. 256:5189 (1981).

149. R. W. Ruddon, R.J. Hartle, B.P. Peters, C. Anderson, R.I. Huat, and K. Stromberg, Biosynthesis and secretion of chorionic gonadotropin subunits by organ cultures of first trimester human placenta, J. Biol. Chem. 256:11389 (1981).

150. L. A. Cole, F. Perini, S. Birken, and R.W. Ruddon, An oligosaccharide of the O-linked type distinguishes the free from the combined form of hCG α subunit, Biochem. Biophys. Res. Commun. 122:1260 (1984).

151. N. H. Behrens and L.F. Leloir, Dolichol monophosphate glucose: an intermediate in glucose transfer in liver, Proc. Natl. Acad. Sci. U.S.A. 66:153 (1970).

152. R. Kornfeld and S. Kornfeld, Assembly of asparagine-linked oligosaccharides, Ann. Rev. Biochem. 54:631 (1985).

153. D. K. Struck and W.J. Lennarz, The function of saccharide-lipids in synthesis of glycoproteins, in: The Biochemistry of Glycoproteins and Proteoglycans., Lennarz, W.J., ed., Plenum Press, New York (1980).

154. T. W. Strickland and J.G. Pierce, The α-subunit of pituitary glycoprotein hormones, Formation of three-dimentsional structure during cell-free biosynthesis, J. Biol. Chem. 258:5927 (1983).

155. J. A. Magner, C. Ronin, and B.D. Weintraub, Carbohydrate processing of thyrotropin differs from that of free α-subunit and total glycoproteins in microsomal subfractions of mouse pituitary tumor, Endocrinology 115:1019 (1984).

156. C. Ronin, B.S. Stannard, I. L. Rosenbloom, J.A. Magner, and B.D. Weintraub, Glycosylation and processing of high-mannose oligosaccharides of thyroid-stimulating hormone subunits: comparison to nonsecretory cell glycoproteins, Biochemistry 23:4503 (1984).

157. C. Ronin, B.S. Stannard, and B.D. Weintraub, Differential processing and regulation of thyroid-stimulating hormone subunit carbohydrate chains in thyrotropic tumors and in normal and hypothyroid pituitaries, Biochemistry 24:5626 (1985).

158. B. S. Stannard, N. Gesundheit, C. Ronin, J. Burnside, and B.D. Weintraub, Differential carbohydrate processing and secretion of thyrotropin and free α subunit, Effects of 1-deo-

xynojirimycin, J. Biol. Chem. 263:8309 (1988).

159. J. A. Magner and E. Papagiannes, Structures of high-mannose oligosaccharides of mouse thyrotropin: differential processing of α- versus β-subunits of the heterodimer, Endocrinology 120:10 (1987).

160. B. P. Peters, R.F. Krzesicki, R.J. Hartle, F. Perini, and R.W. Ruddon, A kinetic comparison of the processing and secretion of the $\alpha\beta$ dimer and the uncombined α- and β-subunits of chronic gonadotropin synthesized by human choriocarcinoma cells, J. Biol. Chem. 259:15123 (1984).

161. C. L. Corless, M.M. Matzuk, T.V. Ramabhadran, A. Krichevsky, and I. Boime, Gonadotropin beta subunits determine the rate of assembly and the oligosaccharide processing of hormone dimer in transfected cells, J. Cell Biol. 104:1173 (1987).

162. R. Sakakibara, Y. Yokoo, K. Yoshikoski, N. Tominaga, K. Eida, and M. Ishiguro, Subcellular localization of intracellular forms of human chorionic gonadotropin in first trimester placenta, J. Biochem. 102:993 (1987).

163. M. M. Matzuk, and I. Boime, The role of the asparagine-linked oligosaccharides of the α-subunit in the secretion and assembly of human chorionic gonadotropin, J. Cell Biol. 106:1049 (1988).

164. M. M. Matzuk and I. Boime, Site-specific mutagenesis defines the intracellular role of the asparagine-linked oligosaccharides of chorionic gonadotropin β-subunit, J. Biol. Chem. 263:17106 (1988).

165. Y. Miura, V.S. Perkel, and J.A. Magner, Rates of processing of the high mannose oligosaccharide units at the three glycosylation sites of mouse thyrotropin and the two sites of free α-subunits, Endocrinology 123:1296 (1988).

166. Y. Miura, V.S. Perkel, and J.A. Magner, Differential susceptibility to N-glycanase at the individual glycosylation sites of mouse thyrotropin and free α-subunits, Endocrinology 123:2207 (1988).

167. C. Ronin, M.J. Papandreou, C. Canonne, and B.D. Weintraub, Carbohydrate chains of human thyrotropin are differentially susceptible to endoglycosidase removal on combined and free polypeptide units, Biochemistry 26:5848 (1987).

168. K. O. Lee, N. Gesundheit, H.C. Chen, and B. D. Weintraub, Enzymatic deglycosylation of thyroid stimulating hormone with peptide-N-glycosidase F and endo-B-N-acetylgucosaminidase F, Biochem. Biophys. Res. Commun. 138:230 (1986).

169. J. R. Swedlow, R.L. Matteri, and H. Papkoff, Deglycosylation of gonadotropins with an endoglycosidase, Proc. Soc. Exp. Biol. Med. 181:432 (1986).

170. Y. Miura, V.S. Perkel, and J.A. Magner, Differential susceptibility to several endoglycosidases at the individual glycosylation sites of mouse thyrotropin and free α-subunits, Manuscript in preparation.

171. E. F. Walborg and D.N. Ward, The carbohydrate components of

ovine luteinizing hormone. Biochim. Biophys. Acta 78:304 (1963).

172. B. Shome, A.F. Parlow, V.D. Ramirez, H. Elrick, and J.G. Pierce, Bovine, Human and porcine thyrotropins: a comparison of electrophoresis and immunological properties with the bovine hormone, Arch. Biochem. Biophys. 126:444 (1968).

173. A. S. Hartree, M. Thomas, M. Graikevitch, E.T. Bell, D.W. Christie, G.V. Spaull, R. Taylor, and J.G. Pierce, Preparation and properties of subunits of human luteinizing hormone, J. Endocrinol. 51:169 (1971).

174. H. J. Grimek, J. Gorski, and B.C. Wentworth, Purification and characterization of bovine follicle-stimulating hormone: Comparision with ovine follicle-stimulating hormone, Endocrinology 104:140 (1972).

175. M. R. Sairam, Role of arginine residues in ovine lutropin: Reversible modification by 1,2-cyclohexanedione, Arch. Biochem. Biophys. 176:197 (1976).

176. J. F. Kennedy and M.F. Chaplin, The structures of the carbohydrate moieties of the α-subunit of human chorionic gonadotrophin, Biochem. J. 155:303 (1976).

177. O. P. Bahl, L. Marz, M.J. Kessler, Isolation and characterization of N- and O-glycosidic carbohydrate units of human chorionic gonadotropin, Biochem. Biophys. Res. Commun. 84:667 (1978).

178. K. Hara, P. Rathnam, and B.B. Saxena, Structure of the carbohydrate moieties of α-subunits of human follitropin, lutropin, and thyrotropin, J. Biol. Chem. 253:1582 (1978).

179. M. J. Kessler, M.S. Reddy, R.H. Shah, and O.P. Bahl, Structures of N-glycosidic carbohydrate units of human chorionic gonadotropin, J. Biol. Chem. 254:7901 (1979).

180. Y. Endo, K. Yamashita, Y. Tachibana, S. Tojo, and A. Kobata, Structures of the asparagine-linked sugar chains of human chorionic gonadotropin, J. Biochem. 85:669 (1979).

181. T. Mizuochi and A. Kobata, Different asparagine-linked sugar chains on the two polypeptide chains of human chorionic gonadotropin, Biochem. Biophys. Res. Commun. 97:772 (1980).

182. M. R. Sairam, Studies on pituitary follitropin. I. An improved procedure for the isolation of highly potent ovine hormone, Arch Biochem. Biophys. 194:63 (1979).

183. M. R. Sairam, Studies on pituitary follitropin. II. Isolation and characterization of the subunits of the ovine hormone, Arch. Biochem. Biophys. 194:71 (1979).

184. O. P. Bahl, M.S. Reddy, and G.S. Bedi, A novel carbohydrate structure in bovine and ovine luteinizing hormones, Biochem. Biophys. Res. Commun. 96:1192 (1980).

185. G. S. Bedi, W.C. French, and O.P. Bahl, Structure of carbohydrate units of ovine luteinizing hormone, J. Biol. Chem. 257:4345 (1982).

186. A. Tolvo, Y. Fujiki, V.P. Bhavanandan, P. Rathnam, and B.B. Saxena, Studies on the unique presence of an N-acetylgalac-

tosamine residue in the carbohydrate moieties of human follicle-stimulating hormone, Biochim. Biophys.Acta 719:1 (1982).

187. Y. R. Jones-Brown, C.Y. Wu, B.D. Weintraub, and S.W. Rosen, Synthesis of chorionic gonadotropin subunits in human choriocarcinoma clonal cell line JEG-3: Carbohydrate differences in glycopeptides from free and combined α-subunits, Endocrinology 115:1439 (1984).

188. E. D. Green, H. van Halbeek, I. Boime and J.V. Baenziger, Structural elucidation of the disulfated oligosaccharide from bovine lutropin, J. Biol. Chem. 260:15623 (1985).

189. E. D. Green, J.U. Baenziger, and I. Boime, Cell-free sulfation of human and bovine pituitary hormones. Comparison of the sulfated oligosaccharides of lutropin, follitropin and thyrotropin, J. Biol. Chem. 260:15631 (1985).

190. B. D. Weintraub, B.S. Stannard, J.A. Magner, C. Ronin, T. Taylor, L. Joshi, R.R. Constant, M. Menezes-Ferreira, P.A. Petrick and N. Gesundheit, Glycosylation and post-translational processing of thyroid-stimulating hormone: Clinical implications, Rec. Prog. Horm. Res. 41:577 (1985).

191. J. A. Magner and B.D. Weintraub, Thyroid-stimulating hormone biosynthesis, in: The Thyroid, Braverman, L.E., and S.H. Ingbar, eds., J.B. Lippincott (1986).

192. B. Nilsson, S.W. Rosen, B.D. Weintraub and D.A. Zopf, Differences in the carbohydrate moieties of the common α-subunits of human chorionic gonadotropin, luteinizing hormone, follicle-stimulating hormone, and thyrotropin: Preliminary structural inferences from direct methylation analysis, Endocrinology 119:2737 (1986).

193. R. J. Ryan, H.T. Keutmann, M.C. Charlesworth, D.J. McCormick, R.P. Milius, F.O. Calvo and T. Vutyanvanich, Structure-function relationships of gonadotropins, Rec. Prog. Horm. Res. 43:383 (1987).

194. W.-K. Liu and D.N. Ward, The purification and chemistry of pituitary glycoprotein hormones, Pharmacol. Ther.1B:545 (1975).

195. H. Tamura-Takahasi and N. Ui, Purification and properties of whale thyroid-stimulating hormone. III. Properties of isolated multiple components, Endocrinol. Jpn 23:511 (1976).

196. K. M. M. Davy, J.S. Fawcett and C.J.O.R. Morris, Chemical differences between thyrotropin isohormones, Biochem. J. 167:279 (1977).

197. L. C. Guidice and J.G. Pierce, Separation of functional and non-functional β-subunits of thyrotropin preparations by polyacrylamide gel electorphoresis, Endocrinology 101:776 (1977).

198. G. Jacobson, P. Roos, and L. Wide, Characterization of five glycoproteins with thyrotropin activity, Biochim. Biophys. Acta 490:403 (1977).

199. T. Yora, S. Matsuzaki, Y. Kondo, and N. Ui, Changes in the

contents of multiple components of rat pituitary thyrotropin in altered thyroid states, Endocrinology 104:1682 (1979).

200. B. R. Webster, B.C.W. Hummel, J.M. McKenzie, G.M. Brown, and J.C. Paice, Isoelectric focusing of human thyrotropin: Identification of multiple components with dissociation of biological and immunological activities, in: Structure-Activity Relationships of Protein and Polypeptide Hormones, Proc. 2nd Inter. Symp., Excerpta Medicia, Amsterdam, Inter. Congr. Series No. 241: 369, (1972).

201. N. A. Takai, S. Filetti, and B. Rapoport, Studies on the bioactivity of radiolabeled highly-purified bovine thyrotropin, Biochem. Biophys. Res. Commun. 97:566 (1980).

202. N. A. Takai, S. Filetti, and B. Rapoport, Studies on the bioactivity of radioiodinated highly purified bovine thyrotropin: Analytical polyacrylamide gel electrophoresis, Endocrinology 109:1144 (1981).

203. F. Pekonen, P. Carayon, S. Amr, and B.D. Weintraub, Heterogeneous forms of thyroid-stimulating hormone in mouse thyrotropic tumor and serum: Differences in receptor binding and adenylate cyclase-stimulating activity, Horm. Metab. Res. 13: 617 (1981).

204. L. R. Joshi and B.D. Weintraub, Naturally occurring forms of thyrotropin with low bioactivity and altered carbohydrate content act as competitive antagonists to more bioactive forms, Endocrinology 113:2145 (1983).

205. T. F. Parsons and J.G. Pierce, Oligosaccharide moieties of glycoprotein hormones: Bovine lutropin resists enzymatic deglycosylation because of terminal O-sulfated N-acetylhexosamines, Proc. Natl. Acad. Sci. U.S.A. 77:7089 (1980).

206. G. Hortin, M. Natowicz, J. Pierce, J. Baenziger, T. Parsons, and I. Boime, Metabolic labeling of lutropin with [^{35}S] sulfate, Proc. Natl. Acad. Sci. U.S.A. 78:7468 (1981).

207. K. R. Anumula and O.P. Bahl, Biosynthesis of lutropin in ovine pituitary slices: Incorporation of [^{35}S] sulfate in carbohydrate units, Arch. Biochem. Biophys. 220:645 (1983).

208. N. Gesundheit, J. A. Magner, T. Chen, and B.D. Weintraub, Differential sulfation and sialylation of secreted mouse thyrotropin (TSH) subunits: Regulation by TSH-releasing hormone, Endocrinology 119:455 (1986).

209. M. Mori, M. Murakami, T. Iriuchijima, H. Ishihara, I. Kobayashi, S. Kobayashi, and K. Wakabayashi, Alteration by thyrotropinreleasing hormone of heterogeneous components associated with thyrotrophin biosynthesis in the rat anterior pituitary gland, J. Endocrinol. 103:165 (1984).

210. L. Wide, Median charge and charge heterogeneity of human pituitary FSH, LH and TSH, Acta Endocrinol. (Copenh.) 109:181 (1985).

211. S. C. Chappel, The presence of two species of FSH within hamster anterior pituitary glands as disclosed by Concanavalin A chromatography, Endocrinology 109:935 (1981).

212. W. D. Peckham and E. Knobil, The effects of ovariectomy, extrogen replacement, and neuraminidase treatment on the properties of the adenohypophysial glycoprotein hormones of the rhesus monkey, Endocrinology 98:1054 (1976).
213. M. Hattori, K. Ozawa, and K. Wakabayashi, Isoelectric properties, lectin binding characteristics and biological activities of neuraminidase-treated rat LH components, Acta Endocrinol. (Copenh.) 117:73 (1988).
214. M. L. Sardanons, A.R. Solano and E.J. Podesta, Gonadotropin-releasing hormone action upon luteinizing hormone bioactivity in pituitary gland: Role of sulfation, J. Biol. Chem. 262:11149 (1987).
215. E. D. Green, I. Boime, and J.U. Baenziger, Differential processing of Asn-linked oligosaccharides on pituitary glycoprotein hormones: implications for biologic function, Mol. Cell. Biochem. 72:81 (1986).
216. E. D. Green and J.U. Baenziger, Asparagine-linked oligosaccharides on lutropin, follitropin, and thyrotropin, I. Structural elucidation of the sulfated and sialylated oligosaccharides on bovine, ovine, and human pituitary glycoprotein hormones, J. Biol. Chem. 263:25 (1988).
217. E. D. Green and J.U. Baenziger, Asparagine-linked oligosaccharides on lutropin follitropin, and thyrotropin. II. Distributions of sulfated and sialylated oligosaccharides on bovine, ovine, and human pituitary glycoprotein hormones, J. Biol. Chem. 263:36 (1988).
218. J. U. Baenziger and E.D. Green, Pituitary glycoprotein hormone oligosaccharides: structure, synthesis and function of the asparagine-linked oligosaccharides on lutropin, follitropin and thyrotropin, Biochim. Biophys. Acta 947:287 (1988).
219. P. L. Smith and J.U. Baenziger, A pituitary N-acetylgalactosamine transferase that specifically recognizes glycoprotein hormones, Science 242:930 (1988).
220. J. A. Magner and E. Papagiannes, The subcellular sites of sulfation of mouse thyrotropin and free alpha subunits: Studies employing subcellular fractionation and inhibitors of the intracellular translocation of proteins, Endocrine Res. 13 (4):337 (1987).
221. E. D. Green, J. Gruenebaum, M. Bielinska, J.U. Baenziger, and I. Boime, Sulfation of lutropin oligosaccharides with a cell-free system, Proc. Nat. Acad. Sci. U.S.A. 81:5320 (1984).
222. J. A. Magner, Assay of sulfotransferase in subcellular fractions of hypothyroid mouse pituitary and liver tissue, Biochemical Medicine and Metabolic Biology 41:81 (1989).
223. Y. Miura, M.J. Johnson, V.S. Perkel, and J.A. Magner (SPON: J. Sheinin), Qualitatively different forms of human TSH in sera of euthyroid, primary and central hypothyroid patients: analyses by ricin and McKenzie bioassay, Program of the 71st Annual Meeting of the Endocrine Society (abstract), 1989.

224. G. S. DeCherney, P.W. Gyves, C.R. Showalter, R.L. Winston, and N. Gesundheit, Hypothyroidism increases the sialylation and decreases the sulfation of secreted mouse thyrotropin, Program of the 70th Annual Meeting of the Endocrine Society, Abstract no. 353. (1988).

225. E. G. Berger, E. Buddecke, J.P. Kamerling, A. Kobata, J.C. Paulson, and J.F.G. Vliengenthart, Structure, biosynthesis and functions of glycoprotein glycans, Experienta 38:1129 (1982).

226. J. Roth, Subcellular organization of glycosylation in mammalian cells, Biochim. Biophys. Acta 906:405 (1987).

227. H. Schachter, Coordination between enzyme specificity and intracellular compartmentation in the control of protein-bound oligosaccharide biosynthesis, Biol. Cell 51:133 (1984).

228. G. D. Longmore and H. Schachter, Product identification and substrate-specificity studies of the GDP-L-fucose: 2-acetamido-2-deoxy-β-D-glucoside (fuc-asn-linked GlcNAc) 6-α-L-fucosyl-transferase in a Golgi-rich fraction from porcine liver, Carbohydr. Res. 100:365 (1982).

229. H. Yoshima, S. Takasaki, S. Ito-Mega and A. Kobata, Purification of almond emulsin α-L-fucosidase I by affinity chromatography, Arch. Biochem. Biophys. 194:394 (1979).

230. O. P. Bahl, Glycosidases of *Aspergillus niger*, J. Biol. Chem. 245:299 (1970).

231. R. A. DiCioccio, J.J. Barlow, and K.L. Matta, Substrate specificity and other properties of α-L-fucosidase from human serum, J. Biol. Chem. 257:714 (1982).

232. D. E. Goldberg and S. Kornfeld, Evidence for extensive subcellular organization of asparagine-linked oligosaccharide processing and lysosomal enzyme phosphorylation, J. Biol. Chem. 258:3159 (1983).

233. A. J. Chapman, J.T. Gallagher, C.G. Beardwell and S.M. Shalet, Variation in the core and branch carbohydrate sequences of serum glycoprotein hormone α-subunit as determined by lectin affinity chromatography, J. Endocrinol. 103:117 (1984).

234. A. Kobata, Structures, function, and transformational changes of the sugar chains of glycohormones, J. Cell. Biochem. 37:79 (1988).

235. G. Pelletier and R. Puviani, Detection of glycoproteins and autoradiographic localization of ^{3}H-fucose in the thyroidectomy cells of rat anterior pituitary gland, J. Cell Biol. 56:600 (1973).

236. G. Pelletier, Autoradiographic studies of synthesis and intracellular migration of glycoproteins in the rat anterior pituitary gland, J. Cell Biol. 62:185 (1974).

237. H. D. Purves and W.E. Griesbach, The site of thyrotrophin and gonadotrophin production in the rat pituitary studied by McManus-Hotchkiss staining for glycoprotein, Endocrinology 49:244 (1951).

238. N. S. Halmi, Two types of basophils in the rat pituitary: Thyrotrophs and gonadotrophs vs. beta and delta cells, Endocrinology 50:140 (1952).

239. N. S. Halmi and W.D. Gude, The morphogenesis of pituitary tumors induced by radiothyroidectomy in the mouse and the effects of their transplantation on the pituitary body of the host, Am. J. Pathol. 30:403 (1954).

240. M. G. Farquhar and J.F. Rinehart, Cytologic alterations in the anterior pituitary gland following thyroidectomy: an electron microscope study, Endocrinology 55:857 (1954).

241. V. B. Kamat, D.F. Hoelzyl Wallach, J. F.Crigler and A.J. Ladman, The intracellular localization of hormonal activity in transplantable thyrotopin-secreting pituitary tumors in mice, J. Biophys. Biochem. Cytol. 7:219 (1960).

242. M. G. Farquhar, Processing of secretory products by cells of the anterior pituitary gland, in: Subcellular Organization and Function in Endocrine Tissues, Heller, H., and K. Lederis, eds., Cambridge University Press, Cambridge (1971).

243. S. Cuerdo-Rocha and D. Zambrano, The action of protein synthesis inhibitors and thyrotropin releasing factor on the ultrastructure of rat thyrotrophs, J. Ultrastruct. Res. 48:1 (1974).

244. S. Cuerdo-Rocha and D. Zambrano, Thyrotrophs of the rat anterior pituitary after different periods of thyroidectomy: a conventional and histochemical electron microscope study, J. Ultrastruct. Res. 49:312 (1974).

245. G. C. Moriarty and R.B. Tobin, An immunocytochemical study of TSH storage in rat thyroidectomy cells with and without D or L thyroxine treatment, J. Histochem. Cytochem. 24:1140 (1976).

246. J. A. Magner, W. Novak and E. Papagiannes, Subcellular localization of fucose incorporation into mouse thyrotropin and free α-subunits: studies employing subcellular fractionation and inhibitors of the intracellular translocation of proteins, Endocrinology 119:1315 (1986).

247. Y. Miura, V. Perkel, and J.A. Magner, Use of lentil lectin and autoradiography to probe for RER-associated fucosylation in mouse thyrotrophs, Manuscript in preparation, (1989).

248. K. Kornfeld, M.L. Reitman, and R. Kornfeld, The carbohydrate-binding specificity of pea and lentil lectins, J. Biol. Chem. 256:6633 (1981).

249. J. A. Magner and E. Papagiannes, Studies of double-labeled mouse thyrotropin and free α-subunits to estimate relative fucose content, Proc. Soc. Exp. Biol. Med. 183:237 (1986).

250. N. Gesundheit, D.L. Fink, L.A. Silverman and B.D. Weintraub, Effect of thyrotropin-releasing hormone on the carbohydrate structure of secreted mouse thyrotropin: analysis by lectin affinity chromatography, J. Biol. Chem. 262:5197 (1987).

251. N. Gesundheit and B.D. Weintraub, Mechanisms and regulation of TSH glycosylation, Adv. Exp. Med. Biol. 205:87 (1986).

252. G. Griffiths, P. Quinn, and G. Warren, Dissection of the Golgi complex. I. Monensin inhibits the transport of viral membrane proteins from medial to trans Golgi cisternae in baby hamster kidney cells infected with Semlike Forest Virus, J. Cell Biol. 96:835 (1983).

253. A. M. Tartakoff, P. Vassali, and M. Detraz, Plasma cell immunoglobulin secretion. Arrest is accompanied by alterations of the Golgi complex, J. Exp. Med. 146:1332 (1977).

254. D. C. Johnson, and M.J. Schlesinger, Vesicular stomatitis virus and sindbis virus glycoprotein transport to the cell surface is inhibited by ionophores, Virology 103:407 (1980).

255. N. Uchida, H. Smilowitz, P.W. Ledger and M.L. Tanzer, Kinetic studies of the intracellular transport of procollagen and fibronectin in human fibroblasts, J. Biol. Chem. 255:8638 (1980).

256. B. P. Peters, M. Brooks, R.J. Hartle, R.F. Krzesicki, F. Perini and R.W. Ruddon, The use of drugs to dissect the pathway for secretion of the glycoprotein hormone chorionic gonadotropin by cultured human trophoblastic cells, J. Biol. Chem. 258:14505 (1983).

257. P. Ring, U. Bjorkman and R. Ekholm, Localization of the incorporation of ^{3}H-galactose and ^{3}H-sialic acid into thyroglobulin in relation to the block of intracellular transport induced by monensin, Cell Tissue Res. 250:149 (1987).

258. A. D. Elbein, Inhibitors of the biosynthesis and processing of N-linked oligosaccharide chains, Ann. Rev. Biochem. 56:497 (1987).

259. G. Ponsin and R. Mornex, Control of thyrotropin glycosylation in normal rat pituitary cells in culture: Effect of thyrotropin-releasing hormone, Endocrinology 113:549 (1983).

260. T. Hayashi, A. Takatsuki and G. Tamura, The action mechanism of brefeldin A. I. Growth recovery of Candida albicans by lipids from the action of brefeldin A, J. Antibiot. 27:65 (1974).

261. A. Takatsuki and G. Tamura, Brefeldin A, a specific inhibitor of intracellular translocation of vesicular stomatitis virus G protein: Intracellular accumulation of high-mannose type G protein and inhibition of its cell surface expression, Agric. Biol. Chem. 49:899 (1985).

262. Y. Misumi, Yu. Misumi, K. Miki, A. Takatsuki, G. Tamura, and Y. Ikehara, Novel blockade by brefeldin A of intracellular transport of secretory proteins in cultured rat hepatocytes, J. Biol. Chem. 261:11398 (1986).

263. K. Oda, S. Hirose, N. Takami, Y. Misumi, A. Takatsuki and Y. Ikehara, Brefeldin A arrests the intracellular transport of a precursor of complement C3 before its conversion site in rat hepatocytes, FEBS Lett. 214:135 (1987).

264. J. A. Magner and E. Papagiannes, Blockade by brefeldin A of intracellular transport of secretory proteins in mouse pituitary cells: Effects on the biosynthesis of thyrotropin

and free α-subunits, Endocrinology 122:912 (1988).

265. V. S. Perkel, A.Y. Liu, Y. Miura and J.A. Magner, The effects of brefeldin A on the high mannose oligosaccharides of mouse thyrotropin, free α-subunits, and total glycoproteins, Endocrinology 123:310 (1988).

266. V. S. Perkel, Y. Miura, and J.A. Magner, Brefeldin A inhibits oligosaccharide processing of glycoproteins in mouse hypothyroid pituitary tissue at several subcellular sites, Proc. Soc. Exp. Biol. Med. 190:286 (1989).

267. T. Fujiwara, K. Oda, S. Yokota, A. Takatsuki and Y. Ikehara, Brefeldin A causes disassembly of the Golgi complex and accumulation of secretory proteins in the endoplasmic reticulum, J. Biol. Chem. 263:18545 (1988).

268. J. F. Wilber and R.D. Utiger, Immunoassay studies of thyrotropin in rat pituitary glands and serum, Endocrinology 81:145 (1967).

269. J. F. Wilber and R.D. Utiger, Thyrotropin incorporation of ^{14}C-glucosamine by the isolated rat adenohypophysis, Endocrinology 84:1316 (1969).

270. J. F. Wilber, Stimulation of ^{14}C-glucosamine and ^{14}C-alanine incorporation into thyrotropin by synthetic thyrotropin-releasing hormone, Endocrinology 89:873 (1971).

271. L. Cacicedo, S.L. Pohl, and S. Reichlin, Effects of thyroid hormones and thyrotropin-releasing hormone on thyrotropin biosynthesis by mouse pituitary tumor cells in vitro, Endocrinology 108:1012 (1981).

272. M. C. Marshall,Jr., D. Williams and B.D. Weintraub, Regulation of de novo biosynthesis of thyrotropin in normal, hyperplastic and neoplastic thyrotrophs, Endocrinology 108:908 (1981).

273. B. D. Weintraub and N. Gesundheit, Thyroid-stimulating hormone synthesis and glycosylation: Clinical inplications, Thyroid Today 10:no. 1 (1987)

274. T. Taylor and B. D. Weintraub, Differential regulation of thyrotropin subunit apoprotein and carbohydrate biosynthesis by thyroid hormone, Endocrinology 116:1535 (1985).

275. T. Taylor and B.D. Weintraub, Thyrotropin (TSH)-releasing hormone regulation of TSH subunit biosynthesis and glycosylation in normal and hypothyroid rat pituitaries, Endocrinology 116:1968 (1985).

276. T. Yora, S. Matsuzaki, Y. Kondo, and N. Ui, Changes in the contents of multiple components of rat pituitary thyrotropin in altered thyroid states, Endocrinology 104:1682 (1979).

277. M. Mori, K. Ohshima, H. Fukuda, I. Kobayashi, K. Wakabayashi, Changes in the multiple components of rat pituitary TSH and TSH β-subunit following thyroidectomy, Acta Endocr. 105:49 (1984).

278. M. Mori, I. Kobayashi and S. Kobayashi, Thytrotrophin-releasing hormone does not accumulate glycosylated thyrotrophin, but changes heterogeneous forms of thyrotrophin within the rat

anterior pituitary gland, J. Endocr. 109:227 (1986).

279. T. Taylor, N. Gesundheit and B.D. Weintraub, Effects of in vivo bolus versus continuous TRH administration on TSH secretion, biosynthesis, and glycosylation in normal and hypothyroid rats, Mol. Cell. Endocr. 46:253 (1986).

280. C. Ronin and C. Caseti, Transfer of glucose in the biosynthesis of thyroid glycoproteins, Biochim. Biophys. Acta 674:58 (1981).

281. T. Osawa and T. Tsuji, Fractionation and structural assessment of oligosaccharides and glycopeptides by use of immobilized lectins, Ann. Rev. Biochem. 56:21 (1987).

282. C. F. Brewer and L. Bhattacharyya, Concanavalin A interactions with asparagine-linked glycopeptides. The mechanisms of binding of oligomannose, bisected hybrid, and complex type carbohydrates, Glycoconjugate J. 5:159 (1988).

283. M. M. Menezes-Ferreira, P.A. Petrick and B.D. Weintraub, Regulation of thyrotropin (TSH) bioactivity by TSH-releasing hormone and thyroid hormone, Endocrinology 118:2125 (1986).

284. T. Taylor, N. Gesundheit, P.W. Gyves, D.M. Jacobowitz and B.D. Weintraub, Hypothalamic hypothyroidism caused by lesions in rat paraventricular nuclei alters the carbohydrate structure of secreted thyrotropin, Endocrinology 122:283 (1988).

285. P. W. Gyves, N. Gesundheit, T. Taylor, J. Butler and B.D. Weintraub, Changes in thyrotropin (TSH) carbohydrate structure and response to TSH-releasing hormone during postnatal ontogeny: analysis by concanavalin A chromatography, Endocrinology 121:133 (1987).

286. N. Gesundheit, P.A. Petrick, T. Taylor, E.H. Oldfield and B.D. Weintraub, Comparison of a pituitary TSH-secreting micro- versus macroadenoma, in: Frontiers in Thyroidology, G. Medeiros-Neto and E. Gaitan, eds., Plenum, New York (1986).

287. H. -Y. Lee, J. Suhl, A.E. Pekary and J.M. Hershman, Secretion of thyrotropin with reduced concanavalin-A-binding activity in patients with severe nonthyroidal illness, J. Clin. Endocrinol. Metab. 65:942 (1987).

288. V. S. Perkel, K.A. Papenberg, Y. Miura and J.A. Magner, Concanavalin A and lentil lectin binding characteristics of human thyrotropin from sera of hypothyroid and euthyroid subjects, Program of the Endocrine Society abstract (1989).

289. P. K. Manasco, D.L. Blithe, S.R. Rose, M.C. Gelato and B.C. Nisula, Evidence that TSH oligosaccharide branching is different in primary and central hypothyroidism, Program of the Endocrine Society (abstract), (1989).

290. E. V. Van Hall, J.L. Vaitukaitis and G.T. Ross, Immunological and biological activity of hCG following progressive desialylation, Endocrinology 88:456 (1971).

291. E. V. Van Hall, J.L. Vaitukaitis, G.T. Ross, J.W. Hickman and G. Ashwell, Effects of progressive desialylation on the rate of disappearance of immunoreactive hCG from plasma in rats, Endocrinology 89:11 (1971).

292. T. Tsuruhara, M.L. Dufau, J. Hickman and K.J. Catt, Biological properties of hCG after removal of terminal sialic acid and galactose residues, Endocrinology 91:296 (1972).
293. B. C. Goverde, F.J.N. Veenkamp and J.D.H. Homan, Studies on human chorionic gonadotrophin. II. Chemical composition and its relation to biological activity, Acta Endocrinol. 59:105 (1968).
294. M. L. Dufau, K.J. Catt and T. Tsuruhara, Retention of in vitro biologic activities by desialylated human luteinizing hormone and chorionic gonadotropin, Biochem. Biophys. Res. Commun. 44:1022 (1971).
295. W. R. Moyle, O.P. Bahl and L. Marz, Role of the carbohydrate of human chorionic gonadotropin in the mechanism of hormone action, J. Biol. Chem. 205:9163 (1975).
296. C. P. Channing, C.N. Sakai and O.P. Bahl, Role of the carbohydrate residues of human chorionic gonadotropin in binding and stimulation of adenosine 3', 5'-monophosphate accumulation by porcine granulosa cells, Endocrinology 103:341 (1978).
297. C. P. Channing and O.P. Bahl, Role of carbohydrate residues of human chorionic gonadotropin in stimulation of progesterone secretion by cultures of monkey granulosa cells, Biol. Reprod. 17:707 (1978).
298. N. R. Thotakura and O.P. Bahl, Role of carbohydrate in human chorionic gonadotropin: Deglycosylation uncouples hormone-receptor complex and adenylate cyclase system, Biochem. Biophys. Res. Commun. 108:399 (1982).
299. J. M. Goverman, T.F. Parsons and J.G. Pierce, Enzymatic deglycosylation of the subunits of chorionic gonadotropin: Effects on formation of tertiary structures and biological activity, J. Biol. Chem. 257:15059 (1982).
300. M. R. Sairam and G.N. Bhargavi, A role for glycosylation of the α-subunit in transduction of biological signal in glycoprotein hormones, Science 229:65 (1985).
301. P. Manjunath and M.R. Sairam, Biochemical, biological and immunological properties of chemically deglycosylated human chorionic gonadotropin, J. Biol. Chem. 257:7109 (1982).
302. H. C. Chen, Y. Shimohigashi, M.L. Dufau and K.J. Catt, Characterization and biological properties of chemically deglycosylated human chorionic gonadotropin, J. Biol. Chem. 257:14446 (1982).
303. N. K. Kalyan and O.P. Bahl, Role of carbohydrate in human chorionic gonadotropin: Effect of deglycosylation on the subunit interaction and on its in vitro and in vivo biological properties, J. Biol. Chem. 258:67 (1983).
304. H. T. Keutmann, P.J. McIlroy, E.R. Bergert and R.J. Ryan, Chemically deglycosylated human chorionic gonadotropin subunits: Characterization and biological properties, Biochemistry 22:3067 (1983).
305. M. R. Sairam and P. Manjunath, Hormonal antagonistic properties

of chemically deglycosylated human choriogonadotropin, J. Biol. Chem. 258:445 (1983).

306. S. Amr, Y. Shimohigashi, P. Carayon, H.-C. Chen and B. Nisula, Sialic acid residues of the α-subunit are required for the thyrotropic activity of hCG, Biochem. Biophys. Res. Commun. 109:146 (1982).

307. M. R. Sairam, Deglycosylation of ovine pituitary lutropin subunits: Effects on subunit interaction and hormone activity, Arch. Biochem. Biophys. 204:199 (1980).

308. J. S. M. Hutchinson, The interpretation of pituitary gonadotrophin assays -- a continuing challenge, J. Endocr. 118:169 (1988).

309. C. Mendelson, M.L. Dufau and K.J. Catt, Gonadotropin binding and stimulation of cAMP and testosterone production in isolated Leydig cells, J. Biol. Chem. 250:8818 (1975).

310. L. A. Cole, L.A. Metsch and H.E. Grotjan, Jr, Significant steroidogenic activity of luteinizing hormone is maintained after enzymatic removal of oligosaccharides, Mol. Endocrinol. 1:621 (1987).

311. P. E. Patton, F.O. Calvo, V.Y. Fujimoto, E.R. Bergert, R.D. Kempers and R.J. Ryan, The effect of deglycosylated human chorionic gonadotropin on corpora luteal funtion in healthy women, Feril. Steril. 49:620 (1988).

312. L. Liu, J.L. Southers, S.M. Banks, D.L. Blithe, R.E. Wehmann, J.H. Brown, H.-C. Chen and B.C. Nisula, Stimulation of testosterone production in the cynomolgus monkey in vivo by deglycosylated and desialylated human choriogonadotropin, Endocrinology 124:175 (1989).

313. N. A. Takai, S. Filetti and B. Rapoport, Studies on the bioactivity of radiolabeled, highly-purified bovine thyrotropin, Biochem. Biophys. Res. Commun. 97:566 (1980).

314. N. A. Takai, S. Filetti and B. Rapoport, Studies on the bioactivity of radioiodinated highly purified bovine thyrotropin: analytical polyacrylamide gel electrophoresis, Endocrinology 109:1144 (1981).

315. P. A. Dahlberg, P.A. Petrick, M. Nissim, M.M. Menezes-Ferreira and B.D. Weintraub, Intrinsic bioactivity of thyrotropin in human serum is inversely correlated with thyroid hormone concentrations: application of a new bioassay using the FRTL-5 rat thyroid cell strain J. Clin. Invest. 79:1388 (1987).

316. M. I. Berman, C.G. Thomas, P. Manjunath, M.R. Sairam and S.N. Nayfeh, The role of the carbohydrate moiety in thyrotropin action, Biochem. Biophys. Res. Commun. 133:680 (1985).

317. S. M. Amir, K. Kubota, D. Tramontano, S.H. Ingbar and H.T. Keutmann, The carbohydrate moiety of bovine thyrotropin is essential for full bioactivity but not for receptor recognition, Endocrinology 120:345 (1987).

318. S. Amr, M.M. Menezes-Ferreira, Y. Shimohigashi, H.C. Chen, B. Nisula and B.D. Weintraub, Activities of deglycosylated

thyrotropin at the thyroid membrane receptor-adenylate cyclase system, J. Endocrinol. Invest. 8:537 (1986).

319. M. Nissim, K.-O. Lee, P.A. Petrick, P.A. Dahlberg and B.D. Weintraub, A sensitive thyrotropin (TSH) bioassay based on iodide uptake in rat FRTL-5 thyroid cells: Comparison with the adenosine 3', 5'-monophosphate response to human serum TSH and enzymatically deglycosylated bovine and human TSH, Endocrinology 121:1278 (1987).

320. S. Costagliola, A.-M. Madec, M.M. Benkirane, J. Orgiazzi and P. Carayon, Monoclonal antibody approach to the relationship between immunological structure and biological activity of thyrotropin, Mol. Endocr. 2:613 (1988).

321. J. M. Bidart, F. Troalen, G.R. Bousfield, C. Bohuon and D. Bellet, Monoclonal antibodies directed to human and equine chorionic gonadotropins as probes for the topographic analysis of epitopes on the human α-subunit, Endocrinology 124:923 (1989).

322. G. Faglia, L. Bitensky, A. Pinchera, C. Ferrari, A. Paracchi, P. Beck-Peccoz, B. Ambrosi and A. Spada, Thyrotropin secretion in patients with central hypothyroidism: Evidence for reduced biological activity of immunoreactive thyrotropin, J. Clin. Endocrinol. Metab. 48:989 (1979).

323. G. Faglia, P. Beck-Peccoz, M. Ballabio and C. Nava, Excess of β-subunit of thyrotropin (TSH) in patients with idiopathic central hypothyroidism due to the secretion of TSH with reduced biological activity, J. Clin. Endocrinol. Metab. 56:908 (1983).

324. P. Beck-Peccoz, G. Piscitelli, S. Amr, M. Ballabio, M. Bassetti, G. Giannattasio, A. Spada, M. Nissim, B.D. Weintraub and G. Faglia, Endocrine, biochemical, and morphological studies of a pituitary adenoma secreting growth hormone, thyrotropin (TSH), and α-subunit: Evidence for secretion of TSH with increased bioactivity, J. Clin. Endocrinol. Metab. 62:704 (1986).

325. I. M. Spitz, D. LeRoith, H. Hirsch, P. Carayon, F. Pekonen, Y. Liel, R. Sobel, Z. Chorer and B. Weintraub, Increased high-molecular-weight thyrotropin with impaired biologic activity in a euthyroid man, N. Eng. J. Med. 304:278 (1981).

326. S. A. D'Angelo, Disappearance rate of exogenous thyrotrophin from the blood of normal and hypophysectomized rats, Endocrinology 48:249 (1951).

327. M. Sonenberg, A.S. Keaton, W.L. Money, R.W. Rawson, Radioactive thyrotropic hormone preparations, J. Clin. Endocrinol. Metab. 12:1269 (1952).

328. A. A. H. Kassenaar, L.D. Lameyer and A. Querido, The distribution of injected heterologous thyrotrophic hormone in the rat, Acta Endocrinol. (Copenh.) 21:32 (1956).

329. H. A. Levey and D.H. Solomon, Studies on the metabolism of thyrotropin, Endocrinology 60:118 (1957).

330. J. L. Bakke and N.L. Lawrence, Disappearance rate and distribu-

tion of exogenous thyrotropin in the rat, Endocrinology 71:43 (1962).
331. A. Kojima, J.M. Hershman, M. Azukizawa and J.J. DiStefano, Quantification of the pituitary-thyroid axis in pregnant rats, Endocrinology 95:599 (1974).
332. E. C. Ridgway, B.D. Weintraub and F. Maloof, Metabolic clearance and production rates of human thyrotropin, J. Clin. Invest. 53:895 (1974).
333. E. C. Ridgway, F.R. Singer, B.D. Weintraub, L. Lorenz and F. Maloof, Metabolism of human thyrotropin in the dog, Endocrinology 95:1181 (1971).
334. M. I. Surks and B.M. Lifschitz, Biphasic thyrotropin suppression in euthyroid and hypothyroid rats, Endocrinology 101:769 (1977).
335. J. E. Silva and P.R. Larsen, Peripheral metabolism of homologous thyrotropin in euthyroid and hypothyroid rats: acute effects of thyrotropin-releasing hormone, triiodothyronine, and thyroxine, Endocrinology 102:1783 (1978).
336. O. Spira, A. Birdenfeld, J. Gross and A. Gordon, TSH synthesis and release in the thyroidectomized rat: a) effect of short- and long-term hypothyroidism, Acta Endocrinol. (Copenh.) 92: 489 (1979).
337. T. Lemarchand-Beraud and C. Berthier, Effects of graded doses of triiodothyronine on TSH synthesis and secretion rates in hypothyroid rats, Acta Endocrinol. (Copenh.) 97:74 (1981).
338. S. Fujimoto and G.A. Hedge, Altered pituitary-thyroid function in the Brattleboro rat with diabetes insipidus, Endocrinology 110:1628 (1981).
339. R. M. Pastor and T. Jolin, Peripheral metabolism and secretion rate of thyrotropin in streptozotocin-diabetic rats, Endocrinology 112:1454 (1983).
340. J. M. Connors, W.J. DeVito and G.A. Hedge, The effects of the duration of severe hypothyroidism and aging on the metabolic clearance rate of thyrotropin (TSH) and the pituitary TSH response to TSH-releasing hormone, Endocrinology 114:1930 (1984).
341. R. B. Constant and B.D. Weintraub, Differences in the metabolic clearance of pituitary and serum thyrotropin (TSH) derived from euthyroid and hypothyroid rats: effects of chemical deglycosylation of pituitary TSH, Endocrinology 119:2720 (1986).
342. A. G. Morell, G. Greogoriadis, H. Scheinberg, J. Hickman and G. Ashwell, The role of sialic acid in determining the survival of glycoproteins in the circulation, J. Biol. Chem. 246:1461 (1971).
343. R. E. Wehmann and B.C. Nisula, Metabolic and renal clearance rates of purified human chorionic gonadotropin, J. Clin. Invest. 68:184 (1981).
344. S. C. Chappel, A. Ulloa-Aguierre and C. Coutifaris, Biosynthe-

sis and secretion of follicle-stimulating hormone, Endocr. Rev. 4:179 (1983).

345. G. P. Lefort, J.M. Stolk and B.C. Nisula, Evidence that desialylation and uptake by hepatic receptors for galactose-terminated glycoproteins are immaterial to the metabolism of human choriogonadotropin in the rat, Endocrinology 115:1551 (1984).

346. D. L. Blithe and B.C. Nisula, Similarity of the clearance rates of free α-subunit and α-subunit dissociated from intact human chorionic gonadotropin, despite differences in sialic acid contents, Endocrinology 121:1215 (1987).

347. C. Rosa, S. Amr, S. Birken, R. Wehmann and B. Nisula, Effects of desialylation of human chorionic gonadotropin on its metabolic clearance rate in humans, J. Clin. Endocrinol. 59:1215 (1984).

348. M. R. Sairam, Gonadotropic hormones: relationship between structure and function with emphasis on antagonists, in: Hormonal Proteins and Peptides, C. H. Li, ed., Academic, New York (1983).

349. W. L. Gordon and D.N. Ward, Structural aspects of luteinizing hormone actions. in: Luteinizing Hormone Action and Receptors, M. Ascoli, ed., CRC Press, Boca Raton (1985).

350. J. A. Weare and L.E. Reichert, Jr, Studies with carbodiimide cross-linked derivatives and implication for interaction with the receptors in testis, J. Biol. Chem. 254:6972 (1979).

351. R. J. Ryan, M.C. Charlesworth, D.J. McCormick, R.P. Milius and H.T. Keutmann, The glycoprotein hormones: recent studies of structure-function relationships. FASEB J. 2:2661 (1988).

352. J. C. Morris, III, N.-S. Jiang, M.C. Charlesworth, D.J. McCormick and R.J. Ryan, The effects of synthetic alpha subunit peptides on thyrotropin interaction with its receptor, Endocrinology 123:456 (1988).

353. J. C. Morris, III, N.-S. Jiang, I.D. Hay, M.C. Charlesworth, D.J. McCormick and R.J. Ryan, The effects of synthetic alpha-subunit peptides on thyroid-stimulating immunoglobulin activity, J. Clin. Endocrinol.Metab. 67:707 (1988).

354. M. M. Matzuk, J.L. Keene and I. Boime, Site specificity of the chorionic gonadotropin N-linked oligosaccharides in signal transduction, J. Biol. Chem. 264:2409 (1989).

355. S. Watanabe, Y. Hayashizaki, Y. Endo, M. Hirono, N. Takimot, M. Tamaki, H. Teraoka, K. Miyai and K. Matsubara, Production of human thyroid-stimulating hormone in Chinese Hamster Ovary Cells, Biochem. Biophys. Res. Commun. 149:1149 (1987).

356. M. C. Murray, V.P. Bhavanandan and E.A. Davidson, Modification of sialyl residues of gonadotropic hormones by reductive amination. Influence on biological activity and circulating half-life, Glycoconjugate J. 5:485 (1989).

CHARACTERIZATION OF RECEPTORS FOR INSULIN AND INSULIN-LIKE GROWTH FACTOR-1 ON FRTL-5 THYROID CELLS

N. Perrotti, C.M. Rotella, F.V. Alvarez, L.D. Kohn and S. Taylor

Diabetes Branch
NIDDK
National Institutes of Health
Bethesda, MD 20892

INTRODUCTION

The development of the FRTL and FRTL-5 thyroid cells (Fig. 1A) by F.S. Ambesi-Impiombato and his colleagues (1,2) moved research in the thyroid area from a concern with the thyrotropin receptor to an examination of receptor interactions or cross-talk. These cells require TSH for their growth (Fig. 1B). However, the TSH action requires the presence of insulin and serum factors, one of which we now know to be IGF-I (Fig. 1B); no single factor, TSH, insulin, or IGF-I, can reproduce the mixture of all. Further it is evident that the insulin and IGF-I actions are not identical; thus when concentrations of insulin as high as 10 micrograms per ml are present, the addition of only 50 or 100 ng/ml of IGF-I is still significantly additive to TSH and insulin in stimulating an increase in cell number.

Several important questions emerged from these observations. For example, how does insulin/IGF-I influence the action of TSH or, conversely, did TSH influence the action of insulin or IGF-I? Were there separate receptors for insulin and IGF-I, could they also modulate thyroid function, and could they act independently? Would

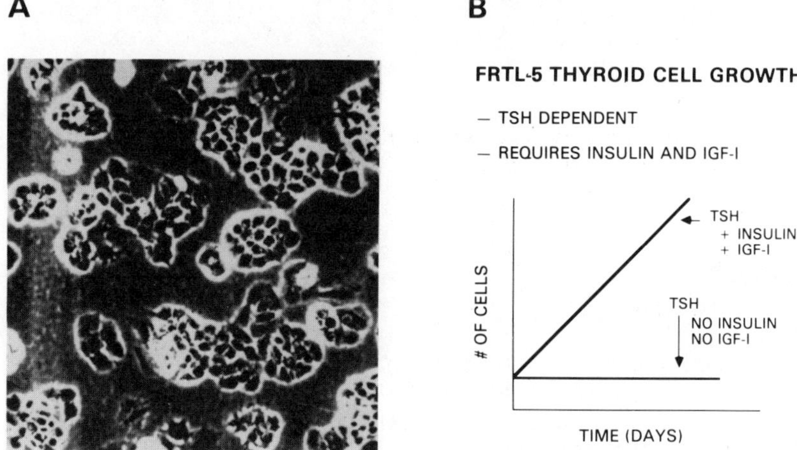

Fig. 1. (A) FRTL-5 rat thyroid cells. (B) Diagramatic representation of the effect of TSH or TSH plus insulin and IGF-I on the growth of FRTL-5 cells in culture. In addition to the noted hormones, cells were in 0.2% serum and in Coons modified F-12 medium with the 4H mixture (somatostatin, transferrin, hydrocortisone, and glycyl-L-histidyl-L-lysine) (1,2).

the relationship between insulin, IGF-I, and TSH receptors extend to relationships with other receptors important for thyroid growth and function? Could knowledge gained in the thyroid be extended to other cells and other tissues to further our ideas as to how receptors communicate with each other to regulate biological activities.

These concerns and some of their answers will be addressed in several reports in this meeting. In the present report, we establish that separate receptors do indeed exist for insulin and IGFs on the FRTL-5 cells and we characterize their structural properties. The report shows further that TSH modulates each differently, increasing the number of insulin receptors but decreasing the number of IGF-I receptors on the surface of the FRTL-5 cells.

INSULIN AND IGF-I BINDING TO FRTL-5 THYROID CELLS

FRTL-5 rat thyroid cells (ATCC CRL# 8305) were grown in Coon's modified Ham's F-12 medium, supplemented with 5% calf serum and a six-hormone mixture (6H), containing bovine TSH, insulin, cortisol, transferrin, glycyl-L-histidyl-L-lysine acetate and somatostatin (1,2). Cells were grown at 37° C in a 5% CO_2 -95% air atmosphere and were passaged every 7 to 10 days (1,2). They maintained a diploid karyotype throughout the course of these experiments and were monitored at least monthly to ensure that, after 10 days of TSH withdrawal, they retained their ability to respond to TSH as follows: elevated cAMP levels (50 to 100 fold), iodide uptake (3 to 6 fold), growth (24 to 48 hr doubling time after a 48-72 hr lag; dependence on insulin and serum), and thyroglobulin synthesis (~2 fold with respect to protein and mRNA).

For insulin and IGF-I binding experiments, cells were seeded at least 7-10 days in advance of each experiment, were grown in the complete media above, and were used when they reached a density of 2 X 10^7 cells per 10 cm culture dish. Cells were then shifted to and maintained for 5 days in medium minus TSH and insulin and containing only 0.2% calf serum and for an additional 2 days in the same medium with 1% 5x recrystallized albumin rather than 0.2% serum. Cells were detached by a 20-30 min exposure at 37° C to 4 mM EGTA in a Hanks' balanced salt solution (HBSS) without calcium or magnesium. Cells were sedimented (500xg) and washed twice in a binding buffer at pH 8.0 consisting of 0.1M Hepes, 0.12M NaCl, 1.2mM $MgSO_4$, 2.5mM KCl, 10mM glucose, 1mM EDTA, and 10 mg/ml 5x recrystallized bovine serum albumin (3). They were then resuspended in the same buffer and a concentration of 1-2x10^7 cells per ml. Binding incubations were in an 0.5 ml volume and included 0.1 ng/ml ^{125}I-porcine insulin

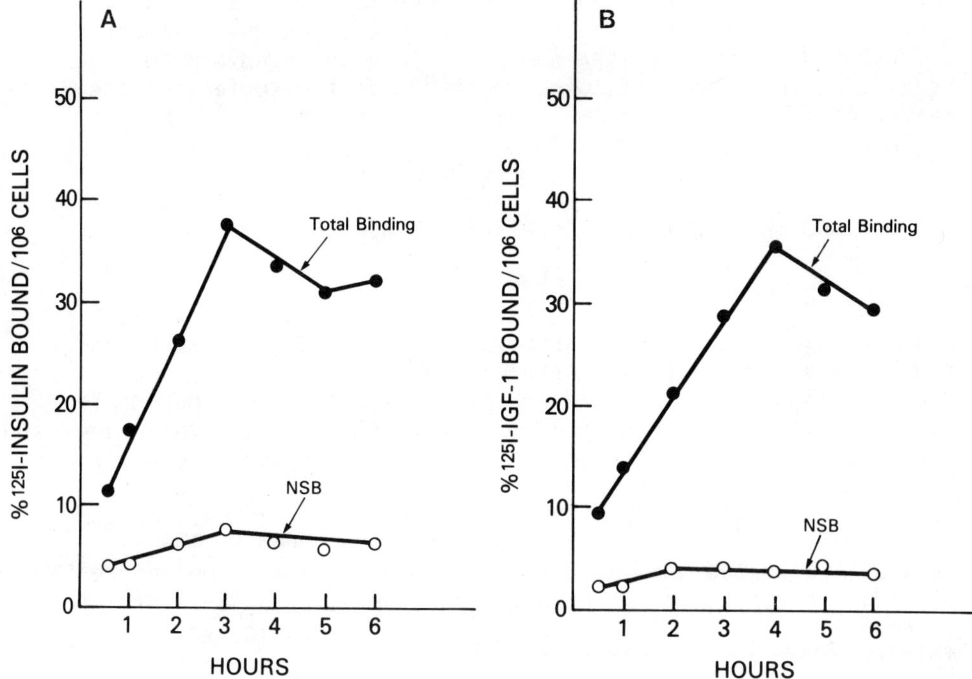

Fig. 2. The time course of insulin (A) and IGF-I (B) binding to FRTL-5 cells at 15° C in a Hepes binding medium. 2.5 X 10^6 cells were incubated with 0.1 ng/ml labeled ligand, (30,000 cpm) in the presence (•) or absence (o) of 10 μg/ml unlabeled ligand. Results were expressed as percent of labeled peptide bound per 10^6 cells.

or ^{125}I-59 threo-IGF-I. At 15°, ^{125}I-insulin binding reached a maximum at 3 h and then decreased with longer periods of incubation (Fig. 2A). ^{125}I-IGF-I binding to the hormone depleted FRTL-5 cells reached a maximum at 4 h, then decreased over the following 2 h (Fig. 2B). Non-specific binding (NSB) of both ligands was significantly lower and did not vary significantly over time (Fig. 2). When cells were incubated at 37° C, steady-state binding of both ligands was achieved more rapidly (within 1-2 h), but the maximal binding was 35-40% lower than at 15° C.

Porcine insulin displaced 50% of ^{125}I-insulin binding at a concentration of approximately 200 ng/ml (Fig. 3A). Porcine proinsulin and IGF-I were both approximately 10% as potent as insulin (Fig. 3A). IGF-I displaced 50% of ^{125}I-IGF-I binding at a concentration of approximately 20 ng/ml (Fig. 3B). Insulin and proinsulin were approximately 0.3% and 0.05% as potent, respectively (Fig. 3B). Even at concentrations of 100,000 ng/ml, neither glucagon nor human growth hormone (hGH) inhibited the binding of ^{125}I-insulin or ^{125}I-IGF-I (Fig. 3A and Fig. 3B).

EFFECTS OF TSH UPON INSULIN AND IGF-I BINDING

Insulin and IGF-I binding were studied in serum depleted cells maintained as above in the absence of TSH and insulin or in serum depleted cells with TSH but no insulin. The Scatchard plots (5) for both insulin and IGF-I binding appear to be linear under these conditions (Fig. 4A and 4B). In comparing the cells, the addition of TSH increased ^{125}I-insulin binding (Fig. 4A), but decreased ^{125}I-IGF-I binding (Fig. 4B). TSH increased the number of insulin binding sites without having a major effect upon receptor affinity (Table I). It decreased the number of ^{125}I-IGF-I sites, again with no apparent change in affinity (Table I). Thus, addition of TSH caused the up-regulation of insulin receptors, but the down regulation of IGF-I receptors.

With relatively few exceptions, insulin receptors exhibit curvilinear Scatchard plots (6). However, the Scatchard plot for insulin binding to FRTL-5 cells is linear (Fig. 4A), as in the case with cultured Fao hepatoma cells (7). Also like cultured Fao hepatoma cells (7), the apparent affinity for insulin binding is relatively low. It is not known what determines whether a particular cell type will exhibit a curvilinear Scatchard plot for insulin binding. The Scatchard plot for IGF-I binding to FRTL-5 cells is also linear (Fig. 4B). However, in the case of IGF-I binding, the Scatchard plot is generally found to be linear (8).

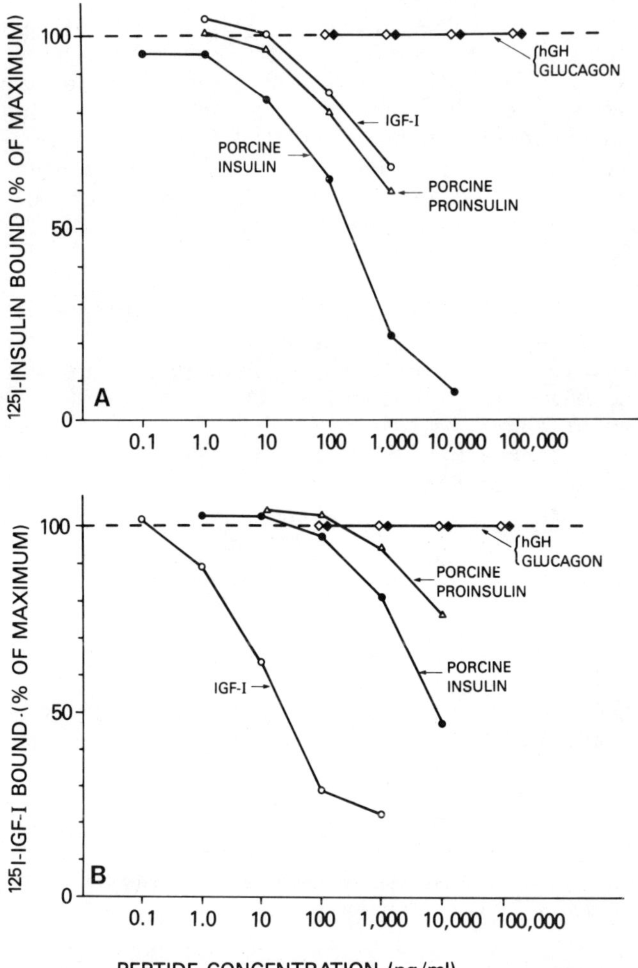

Fig. 3(A). Displacement of ^{125}I-insulin binding to FRTL-5 cells by unlabeled porcine insulin, porcine proinsulin, IGF-I and two polypeptide hormones devoid of insulin bioactivity, glucagon and human growth hormone (hGH). Cells, 4.5 X 10^6 in number, were incubated at 15° C for 3 hr in a Hepes binding buffer with radiolabeled insulin in the presence or in the absence of unlabeled peptides. Results are expressed as percent of maximum ^{125}I insulin bound. (B) Displacement of ^{125}I-IGF-I binding to FRTL-5 cells by unlabeled IGF-I, porcine insulin, porcine proinsulin and other polypeptide hormones devoid of insulin bioactivity. 5.0 X 10^6 cells were incubated at 15° C for 3 hr in a Hepes binding buffer with radiolabeled IGF-I in the presence or in the absence of unlabeled peptides and results expressed as percent of maximum ^{125}I IGF-I bound.

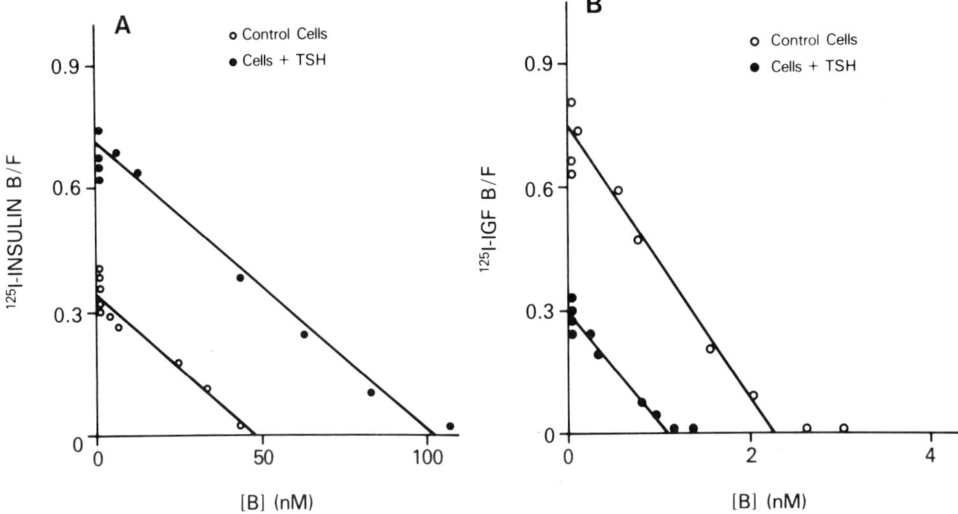

Fig. 4(A). Scatchard plot (5) of ^{125}I-insulin binding in the presence of graded amounts (0.1 ng/ml to 10μg/ml) of porcine insulin in serum depleted FRTL-5 cells either maintained in the presence of $1X10^{-10}$ M TSH (•) or kept for 7 days in a medium without TSH (o). $7.5X10^{6}$ cells were incubated at 15°C for 3 hr according to the procedure described in the text and data were analyzed by means of the program "LIGAND" according to Munson and Rodbard (4). (B) Scatchard plot (5) of ^{125}I-IGF-I binding in the presence of graded amounts (0.1 ng/ml to 5 μg/ml) of unlabeled IGF-I in FRTL-5 cells maintained in the presence of $1X10^{-10}$ M TSH (•) or kept for 7 days in a medium lacking TSH (o). 7.5 x 10^{6} cells were incubated at 15°C for 3 hr according to the procedure described in the text and data were analyzed by means of the program "LIGAND" according to Munson and Rodbard (4).

TABLE 1. Dissociation constant (Kd) and number of binding sites (R_1) for insulin and IGF-I in FRTL-5 cells continuously kept in the control, serum depleted medium with no TSH and no insulin or in serum depleted medium containing $1X10^{-10}$ M TSH. Results were derived from data such as those reported in Figures 4A and 4B by means of the program "LIGAND" (4).

	Control Cells				Cells + TSH			
	Kd (nM)	CV[a]	R_1 (picomoles/ 10^6 cells)	CV	Kd (nM)	CV	R_1 (picomoles/ 10^6 cells)	CV
INSULIN	140.8	24%	3.2	21%	145.0	18%	7.3[c]	14%
IGF-I	3.0	20%	0.16	14%	3.5	25%	0.06[d]	20%

[a] CV, coefficient of variation.
[b] The mixture of 6 hormones of growth factors detailed (1,2).
[c] significantly ($p<0.02$) higher than that of control cells, as assessed by F test (4).
[d] significantly ($p<0.0001$) lower than that of control cells, as assessed by F test (4)..

STUDIES OF RECEPTOR SUBUNIT STRUCTURE

We have applied the method of Czech and his colleagues (9,10) to identify the receptor subunits responsible for binding ^{125}I-insulin and ^{125}I-IGF-I in these cells. FRTL-5 cells were maintained in serum depleted medium without TSH or insulin for 7 days before membranes were prepared from 60 plates of cells. Membrane pellets were resuspended in assay binding buffer, as previously described, at a protein concentration of approximately 2 mg/ml. Each membrane preparation was divided into 18 one ml aliquots which were used for binding and displacement with the appropriate hormones after their addition to 1.5 ml Eppendorf tubes. ^{125}I-59 threo-IGF-I or ^{125}I-insulin were used at a concentration of 2 ng/ml; incubations were performed overnight at 4° C in a shaker and in the presence of phenylmethylsulfonyl fluoride (2 nM), leupeptin (10 µg/ml), and the different hormones specified in the legends of Figures 5A and 5B. After incubation, the membranes were centrifuged in a Beckman microfuge and resuspended in 0.5 ml of 50 mM Hepes buffer, pH 7.8, containing 150 mM NaCl. Disuccinimdyl suberate, dissolved in dimethyl sulfoxide, was added to a final concentration 0.1 mM and the reaction allowed to proceed for 15 min on ice. The reaction was stopped by 1:1 dilution with quenching solution (10 mM Tris and 1 mM ETDA in PBS at pH 7.8).

The membranes were then centrifuged in a Beckman microfuge washed three times in Hepes 50 mM, pH 7.8, containing 150 mM NaCl, and resuspended in 0.15 ml of Laemmli (11) sample buffer containing 0.1 M dithiothreitol. After being boiled for 5 min at 100° C, the incubation mixtures were centrifuged in the microfuge to remove insoluble material, and 0.075 ml from each tube were applied to a 7.5% polyacrylamide gel, containing sodium dodecyl sulfate (SDS) (11).

Using this affinity-labeling technique, both radioligands were chemically cross-linked to proteins with apparent molecular weight of 120 KD (Figs. 5A and 5B). When ^{125}I-insulin was cross-linked to the insulin receptor, unlabeled insulin at a concentration of 50-100 ng/ml inhibited affinity labeling by approximately 50% (Fig. 5A). IGF-I was approximately 2- to 5-fold less potent than insulin in this respect (Fig. 5B). When ^{125}I-IGF-I was cross-linked to the type I IGF-receptor, half maximal inhibition of affinity-labeling was accomplished at an IGF-I concentration of 40-80 ng/ml (Fig. 5B) whereas unlabeled insulin was approximately 50-fold less effective.

To determine the size of the ß-subunit of the insulin and IGF-I receptors, membranes from 60 10 cm dishes were suspended in 5 ml of 50 mM Hepes, pH 7.8, containing 150 mM NaCl, 1% Triton X-100 and 2 mM phenylmethylsulfonyl fluoride. Solubilization was performed for 1 h at 0° C. The solubilized material was clarified by

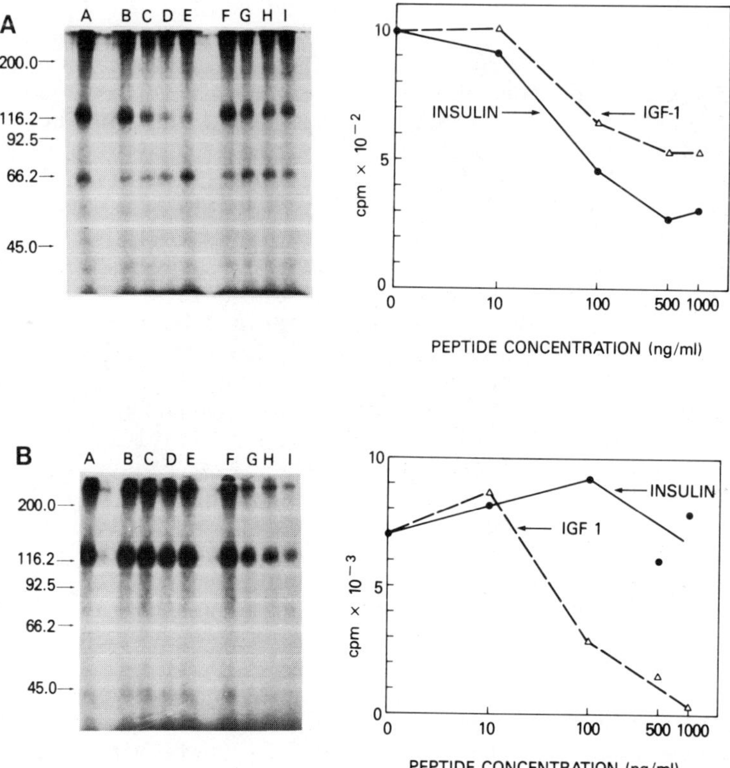

Fig. 5(A) Affinity labeling of insulin receptor with ^{125}I-insulin. ^{125}I-insulin (receptor grade) was used at concentration of 2 ng/ml. Incubation with FRTL-5 cell membranes was performed overnight at 4° C in a shaker in the presence of 2 mM PMSF, 10 μg/ml Leupeptin, and the following: A: no addition control; B: insulin 10 ng/ml; C: insulin 100 ng/ml; D: insulin 500 ng/ml; E: insulin 1000 ng/ml; F: IGF-I, 10 ng/ml; G: IGF-I 100 ng/ml; H: IGF-I 500 ng/ml; I: IGF-I 1000 ng/ml. An autoradiograph of the SDS polyacrylamide gels is presented in the left panel. The parts of the gel corresponding to the 120K bands were cut and counted in a γ-counter for 50 min. Portions of the gel where no discrete bound was detectable were also cut from each lane and counted in the same way to give a measure of the background. Values reported in the right panel refer to CPM recovered in the lane after subtraction of background radioactivity. (B) Affinity labeling of IGF-I receptor with ^{125}I-IGF-I. The same method was followed as for insulin, except that ^{125}I-IGF-I was used as a label at a concentration of 2 ng/ml and displacement was performed with the same hormones in the same order as reported in legend of Fig. 5A. An autoradiograph of the SDS polyacrylamide gels is presented in the left panel; values of CPM recovered in the 120K bands, after subtraction of background radioactivity, are presented on the right.

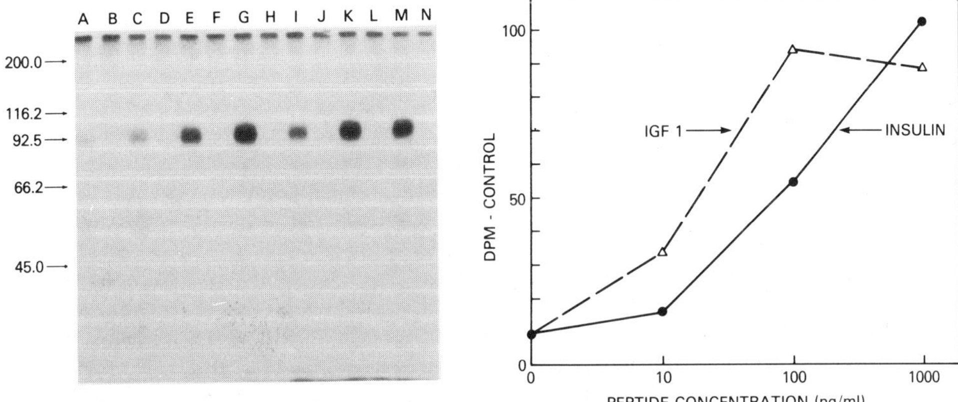

Fig. 6. Phosphorylation of the ß-subunit of the insulin and IGF-I receptors. The polyacrylamide gels of the wheat germ affinity column purified receptor preparations (see text) are presented on the left. Partially purified receptors were incubated with the following: Buffer: (A and B); insulin 10 ng/ml (C and D); insulin 100 ng/ml (E and F); insulin 1000 ng/ml (G and H); IGF-I 10 ng/ml: (I and J); IGF-I 100 ng/ml: (K and L); IGF-I 1000 ng/ml (M and N). Immunoprecipitation was performed using the B-8 antibody at a dilution of 1:100 (lanes A, C, E, G, I, K and M) or normal human serum at the same dilution (Lanes B, D, F, H, J, L, N). The portions of the gel corresponding to the band were cut, swollen in water, digested with protosol, resuspended in 15 ml of Econofluor and counted in a ß-counter for 20 min. ^{32}P was incorporation is expressed as DPM in the 95K band, where antireceptor antibody was used, less the radioactivity in the same region of the gel where normal human serum was used (right panel).

ultracentrifugation at 200,000 xg for 45 min. The pellet was discarded and the supernatant solution subjected to partial purification by chromatography over wheat germ agglutinin-agarose according to previously described methods (12). Optical density of the eluate was used to pool peak fractions, aliquots of which were used in the phosphorylation assay which was performed as previously detailed (13,14). The partially purified receptor preparation in a final volume of 0.4 ml, was incubated with different hormones as specified in the legend of Figure 6. After a 1 h incubation at 22° C, phosphorylation was started by adding 0.25 ml of a solution containing 0.2 mCi [γ^{32}p]ATP, 25 mM ATP, 5 mM CTP, and 25 mM manganese acetate. The reaction was terminated after 20 min by addition of 0.1875 ml of a stopping solution consisting of 16 mM EDTA, 32 mM sodium pyrophosphate, 320 mM NaF and 3.2 mM sodium vanadate.

Immunoprecipitation was performed in an 0.3 ml volume using a human anti-receptor antibody [patient B-8 (15)] at a dilution of 1:100 or normal human serum at the same dilution. After an incubation for 16 h the immune complexes were separated by adding 0.15 ml of 20% pansorbin. The pellet was washed three times in 50 mM Hepes buffer, pH 7.8 containing 150 mM NaCl and 0.1% Triton X-100, then resuspended in Laemmli sample buffer (11) and applied to a 7.5% SDS polyacrylamide gel prepared according to Laemmli (11). Gels were dryed and autoradiographed.

Both insulin and IGF-I caused a ten-fold stimulation of phosphorylation of 95KD phosphoproteins which can be immunoprecipitated by anti receptor antiserum B-8 containing antibodies to both insulin and IGF-I receptors (Fig. 6). These phosphoproteins correspond to the beta subunits of the receptors for insulin and IGF-I, respectively. Half maximal stimulations of phosphorylation were observed at peptide concentrations of 50 ng/ml of insulin and 20 ng/ml of IGF-I. Similar observations were made when the phosphoproteins were analyzed by SDS-polyacrylamide electrophoresis without prior immunoprecipitation.

In FRTL-5 cells, the subunit structure of the receptors for insulin and IGF-I is generally similar to that described in other cell types (8,10,15, 12-14, 16-23). Both types of receptors have alpha-subunits which appear to contain the ligand binding sites and can, therefore, be labeled by an affinity cross-linking technique. In addition, both receptors possess beta-subunits which are the sites for ligand-stimulated autophosphorylation. However, unlike what has been reported in most other cells (8,16,23), in FRTL-5 cells, we could not detect any difference between the apparent molecular weights of the subunits of the insulin receptor and IGF-I receptor (Figs. 5,6). Moreover, the alpha-subunits resembled those found in the brain insulin receptor (24,25) in that the apparent molecular weight of the affinity-labeled alpha-subunit was approximately 120,000 rather than the 135,000 observed in most other cells and tissues (26-31).

SUMMARY

FRTL-5 rat thyroid cells have receptors for both insulin and IGF-I which can be distinguished in binding studies. The ability of TSH to regulate each in an antiparallel manner is atypical. If these receptors are shown to have independent as well as coordinate activities, studies of the mechanisms of their receptor cross-talk in these cells will be relevant to understanding IGF-I and insulin receptors in other tissues.

REFERENCES

1. F. S. Ambesi-Impiombato, L. A. M. Parks, and H. G. Coon, Culture of hormone dependent epithelial cells from rat thyroids, Proc. Natl. Acad. Sci. USA, 77: 3455 (1980).
2. F. S. Ambesi-Impiombato, Living, fast-growing thyroid cell strain FRTL-5. U.S. Patent #4,608,341, (1986).
3. J. M. Podskalny, J. Y. Chou, and M. M. Rechler, Insulin receptors in a new human placenta cell line: demonstration of negative cooperativity, Arch Biochem. Biophys., 170: 507 (1975).
4. R. Munson and D. Robbard, Ligand: A versatile computerized approach for characterization of ligand-binding systems, Anal. Biochem., 107: 220 (1980).
5. G. Scatchard, The actractions of proteins for small proteins and ions, Ann. N.Y. Acad. Sci., 51: 660 (1949).
6. B. H. Ginsburg, The insulin receptor: properties and regulation, In: "Biochemical Actions of Hormones" G. Litwack, ed., Academic Press, New York (1977).
7. M. Crettaz and C. R. Kahn, Analysis of insulin action using differentiated and dedifferentiated hepatoma cells, Endocrinology 133: 1201 (1983).
8. M. M. Rechler and S. P. Nissley, Receptors for insulin-like growth factors, In: "Polypeptide Hormone Receptors", B. L. Posner, ed., Marcel Dekker, Inc., New York and Basel (1985).
9. T. Massague, B. J. Guillette and M. P. Czech, Affinity labeling of multiplication stimulating activity receptors in membrances from rat and human tissues, J. Biol. Chem. 256: 2122 (1980).
10. P. F. Pilch and M. Czech, Interaction of cross-linking agents with the insulin effector system of isolated fat cells, J. Biol. Chem., 254: 3375 (1979).

11. U. K. Laemmli, Cleavage of structural proteins during the assembly of the head of bacteriophate T4, Nature, 227: 680 (1970).
12. J. A. Hedo, L. C. Harrison and J. Roth, Binding of insulin receptors to lectins: evidence for common carbohydrate determinants on several membrane receptors, Biochemistry, 20: 3385, (1981).
13. R. W. Rees-Jones and S. I. Taylor, An endogenous substrate for the insulin receptor-associated tyrosine kinase, J. Biol. Chem., 260: 4461 (1985).
14. Y. Zick, M. Kasuga, C. R. Kahn and J. Roth, Characterization of insulin-mediated phosphorylation of the insulin receptor in a cell-free system, J. Biol. Chem., 258: 75 (1983).
15. S. Taylor, T. A. Schroer, B. Marcus-Samuels, A. McElduff and T. P. Bender, Binding of insulin to its receptor impairs recognition by monoclonal anti-insulin antibodies, Diabetes, 33: 778 (1984).
16. E. R. Froesch, C. Schmid, J. Schwander and J. Zapf, Actions of insulin-like growth factor, Ann. Rev. Physiol. 47: 443 (1985).
17. S. D. Chernausek, S. D. Jacobs and J. J. VanWyk, Structural similarities between human receptors for somatomedin-C and insulin: analyses by affinity labeling, Biochemistry, 20: 7345 (1981).
18. B. Bhaumick, R. M. Bala and M. D. Hollenberg, Somatomedin receptor of human placenta: solubilization, photolabeling, partial purification and comparison to insulin receptor, Proc. Natl. Acad. Sci. USA, 78: 4279 (1981).
19. J. Massaque and M. P. Czech, The subunit structure of two distinct receptors for insulin-like growth factors I and II and their relationship to the insulin receptor, J. Biol. Chem. 257: 5038 (1982).
20. F. C. Kull Jr., S. Jacobs, F. Y. Su, M. E. Svoboda, J. J. Van Wyk and P. Cuatrecasas, Monoclonal antibodies to receptors for insulin and somatomedin-C, J. Biol. Chem., 258: 6561 (1983).
21. G. V. Ronnett, V. P. Knutson, R. A. Kohanski Ra, T. L. Simpson and M. D. Lane, Role of glycosylation in the processing of newly translated insulin proreceptor in 3T3-L1 adipocytes, J. Biol. Chem., 259: 4566 (1984).
22. S. Jacobs, F. C. Kull and P. Cuatrecasas, Monensin blocks the maturation of receptors for insulin and somatomedin-C: Identification of receptor precursors, Proc. Natl. Acad. Sci. USA, 80: 1228 (1983).
23. A. Ulrich, A. Gray, A. W. Tam, T. Yang-Feng, M. Tsubokawa, C. Collins, W. Henzel, T. LeBon, S. Kathuria, E. Chen, S. Jacobs, V. Francke, J. Ramachandran and Y. Fujita-Yamaguchi, Insulin-like growth factor I receptor primary structure: comparison with insulin receptor suggests structural determinants that define functional specificity, The EMBO Journal, 5: 2503 (1986).

24. K. Heidenreich, N. R. Zahniser, R. Berhanu, D. Brandenburg and J. M. Olefsky, Structural differences between insulin receptors in the brain and peripheral target tissues, J. Biol. Chem. 258: 8527 (1983).
25. S. A. Hendricks, C. D. Agardh, S. T. Taylor and J. Roth, Unique features of the insulin receptor in rat brain, J. Neurochem., 43: 1302 (1984).
26. S. Jacobs, E. Hazum and P. Cuatrecasas, The subunit structure of rat liver insulin receptor, J. Biol. Chem., 255: 6937 (1980).
27. S. Jacobs, E. Hazum and P. Cuatrecases, Digestion of insulin receptors with proteolytic and glycosidic enzymes: effects on purified and membrane-associated receptor subunits, Biochem. Biophys, Res. Commun., 94: 1066 (1980).
28. P. Pilch and M. P. Czech, The subunit structure of the high affinity insulin receptor, J. Biol. Chem., 255: 1722 (1980).
29. C. C. Yip, M. L. Moule and C. W. T. Yeung, Characterization of insulin receptor subunits in brain and other tissues by photoaffinity labeling, Biochem. Biophys. Res. Commun., 96: 1671 (1980).
30. M. Kasuga, E. Van Obberghen, K. M. Yamada and L. C. Harrison, Autoantibodies against the insulin receptor recognize the insulin binding subunits of an oligomeric receptor, Diabetes, 30: 354 (1981).
31. M. Kasuga, J. A. Hedo JA, K. M. Yamada and C. R. Kahn, The structure of insulin receptor and its subunits, J. Biol. Chem., 257: 10392 (1982).

REGULATORY PEPTIDES IN THE THYROID GLAND

Torsten Grunditz[1], Frank Sundler[2]
Rolf Håkanson[3] and Rolf Uddman[1]

Departments of Otolaryngology[1] (Malmö)
Medical Cell Research[2] and Pharmacology[3]
University of Lund, Lund, Sweden

BACKGROUND

The mammalian thyroid gland harbours two different endocrine cell types: follicular and parafollicular (C) cells. The follicle cells are of entodermal origin and develop from the thyroglossus duct in the floor of the pharyngeal cavity(1,2). The C cells are thought to derive from the neuroectoderm(3). The C cell precursors migrate to form the ultimobranchial bodies which persist as separate organs throughout life in submammalian vertebrates(4,5). In mammals the ultimobranchial bodies fuse with the thyroid anlage during the fetal development (6-8). The follicle cells synthesize and secrete triiodothyronine (T_3) and tetraiodothyronine or thyroxine (T_4), which control energy metabolism and are necessary for normal growth(9). The C cells synthesize, store and secrete calcitonin (CT), which is thought to be involved in the regulation of serum Ca by suppressing bone resorption(10,11).

The thyroid gland receives its blood supply from the carotid artery via the thyroid arteries which divide into smaller branches before penetrating the upper and lower poles of the gland(12). Within the thyroid, the blood vessels ramify in the connective tissue between the follicles(12-15). Capillaries form a dense network around each follicle(16). The follicles are the most conspicuous feature of the thyroid gland and form the major portion of the parenchyma. A thin basement membrane surrounds each follicle, which is composed of a single layer of epithelial cells (follicle cells) enclosing the follicle lumen. The C cells are generally larger than the follicle cells and occur scattered in the follicle wall or in small clusters in the interfollicle space(17). They are located predominantly in the central and dorsolateral parts of the thyroid lobes(18). As a rule the C cells do not reach the follicle lumen(17).

The activity of the follicle cells is controlled by the thyroid stimulating hormone (TSH) from the pituitary gland(19-21). Although TSH is thought to be the principal regulator of thyroid function, an involvement of the autonomic nervous system has been suggested(22,23). Such an involvement is likely in view of the rich supply of noradrenaline (NA)-storing and acetylcholinesterase (AChE)-positive nerve fibres in the thyroid gland(24,25). The adrenergic innervation of the thyroid has been examined by histofluorescence techniques in several species (26,27). Adrenergic nerve fibres occur both around blood vessels and follicles. The fibres derive from the superior cervical and stellate ganglia and seem to enter the thyroid gland via the blood vessels(24,27-32). As studied by electron microscopy adrenergic nerve terminals are sometimes in close apposition to follicle cells(24). Exogenous catecholamines and electrical stimulation of sympathetic branches to the thyroid gland cause colloid droplet formation and thyroid hormone secretion in mice (24). Interestingly, catecholamines inhibit TSH-induced secretion of thyroid hormones(24,33,34). The sympathetic nerves are thought to interact with TSH in the regulation of thyroid hormone secretion(24). In addition, catecholamine-induced vasoconstriction reduces the thyroid blood flow and indirectly the capacity of the thyroid gland to release its hormones(30). There is also evidence that the sympathetic nervous system may play a role in the control of thyroid growth(35).

In the parasympathetic nervous system the classical postganglionic neurotransmitter is acetylcholine(36). Acetylcholinesterase (AChE)-positive nerve fibres are present in the thyroid gland(25,37). It is generally assumed that these fibres represent cholinergic, presumably postganglionic parasympathetic fibres. However, AChE may occur also in adrenergic and sensory neurones(38-40). Whatever the nature of the AChE-positive fibres, their distribution around blood vessels and follicles suggests a role in the regulation of local blood flow and thyroid hormone secretion(25,41-44).

Until fairly recently our knowledge of the morphological and functional aspects of the parasympathetic and sensory innervation of the thyroid could be summarized as follows: Parasympathetic fibres (and possibly sensory fibres) in the thyroid gland originate in the vagal jugular-nodose ganglionic complex(14,28). The thyroid gland receives its vagal innervation mainly via the superior laryngeal nerve(28). There is a minor vagal contribution from the recurrent nerve (the inferior laryngeal nerve) which anastomoses with the superior laryngeal nerve(28,45). In mice the cholinergic agonist carbachol impairs TSH-induced thyroid hormone release, suggesting an inhibitory influence of parasympathetic cholinergic nerves via muscarinic receptors(25). Studies in rats suggest a stimulatory role of the parasympathetic innervation on thyroid function(46). Electrical stimulation of vagal nerves in rats, cats, and rabbits stimulates thyroid blood flow(30,44). In dogs the response involves also an increase of thyroid hormone secretion (41).

NEUROPEPTIDES IN THE THYROID GLAND

During the last decade many regulatory peptides have been demonstrated in neurones suggesting that they have a neurotransmitter/neuromodulator role(47-49). Advances in chemistry have made it possible to detect, isolate and sequence small amounts of such peptides and to synthesize large quantities. Radioimmunochemical methods can be used to measure blood and tissue concentrations of the different peptides and immunocytochemical techniques have made it possible to localize them in their cells of origin(50,51). A neurovesicular localization has been established for some of these peptides(52-57); it is likely that they all have such a localization. Although peptides may function as neurotransmitters (58), the lack of specific blockers makes it difficult to define their functional roles.

The first neuropeptide to be described in the thyroid gland was vasoactive intestinal peptide (VIP)(59). VIP-containing nerve fibres occur around blood vessels and close to follicles(60,61). VIP elevates cyclic AMP concentration, causes colloid droplet formation and stimulates thyroid hormone secretion(59,61-63). The VIP response is unaffected by α- and β-adrenoceptor blockade (62,64). However, carbachol inhibits VIP-induced thyroid hormone secretion(65). This observation suggests that a non-adrenergic, non-cholinergic nervous mechanism may participate in the modulation of thyroid blood flow and

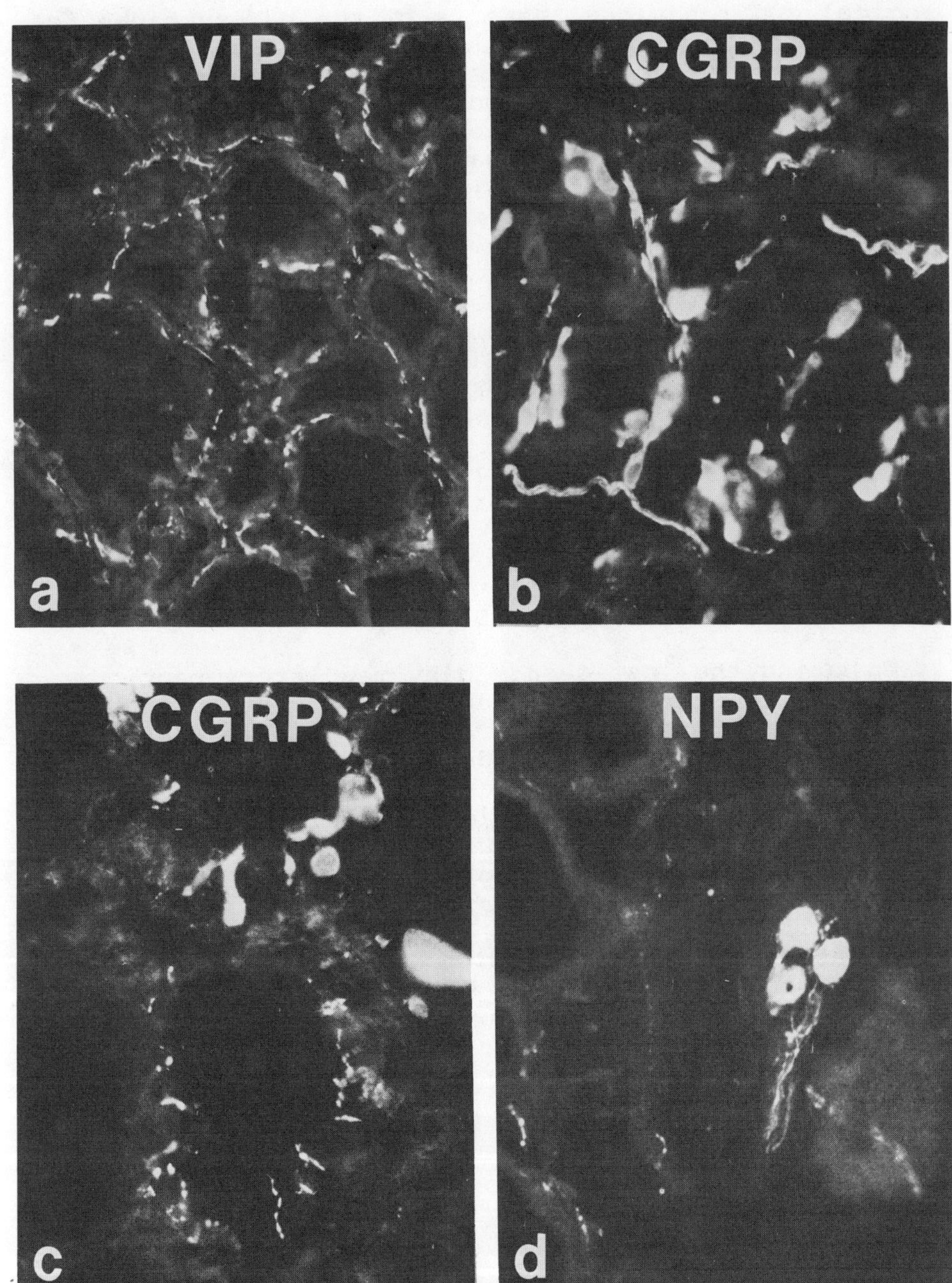

Fig 1 a. VIP-immunoreactive nerve fibres around blood vessels and follicles in the rat thyroid. b, CGRP-immunoreactive nerve fibres in nerve bundles running between follicles in the rat thyroid. In addition, numerous C cells display CGRP immunofluorescence. c. CGRP-immunoreactive nerve fibres in rat thyroid are seen to penetrate the basal membrane of the follicle cell; they appear to reach the follicle lumen. d. NPY-immunoreactive nerve cell bodies and nerve fibres in a small intrathyroid ganglion in calf thyroid gland.

follicle cell activity. Since then, other peptides have been demonstrated in thyroid nerve fibres, e.g. neuropeptide Y (NPY), peptide histidine isoleucine (PHI), galanin (GAL), substance P (SP), neurokinin A (NKA), calcitonin gene-related peptide (CGRP) and cholecystokinin (CCK)(23,27,61,66-68). Nerve fibres storing these peptides have a fairly uniform distribution in the thyroid parenchyma (Fig 1a). They are usually fine-varicose and located around blood vessels and between the follicles. Sometimes, GAL, SP, NKA and CGRP occur in nerve bundles running between the follicles (Fig 1b). Occasionally, single beaded GAL-, SP-, NKA- and CGRP-containing fibres are seen to penetrate the basal membrane, passing between the follicle cells, at times apparently reaching the follicle lumen (Fig 1c). Nerve fibres displaying CCK-like immunoreactivity are few and occur scattered between the follicles(69). Peptide-containing nerve fibres form networks around arteries. Nerve fibres around veins are few. The frequency of the peptide-containing nerve fibres decreases with age (Grunditz, unpublished observations), which brings to mind similar observations on the adrenergic innervation(24,26,68). Interestingly, there are notable species differences with respect to the occurrence and frequency of different peptide-containing nerve fibres in the thyroid gland (Table 1). This may be a true quantitative species difference or reflect the inability of the antibody to detect the antigen (or modified forms of the antigen) in certain species.

Table 1. The relative frequency of NA-containing nerve fibers and of nerve fibers containing various peptides in the thyroid gland of several mammals.

Species	NA	NPY	VIP	GAL	SP	CGRP	CCK
Mouse	+++	++	+++	++	+++	+++	+
Rat	+++	++	+++	+	++	++	+
Guinea pig	++	++	++	0	+++	+++	0
Cat	+++	++	++	0	+	+	0
Dog	++	+	+	0	+	+	0
Pig	+	+	+	0	+	+	0
Sheep	+++	+++	+	0	+	+	0
Cow	+++	+++	+	0	+	+	0
Man	++	++	+	0	+	+	0

The relative frequency of nerve fibers was graded arbitrarily: 0, no fibers; +, few, scattered; ++, moderate in number; +++, numerous. NA demonstrated by histofluorescence.

COEXISTENCE OF NEUROMESSENGERS

It is not unusual to find that peptides coexist with "classical" transmitters or that one and the same neurone or endocrine cell harbours more than one regulatory peptide(47-49,70). Such coexistence can be anticipated when the peptides demonstrated arise from the same precursor, which is processed to generate several small peptide fragments. The complexity is increased by the fact that some neurones and endocrine cells can produce regulatory peptides, which do not derive from the same precursor(49,70). The identification of two or more antigens in one and the same neurone or endocrine cell can be made by sequential or simultaneous double immunostaining(71,72)(Fig 2).

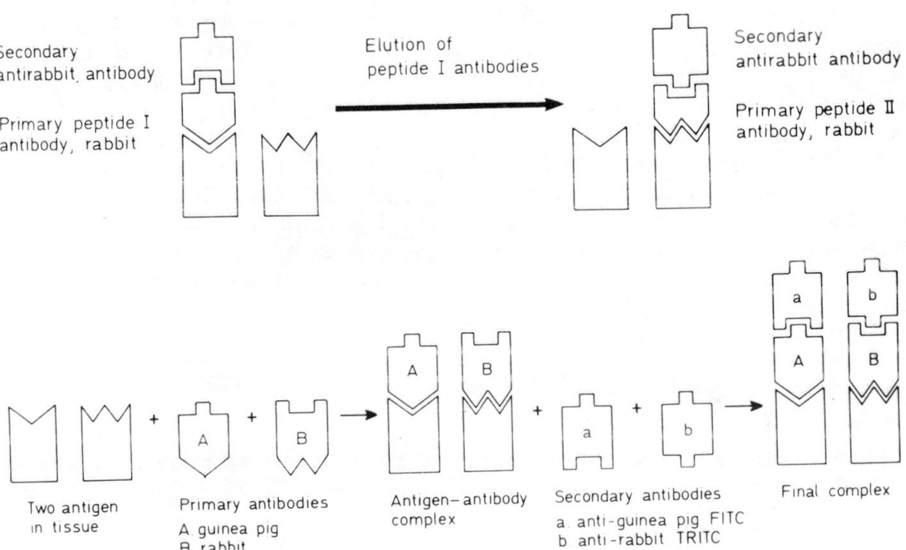

Fig 2. Sequential double immunostaining (top): After photographic documentation of the immunofluorescence produced by the first set of antibodies, the sections are exposed to a potassium permanganate solution for 15-60 sec. It is essential to verify that both the primary antibodies and the fluoresceinated anti-IgG antibodies have been eliminated by this treatment (to avoid false positive results). This is tested by application of fluoresceinated anti-IgG antibodies. If no immunofluorescence can be detected, the sections are exposed to the second set of antibodies. The resulting immunofluorescence is then examined and photographed. The details of the elution procedure must be tested individually for each antiserum and each tissue. The fact that antigens can be destroyed by treatment with potassium permanganate represents a problem. Thus attempt to demonstrate a second antigen may fail for technical reasons (false negative results). Simultaneous double immunostaining (below): The basic requirement in this technique is that the two primary antisera are raised in different species. Also the second antibodies, which must be labelled with two different markers, such as fluorescein isothiocyanate (FITC) and tetramethyl rhodamine isothiocyanate (TRITC), have to be raised in different species. The site of the antigen-antibody reaction is examined in a fluorescence microscope equipped with a combination of filters that can be shifted to demonstrate selectively each of the two fluorophores.

Nucleotide sequencing has indicated a common precursor for VIP and PHI(73) and for SP and NKA(74), respectively. This explains the coexistence of VIP and PHI on one hand and of SP and NKA on the other, as demonstrated e.g. in nerve fibres in the thyroid(66,67). There is reason to assume that the peptides coexist in the same vesicles and that they are released together upon nerve stimulation. Also neuropeptides arising from separate precursors seem to coexist in nerve fibres in the thyroid e.g. NPY with VIP/PHI and CGRP with SP/NKA (66-68). The finding that neurones can produce, store and release more than one messenger compound has attracted much attention(48,58,75,76). The coexistence and possible corelease of a regulatory peptide and a "classical" transmitter or of several peptides challenges the old concept that each neurone produces and releases only one transmitter. In fact, each neurone probably represents a multimessenger system(77,78). Our knowledge of the chemical coding of the various neurones, the information content of the transmitted signals and the significance of the different peptide constellations is still incomplete. The messengers released may interact closely in evoking a response, or they may have completely different postjunctional effects exerted through separate receptor populations: one messenger, for instance, may elicit immediate responses (excitation/inhibition), another may have long-term trophic effects.

NPY has been demonstrated in a population of dopamine-β-hydroxylase (DBH)-containing (and hence probably NA-storing) neurones(79-82). In the thyroid gland most of the NA-storing nerve fibres around blood vessels and follicles contain NPY(27,68). NA released from intrathyroid sympathetic nerve terminals stimulates thyroid hormone secretion, while NPY affects neither basal nor NA-induced I release. The coexistence of NPY and NA in intrathyroid perivascular nerve fibres suggests that NPY might be important for the regulation of local blood flow. In fact, studies on peripheral blood vessels in vitro have indicated that NPY may evoke vasoconstriction and that the NA-induced vasoconstriction elicted by electrical stimulation of sympathetic fibres is markedly enhanced by NPY(80,81,83). A subpopulation of the NPY-immunoreactive fibres in the thyroid gland lacks DBH and contains VIP instead(68)(Fig 3a-d). The coexistence of NPY and VIP in non-adrenergic nerve fibres is interesting in view of the fact that NPY enhances VIP-induced thyroid hormone secretion(27).

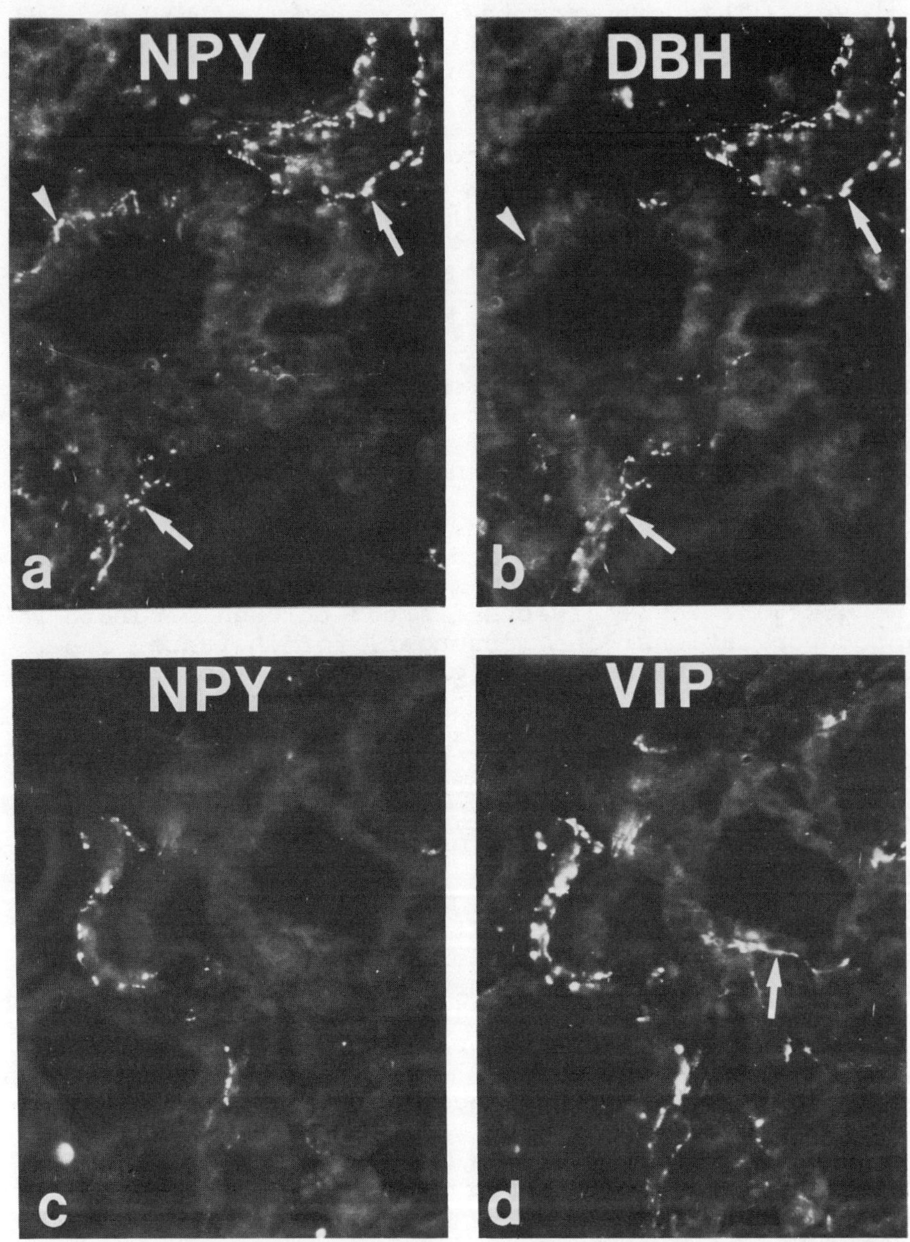

Fig 3 a and b. Simultaneous double immunostaining of the rat thyroid for NPY (a) and DBH (b) reveals coexistence of NPY and DBH in a population of nerve fibres (arrows). One NPY-immunoreactive fibre lacks DBH (arrowhead). c and d. Simultaneous double immunostaining for NPY (c) and VIP (d) in the rat thyroid gland. A few scattered NPYimmunofluorescent fibres contain VIP. Additional VIP-immunofluorescent fibres lack NPY (arrows).

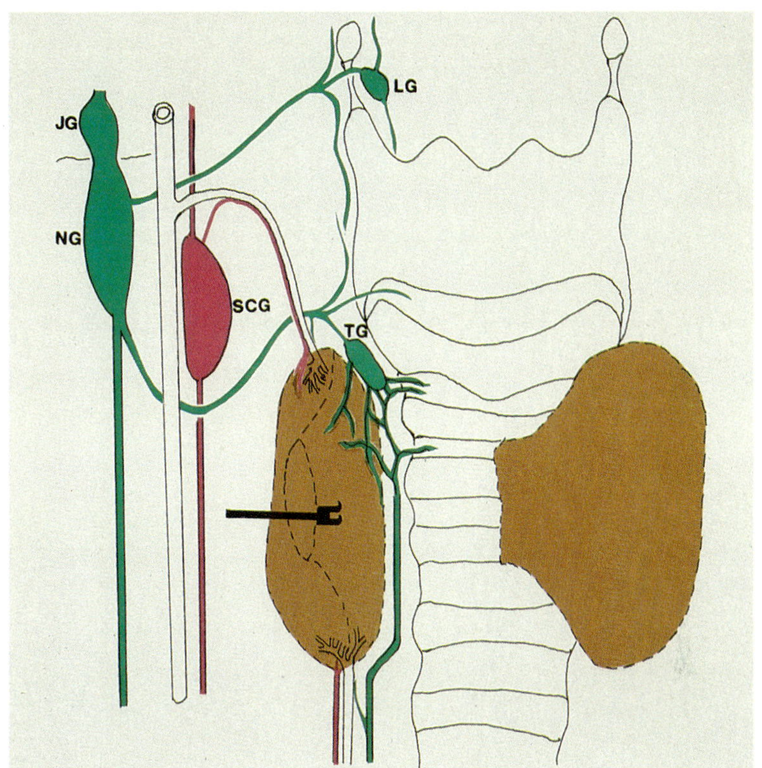

Fig 4. Front view of the thyroid-larynx region in the rat. The thyroid isthmus is cut and the right lobe is mobilized. The superior cervical ganglion (SCG) and its branches to the thyroid (carried by the thyroid arteries) are indicated in red and the vagal jugular (JG) and nodose (NG) ganglia with branches to the thyroid in green. The thyroid ganglion (TG) is located in the nerve plexus close to the thyroid gland and the laryngeal ganglion (LG) in the upper part of the larynx.

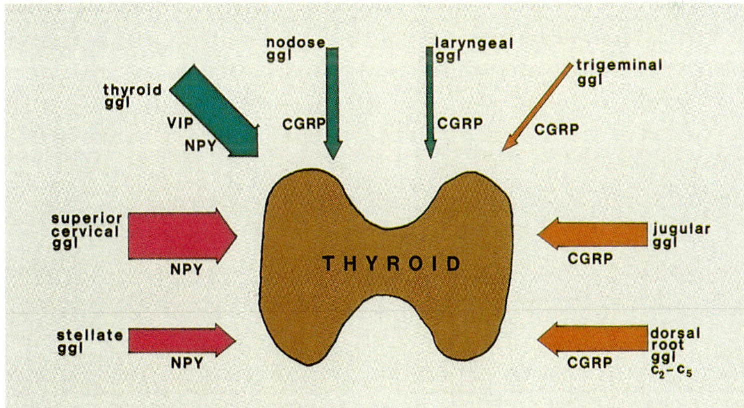

Fig 7. The various ganglia that supply the thyroid gland are provisionally classified as sympathetic = red, parasympathetic = green and sensory = yellow. The chemical coding of the neurones in these ganglia is summarized in Tables 3 and 4. The scheme illustrates the contributions made by NPY-, VIP- and CGRP-containing neurones in the different ganglia to the thyroid innervation. The magnitude of each contribution (assessed from the number of neurones labelled with True Blue) is reflected in the thickness of the arrows.

SP and CGRP are known to coexist in a population of primary sensory neurones of the C (unmyelinated) type (84-87). CGRP occurs together with SP in numerous thyroid nerve fibres, presumably of sensory nature(66). However, many CGRP-containing fibres lack SP while only a few SP-containing fibres are devoid of CGRP. A minor population of SP/CGRP-containing thyroid nerve fibres harbours also GAL(67). The major population of GAL-containing fibres harbours SP/CGRP. A subpopulation of GAL-containing fibres stores VIP instead of SP and CGRP(67). GAL, SP and CGRP have no effect on basal and TSH-induced ^{125}I release(66,67).

NEURONAL PATHWAYS TO THE RAT THYROID GLAND

Little information was available concerning neuronal pathways to the thyroid and the ganglia that project to the thyroid gland. We therefore found it of interest to examine the origin of the thyroid innervation in rats and to study the contributions made by different ganglia in order to better understand the nervous influence on thyroid blood flow and follicle cell activity. Neuronal pathways to the rat thyroid gland were identified by immunocytochemistry (using the many different neuropeptides as markers) in combination with 1. serial sectioning of the thyroid-larynx region, 2. selective denervations of the thyroid or 3. retrograde tracing of thyroid nerve fibres.

Microanatomy of nervous pathways

Serial sectioning of the entire thyroid-larynx region enables examination of nerve trunks and their projections to the thyroid and larynx(61,66)(Fig 4). The superior laryngeal nerve (henceforth referred to as the thyroid nerve) passes close to the upper pole of the thyroid gland and harbours a ganglionic formation, the thyroid ganglion, located just outside the thyroid capsule at the dorsomedial aspect of the gland(61,66) (Fig 4). From this ganglion nerve fibers penetrate the capsule in nerve bundles with or without association with blood vessels. Thus, this ganglion seems to contribute greatly to the thyroid innervation in the rat. Higher mammals seem to lack such a ganglion. Instead, nerve cell bodies have been described within the thyroid parenchyma of dogs and calves(13,27)(Fig 1d). The vagal branch from the middle part of the nodose ganglion innervates the upper larynx. This branch harbours the laryngeal ganglion, which is located slightly medially and cranially to the lateral wing of the thyroid cartilage at the dorsal aspect of the larynx close to the paraesophageal space(61,66)(Fig 4). The laryngeal ganglion has been observed in the human larynx(88). Small clusters of nerve cell bodies occur along vagal branches within the larynx(23).

Denervations

The origin and distribution of the various nerve fibre populations were studied following sympathectomy, cervical vagotomy and local denervation(23,27,68) and the results are summarized in Table 2.

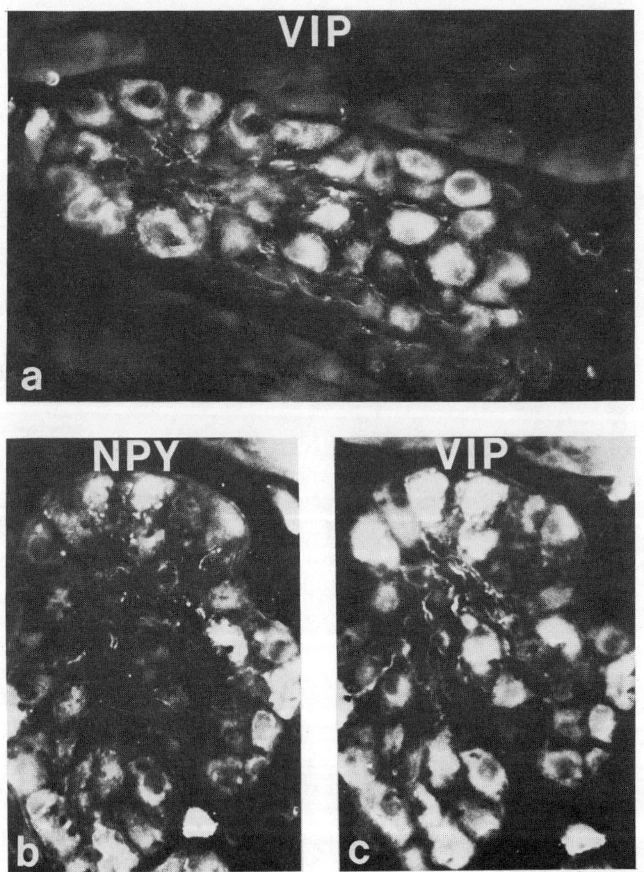

Fig. 5. Thyroid ganglion in the rat. Longitudinal (a) and cross (b and c) sections of the ganglion showing numerous VIP-immunoreactive nerve cell bodies and nerve fibres (a and c). Sequential double immunostaining for NPY (b) and for VIP (c). All NPY-immunoreactive cell bodies contain VIP and additional cell contain VIP alone. Some NPY-immunoreactive fibres (b) and numerous VIP-immunofluorescent fibres (c) are seen among the cell bodies.

<u>Cervical sympathectomy</u>, i.e. removal of the superior cervical ganglia, rich in NA- and NPY-containing cell bodies, eliminates all NA-containing nerve fibres in the thyroid gland(24,27,32). Following sympathectomy the majority of the NPY-containing nerve fibres in the thyroid gland disappears, suggesting that these fibres emanate from or pass through the superior cervical ganglion. The remaining NPY-containing nerve fibres, located close to follicles and occasionally around blood vessels, do not contain NA(68). VIP-, SP-, CGRP- and GAL- immunoreactive fibres in the thyroid gland are unaffected by surgical sympathectomy.

<u>Cervical vagotomy</u> is performed by removal of the right nodose ganglion including the vagal branches to the larynx-thyroid region and approx. 4 mm of the vagal trunk(23,66). Bilateral extirpation of the nodose ganglion is not possible because of the subsequent respiratory insufficiency. Unilateral vagotomy eliminates approx. 50% of the SP-, CGRP- and GAL-containing fibres in the ipsilateral (but not the contralateral) thyroid lobe(66,67). The number of NPY- and VIP-containing fibers in the thyroid gland is not overtly affected(68).

<u>Local denervation</u> is achieved by unilateral removal of the superior laryngeal nerve (thyroid nerve) including the thyroid ganglion(23,68). The thyroid ganglion is rich in VIP-containing nerve cell bodies (Fig 5). The majority of them harbours also NPY(68). As could be expected, local denervation eliminates most of the NPY- and VIP-containing nerve fibres in the ipsilateral thyroid lobe. In addition, it causes the disappearance of all GAL- and SP- containing fibres and reduces the number of NA- and CGRP-containing fibres(68). The elimination and reduction of nerve fibres other than those containing NPY and VIP probably reflect the effect of the operation on nerve fibres that pass through or close to the thyroid ganglion.

Table 2. The relative frequency of NA-containing nerve fibres (DBH as marker) and of nerve fibres containing various peptides in intact, sympathectomized, vagotomized or locally denervated rat thyroid.

Types of denervation	Relative frequency of nerve fibres containing NA	NPY	VIP	GAL	SP	CGRP
Control	+++	++	+++	+	++	++
Sympathectomy	0	+	+++	+	++	++
Vagotomy	+++	++	+++	(+)	+	+
Local denervation	+	+	+	0	0	+

The relative frequency of nerve fibres was graded arbitrarily: 0, no fibres; (+), rare; +, few; ++, moderate in number; +++, numerous.

Tracing of neuronal pathways

Another way of identifying neuronal pathways is by anterograde and retrograde tracing. In principle, retrograde tracing in combination with immunocytochemistry makes it possible to define the origin and identity of all nerve fibres in a tissue(89,90). We have used a fluorescent marker, True Blue (TB), for retrograde tracing of thyroid nerve fibres(23). The results support the view that the thyroid gland receives innervation from several ganglia.

Injection of TB into one thyroid lobe labelled neurones in the ispsilateral superior cervical ganglion, the stellate ganglion, the thyroid ganglion, the laryngeal ganglion the jugular-nodose ganglionic complex, the cervical dorsal root ganglia and the trigeminal ganglion. TB-labelled nerve cell bodies were numerous in the superior cervical ganglion and the thyroid ganglion, suggesting that these two ganglia contribute greatly to the thyroid innervation. A moderate number of labelled cell bodies was seen in the stellate ganglion, the jugular-nodose ganglionic complex and the cervical dorsal root ganglia at the level C_2- C_5, whereas such cell bodies were few in the trigeminal and laryngeal ganglia. The major contribution is ipsilateral, but there are also minor contributions from the contralateral superior cervical ganglion, stellate ganglion, thyroid ganglion and dorsal root ganglia at the level C_2- C_3.

By combining retrograde tracing and immunocytochemistry we examined the TB-labelled nerve cell bodies in the various ganglia for NPY, VIP and CGRP(23)(Fig 6,7). The results support the view that NPY-immunoreactive fibres in the thyroid are of two types; one (adrenergic) emanates from the superior cervical and stellate ganglia and the other (non-adrenergic) from the thyroid gangli on. The VIP-immunoreactive fibres seem to derive from the thyroid ganglion(68). The CGRP-immunoreactive fibres in the thyroid gland emanate mainly from the jugular and dorsal root ganglia (C_2- C_5). Additional CGRP-containing fibres may derive from the nodose, laryngeal and/or trigeminal ganglia(23). The majority of the CGRP-containing fibres reaches the thyroid gland from behind and enters the lobe from its medial aspect. Most of them seem to pass through the thyroid ganglion on their way to the thyroid. Hence, it appears conceivable that the neuronal activity of the thyroid ganglion is affected by the vagus. Sympathetic (NA-containing) nerve fibres run just outside the ganglion.

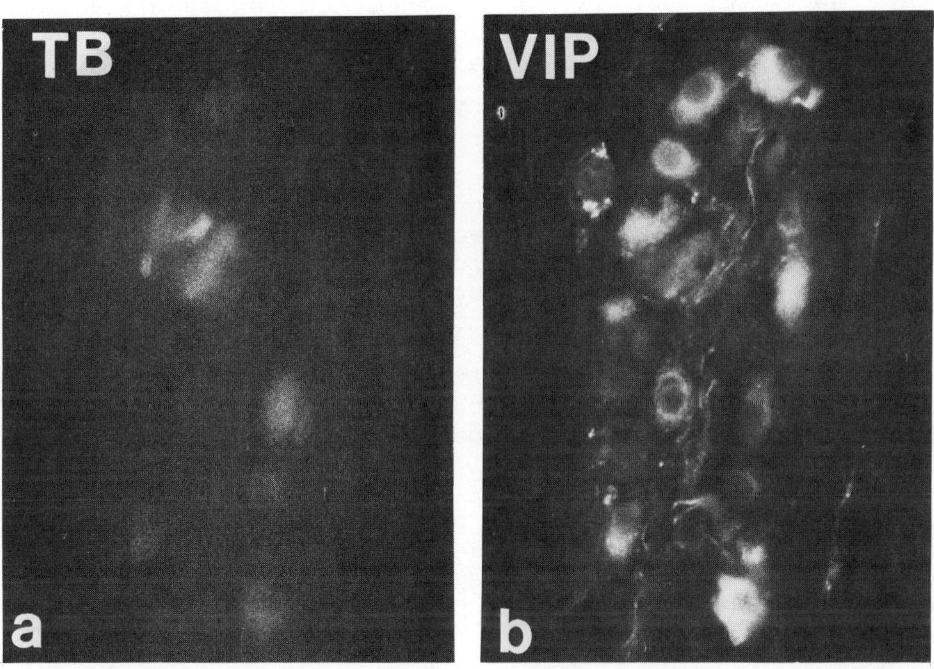

Fig 6. Thyroid ganglion. Concomitant vizualization of True Blue (TB) (a) and VIP (b). VIP- containing nerve cell bodies are numerous; TB-labelled cell bodies fewer. All TB-labelled cell bodies are immunostained for VIP.

Fig 7. See color plate facing page 128.

CHEMICAL CODING OF NEURONES PROJECTING TO RAT THYROID

The results are summarized in Tables 3 and 4. The superior cervical and stellate ganglia harbour numerous NA/NPY- and NA-containing neurones, some of which project to the thyroid gland. Activation of adrenergic neurones is known to evoke thyroid hormone secretion and to reduce thyroid blood flow(24,30). Conceivably therefore, these ganglia are involved in the sympathetic control of thyroid activity.

The jugular-nodose ganglionic complex is a mixed sensory and parasympathetic ganglion(91). There is a marked difference in peptide content between the jugular and the nodose ganglia. The jugular (sensory) portion contains GAL-, SP- and CGRP-immunoreactive cell bodies (Fig 8), some of which project to the thyroid, whereas neurones in the nodose (parasympathetic) portion harbour mainly GAL and VIP; these neurones do not seem to project to the thyroid(23). However, a few, scattered nerve cell bodies storing CGRP occur also in the nodose ganglion and some of them project to the thyroid gland. The two ganglia differ in their projections in that the nodose ganglion innervates viscera in the thorax and abdomen, while the jugular ganglion supplies the pharynx, larynx and thyroid(92). In the thyroid, GAL, SP and CGRP coexist in a population of nerve fibres around blood vessels and follicles. In view of the known coexistence of these peptides in sensory neurones elsewhere(87,93), it is tempting to speculate that GAL, SP and CGRP occur in sensory fibres also in the thyroid and that they cooperate. CGRP, like SP, is a potent vasodilator(94). CGRP enhances VIP-stimulated ^{125}I release, an effect which may reflect an action on the blood flow.

The thyroid ganglion contributes significantly to the thyroid innervation. Thus, all VIP and NPY/VIP-containing nerve fibres in the rat thyroid seem to emanate from the thyroid ganglion(68)(Fig 5). Scattered and clustered VIP-containing nerve cell bodies occur in the superior laryngeal nerve just proximally to the thyroid ganglion(68). Both VIP and PHI stimulate thyroid hormone secretion in mice, VIP being more potent than PHI(61). Direct application of VIP to the rat thyroid evokes vasodilation and increased thyroid blood flow but does not result in elevated levels of circulating thyroid hormone levels(95,96).

The laryngeal ganglion harbours numerous VIP-containing nerve cell bodies, most of which contain NPY(23).

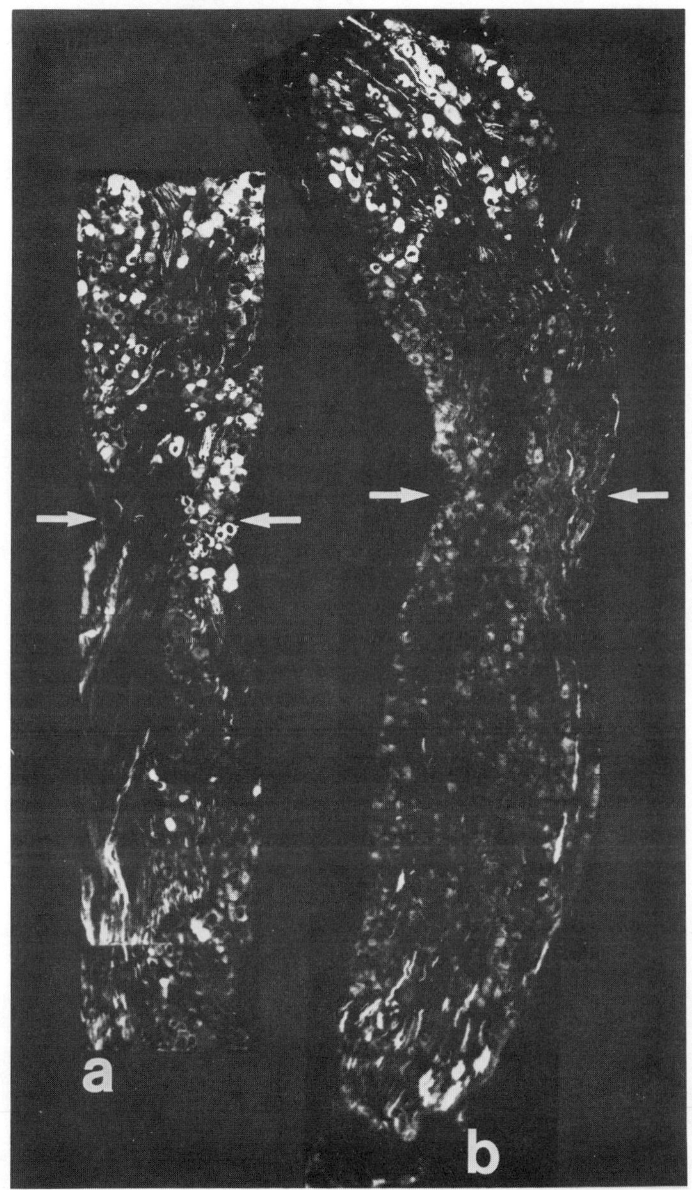

Fig 8. The jugular-nodose ganglionic complex in the mouse (a) and rat (b). Numerous CGRP- immunoreactive nerve cell bodies are seen in the jugular portion (above the arrows) whereas the nodose portion (below arrows) contains only few. Immunoreactive nerve fibres are numerous within both ganglia.

Table 3. The relative frequency of NA- and peptide-containing nerve fibres in the rat thyroid and of NA- and peptide-containing nerve cell bodies in the ganglia that project to the thyroid.

Neuronal markers	Nerve fibres in thyroid gland	Nerve cell bodies in: Superior cervical ganglion	Stellate ganglion	Thyroid ganglion	Nodose ganglion	Laryngeal ganglion	Jugular ganglion	Dorsal root ganglion	Trigeminal ganglion
NA	+++	+++	+++	0	0	0	0	0	0
NPY	++	+++	+++	++	0	++	0	0	0
VIP	+++	0*	+	+++	+++	+++	0*	0	0
GAL	+	0	0	+	+++	+	+	+	+
SP	++	0	0	0	+	+	++	++	++
CGRP	++	0	0	0	+	+	+++	+++	+++

The relative frequency was graded arbitrarily: 0, no fibres or cell bodies; +, few; ++, moderate in number; +++, numerous. * indicates occasional occurrence of VIP-containing cell bodies.

Table 4. Estimated frequency of different subpopulations of nerve fibres in the rat thyroid and of nerve cell bodies in the ganglia that project to the thyroid.

Chemical coding	Nerve fibres in thyroid gland	Nerve cell bodies in: Superior cervical ganglion	Stellate ganglion	Thyroid ganglion	Nodose ganglion	Laryngeal ganglion	Jugular ganglion	Dorsal root ganglion	Trigeminal ganglion
NA	+	+	+	0	0	0	0	0	0
NPY/NA	++	+++	+++	0	0	0	0	0	0
NPY/VIP	+	0	0	++	0	++	0	0	0
VIP	++	0*	+	++	+	+	0*	0	0
GAL/VIP	(+)	0	0	+	+++	++	0	0	0
GAL	0	0	0	0	+	+	+	+	+
SP	+	0	0	0	+	+	+	+	+
CGRP	+	0	0	0	+	+	++	++	++
SP/CGRP	++	0	0	0	+	+	++	++	++
GAL/SP/CGRP	+	0	0	0	0	0	+	+	+

The relative frequency was graded arbitrarily : 0, no fibres or cell bodies; (+), very few; +, few; ++, moderate in number; +++, numerous. * indicates occasional occurrence of VIP-containing cell bodies.

Nerve cell bodies storing CGRP are few and scattered and some of them project to the thyroid gland(23).

The dorsal root ganglia and the trigeminal ganglion are thought to be purely sensory. The cervical dorsal root ganglia (C_2- C_7) innervate structures of the neck, while the trigeminal ganglion supplies structures of the head. Both ganglia are rich in GAL-, SP-, NKA- and CGRP-immunoreactive cell bodies(23). Retrograde tracing in combination with immunocytochemistry showed CGRP-containing neurones in the two ganglia to project to the thyroid(23). The functional role of the prominent sensory innervation of the thyroid is unclear.

C CELL HORMONES

It cannot be ruled out that the control of thyroid activity involves not only TSH and neuronal stimuli but also peptides manufactured, stored and released by the C cells. The close spatial relationship between C cells and follicle cells in the mammalian thyroid has stimulated speculations about a possible interaction between these two cell systems(97). So far, there is no satisfactory explanation for the fact that these two cell types, which have different embryological origin, occur together. Besides CT, the thyroid C cells produce CGRP, and in some species also somatostatin and gastrin releasing peptide(66,98,99). Recently, helodermin-like immunoreactivity was demonstrated in thyroid C cells in several species and in the C cell homologues of the chicken ultimobranchial gland(100)(Fig 9). In addition, there is immunocytochemical evidence for the production of helodermin-like peptides in cells in medullary thyroid carcinomas and in C cell adenomas. The helodermin-like material was found to coexist with CT in normal and neoplastic C cells(100,101)(Fig 9). Thus, the C cells seem capable of producing many regulatory peptides arising from different precursors.

Helodermin, originally isolated from the salivary gland venom of the lizard Heloderma suspectum, displays sequence homologies with peptides of the secretin family and exerts VIP-like actions in several biological systems(102,103). Like VIP, helodermin induces colloid droplet formation and stimulates basal thyroid hormone release in mice(100)(Fig 10,11) and is also a potent vasodilator(104). However, the thyroid response to helodermin is more long-lasting and powerful than that to VIP (Fig 11). Unlike VIP, helodermin does not potentiate

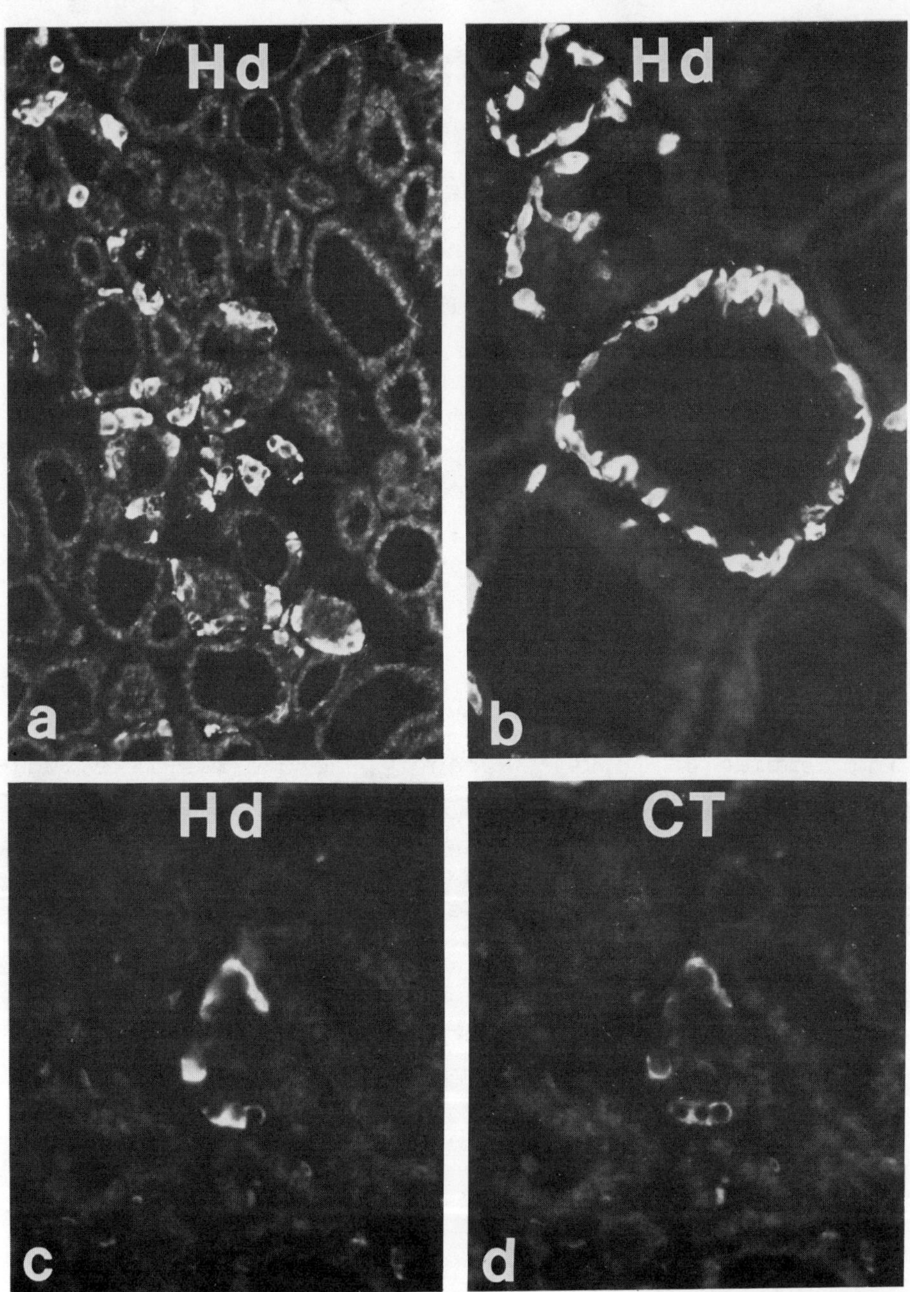

Fig 9. Helodermin-like immunofluorescence in the parafollicular cells in the thyroid of rat (a) and pig (b). Simultaneous double immunostaining for helodermin (Hd)(c) and CT (d) in parafollicular cells of the rat. Note that the same parafollicular cells are stained for both Hd and CT.

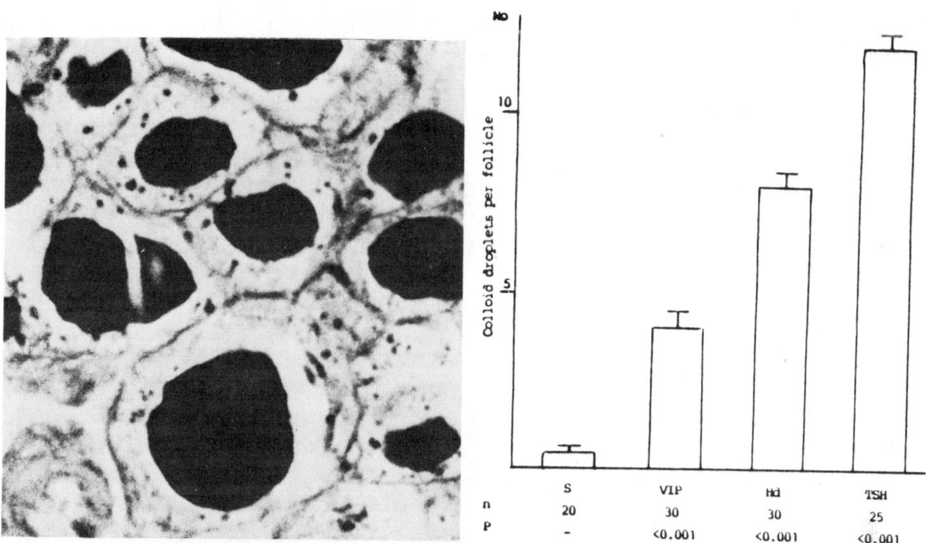

Fig 10. a. Mouse thyroid stained by periodic acid-Schiff (PAS) technique. The colloid in the lumen and numerous colloid droplets in the follicle cells are stained. b. Colloid droplets in thyroid follicle cells in mouse 30 min after an i.v. injection of saline (S), VIP (1.5 nmol), helodermin (Hd)(0.375 nmol) or TSH (70 uU). Values are the mean ± s.e.m.. n = number of follicles counted. P = Probability level of random difference.

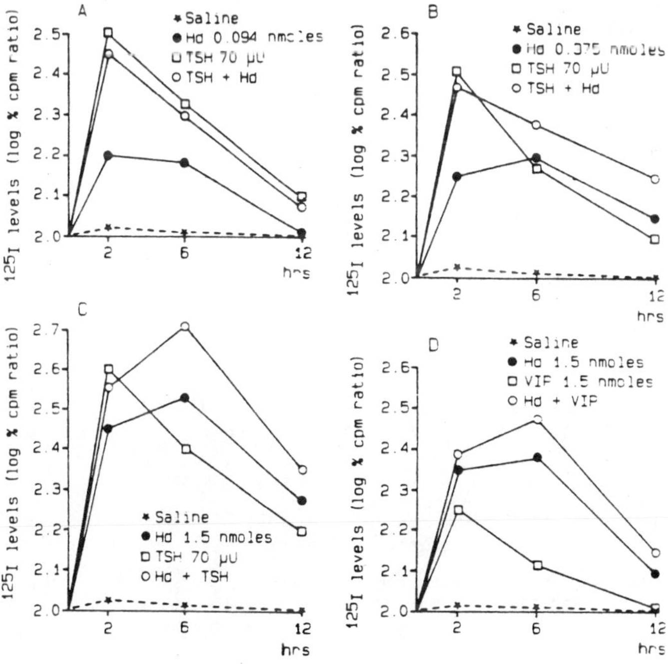

Fig 11. Thyroid hormone (radioiodine) release in the mouse 2, 6 and 12 hrs after an i.v. injection of helodermin (Hd) (dose range 0.094 - 1.5 nmol) alone or together with TSH (70 uU) and VIP (1.5 nmol). Hd stimulates ^{125}I-release but has no effect on TSH- and VIP-induced ^{125}I-release. Hd has a more long-lasting effect than VIP.

TSH-induced thyroid hormone release. Nonetheless, the structural similarity between VIP and helodermin suggests that the two peptides act on the same receptor. Like the response to VIP, that to helodermin is unaffected by α- and β-adrenoceptor blockade(105). Although CT and CGRP are without effect on thyroid hormone secretion(66), it can not be excluded that C cell peptides, such as helodermin-like peptides, are involved in the regulation of thyroid activity and blood flow.

CONCLUSION

The thyroid gland is richly innervated and the activity of the thyroid may be influenced by many ganglia of sympathetic, parasympathetic and sensory nature. The characteristic chemical coding of the neurones that project to the thyroid gland suggests important and diverse roles for neuropeptides as mediators in the regulation of thyroid functions. Direct evidence for such roles is still lacking. In addition to the influence exerted by TSH and by the autonomic nervous system it cannot be excluded that C cells exert a paracrine function and that C cell hormones act as local modulators of follicle cell activity and/or blood flow.

ACKNOWLEDGEMENTS

Grant support from the Swedish Medical Research Council (projects no 6859, 4499 and 1007) and from the Swedish Society of Medicine.

REFERENCES

1. J. D. Boyd, Development of the human thyroid gland, in: "The Thyroid Gland, Vol 1", R. Pitt-Rivers and W. R. Trotter, eds., Butterworths, London (1964).
2. R. Ekholm, Thyroid physiology: Anatomy and development, in: "Endocrinology, Vol 1", L. J. DeGroot, ed., Grune & Stratton, New York (1979).
3. N. Le Douarin, "The Neural Crest". Cambridge University Press, Cambridge (1982).
4. J. M. Polak, A. G. E. Pearse, C. Le Liévre, J. Fontaine, and N. Le Douarin, Immunocytochemical confirmation of the neuronal crest origin of avian calcitonin-producing cells, Histochemistry 40:209 (1974).

5. N. Le Douarin, J. Fontaine, and C. Le Lievre, New studies on the neural crest origin of the avian ultimobranchial glandular cells - Interspecific combinations and cytochemical characterization of C cells based on the uptake of biogenic amine precursors, Histochemistry 38:297 (1974).
6. A. G. E. Pearse, and A. F. Carvalheira, Cytochemical evidence for an ultimobranchial origin of rodent thyroid C cells, Nature 214:929 (1967).
7. A. G. E. Pearse, and J. M. Polak, Cytochemical evidence for the neural crest origin of mammalian ultimobranchial C cells, Histochemie 27:96 (1971).
8. A. G. E. Pearse, The diffuse neuroendocrine system: Falsification and verification of a concept, in: "Cellular Basis of Chemical Messengers in the Digestive System", M. I. Grossman, M. A. B. Brazier and J. Lechago, eds., Academic Press, New York (1981).
9. L. J. DeGroot, and H. Niepomniszcze, Biosynthesis of thyroid hormone: Basic and clinical aspects, Metabolism 26:665 (1977).
10. A. D. Care, and R. F. L. Bates, The secretion of parathyroid hormone and calcitonin, Hormones 1:364 (1970).
11. D. H. Copp, Endocrine regulation of calcium metabolism, Ann Rev Physiol 32:61 (1970).
12. W. J. Cunliffe, The innervation of the thyroid gland, Acta Anat 46:135 (1961).
13. J. F. Nonidez, Innervation of the thyroid gland. I. The presence of ganglia in the thyroid of the dog, Arch Neurol Phychiat (Chicago) 25:1175 (1931).
14. J. F. Nonidez, Innervation of the thyroid gland. III. Distribution and termination of the nerve fibers in the dog, Am J Anat 57:135 (1935).
15. S. L. Wissig, Morphology and cytology, in: "The Thyroid Gland, Vol 1", R. Pitt-Rivers and W. R. Trotter, eds., Butterworths, London (1964).
16. H. Fujita, Fine structure of the thyroid follicle, in: "Ultrastructure of Endocrine Cells and Tissues", P. M. Motta, ed., Martinus Nijhoff Publ, Boston (1984).
17. R. Ekholm, and L. E. Ericson, The ultrastructure of the parafollicular cells of the thyroid gland in the rat, J Ultrastruct Res 23:378 (1968).
18. L. E. Ericson, and F. Sundler, Thyroid parafollicular cells: Ultrastructural and functional correlations, in: "Ultrastrucure of Endocrine Cells and Tissues", P. M. Motta, ed., Martinus Nijhoff Publ, Boston (1984).

19. S. Reichlin, Regulation of pituitary thyrotropin release, in: "Thyrotropin", S. C. Werner, ed., Thomas, Springfield, Illinois (1963).
20. L. E. Ericson, and B. R. Johansson, Early effects of thyroid stimulating hormone (TSH) on exocytosis and endocytosis in the thyroid, Acta Endocrinol (Copenh) 86:112 (1977).
21. J. E. Dumont, and G. Vassart, Thyroid gland metabolism and the action of TSH, in: "Endocrinology, Vol 1", L. J. DeGroot, ed., Grune & Stratton, New York. 1979,
22. S. T. Green, Intrathyroidal autonomic nerves can directly influence hormone release from rat thyroid follicles: a study in vitro employing electrical field stimulation and intracellular microelectrodes, Cli Sci 72:233 (1987).
23. T. Grunditz, R. Håkanson, F. Sundler, and R. Uddman, Neuronal pathways to the rat thyroid gland revealed by retrograde tracing and immunocytochemistry, Neuroscience 24:321 (1988).
24. A. Melander, L. E. Ericsson, F. Sundler, and U. Westgren, Intrathyroidal amines in the regulation of thyroid activity, Rev Physiol Biochem Pharmacol 73:39 (1975).
25. A. Melander, and F. Sundler, Prescence and influence of cholinergic nerves in the mouse thyroid, Endocrinology 105:7 (1979).
26. A. Melander, F. Sundler, and U. Westgren, Sympathetic innervation of the thyroid: Variation with species and with age, Endocrinology 96:102 (1975).
27. T. Grunditz, R. Håkanson, C. Rerup, F. Sundler, and R. Uddman, Neuropeptide Y in the thyroid gland: Neuronal localization and enhancement of stimulated thyroid hormone secretion, Endocrinology 115:1537 (1984).
28. J. F. Nonidez, Innervation of the thyroid gland. II. Origin and course of the thyroid nerves in the dog, Am J Anat 48:299 (1931).
29. H. Holmgren, and B. Naumann, A study of the nerves of the thyroid gland and their relationship to glandular function, Acta Endocrinol (Copenh) 3:215 (1949).
30. U. Söderberg, Short term reactions in the thyroid gland, Acta Physiol Scand, Suppl 147, 42 (1958).
31. Y. Mikhail, Intrinsic nerve supply of the thyroid and parathyroid glands, Acta Anat (Basel) 80:152 (1971).
32. H. E. Romeo, C. Gonzales-Solveyra, M. I. Vacas, R. E. Rosenstein, M. Barontini, and D. P. Cardina-

li, Origins of the sympathetic projections to the rat thyroid and parathyroid glands, J Auton Nerv Syst 17:63 (1986).

33. M. L. Maayan, A. F. Debons, E. M. Volpert, and I. Krimsky, Catecholamine inhibition of thyrotrophin-induced secretion of thyroxine: Mediation by an α-adrenergic receptor, Metabolism 26:473 (1977).
34. T. Muraki, H. Uzumaki, T. Nakadate, and R. Kato, Involvement of α_1-adrenergic receptors in the inhibitory effect of catecholamines on the thyrotropin-induced release of thyroxine by the mouse thyroid, Endocrinology 110:51 (1982).
35. H. E. Romeo, R. J. Boado, and D. P. Cardinali, Role of the sympathetic nervous system in the control of thyroid growth of normal and hypophysectomized rats, Neuroendocrinology 40:309 (1985).
36. H. H. Dale, Nomenclature of fibers in the autonomic system and their effects, J Physiol (Lond) 80:10, (1933).
37. F. Amenta, D. Caporuscio, F. Ferrante, F. Porcelli, and Zomparelli, M., Cholinergic nerves in the thyroid gland, Cell Tissue Res 195:367 (1978).
38. A. Silver, Do cholinesterases have a function other than in transmission? in: "The biology of cholinesterases", A. Silver, ed., North-Holland Publ., Amsterdam (1974).
39. N. Cauna, and N. T. Naik, The distribution of cholinesterases in the sensory ganglia of man and of some mammals, J Histochem Cytochem 11:129, (1963).
40. O. Eränkö, and M. Härkönen, Noradrenaline and acetylesterase in sympathetic ganglion cells in the rat, Acta Physiol Scand 61:299 (1964).
41. J. Ishii, K. Shizume, and S. Okinaka, Effect of stimulation of the vagus nerve on the thyroidal release of ^{131}I-labeled hormones, Endocrinology 82:7 (1968).
42. J. Van Sande, C. Erneux, and J. Dumont, Negative control of TSH action by iodide and acetylcholine: mechanism of action in intact thyroid cells, J Cyclic Nucleotice Res 3:335 (1977).
43. J. Van Sande, J. E. Dumont, A. Melander, and F. Sundler, Presence and influence of cholinergic nerves in the human thyroid, J Clin Endocrinol Metab 51:500 (1980).
44. H. Ito, K. Matsuda, A. Sato, and H. Tohgi, Cholinergic and VIPergic vasodilator actions of parasympathetic nerves on the thyroid blood flow in rats, Jap J Physiol 37:1005 (1987).

45. F. Lemere, Innervation of the larynx. I. Innervation of laryngeal muscles, Am J Anat 51:417 (1932).
46. H. E. Romeo, M. C. Diaz, J. Ceppi, A. Zaninovich, and D. P. Cardinali, Effect of inferior laryngeal nerve section on thyroid function in rats, Endocrinology 122:2527 (1988).
47. T. Hökfelt, O. Johansson, Å. Ljungdahl, J. M. Lundberg, and M. Schultzberg, Peptidergic neurones, Nature 284:515 (1980).
48. J. M. Lundberg, and T. Hökfelt, Coexistence of peptides and classical neurotransmitters, Trends Neurosci 6:325 (1983).
49. F. Sundler, E. Ekblad, G. Böttcher, J. Alumets, and R. Håkanson, Coexistence of peptides in the neuroendocrine system, in: "Biogenetics of neurohormonal peptides", R. Håkanson and J. Thorell, eds., Academic press, London (1985).
50. A. H. Coons, E. H. Leduc, and J. M. Connolly, Studies on antibody production. I. A method for the histochemical demonstration of specific antibody and its application to a study of the hyperimmune rabbit, J Exp Med 102:49 (1955).
51. L. A. Sternberger, "Immunocytochemistry", 2nd edn., Wiley, New York, (1979).
52. L- I. Larsson, Ultrastructural localization of a new neuronal peptide (VIP), Histochemistry 54:173 (1977).
53. F. Sundler, R. Håkanson, and S. Leander, Peptidergic nervous systems in the gut, Clin Gastoenterol 9:517 (1980).
54. R. Håkanson, S. Leander, F. Sundler, and R. Uddman, P-type nerves Purinergic or peptidergic? in: "Cellular Basis of Chemical Messengers in the Digestive System, " M. I. Grossman, M. A. B. Brazier and J. Lechago, eds., Academic Press, New York (1981).
55. L. Probert, J. De Mey, and J. M. Polak, Ultrastructural localization of four different neuropeptides within separate populations of p-type nerves in the guinea pig colon, Gastroenterology 85:1094 (1983).
56. S. Gulbenkian, A. Merighi, J. Warthon, I. Varndell, and J. M. Polak, Ultrastructure evidence for the coexistence of calcitonin gene-related peptide and substance P in secretory vesicles of peripheral nerves in the guinea pig, J Neurocytol 15:535 (1986).
57. A. Merighi, J. M. Polak, S. J. Gibson, S. Gulbenkian, K. L. Valentino, and S. M. Peirone, Ultrast-

ructural studies on calcitonin gene-related peptide-, tachykinins- and somatostatin-immunoreactive neurones in rat dorsal root ganglia: Evidence for the colocalization of different peptides in single secretory granules, Cell Tissue Res 254:101 (1988)

58. R. Håkanson, and F. Sundler, The role of peptide messengers in the neuroendocrine system: hormones, neurotransmitters or neuromodulators? in: Drug Receptors and Dynamic processes in Cells, J. S. Schou, A. Glister and S. Norn, eds., Munkgaard, Copenhagen (1986).

59. B. Ahrén, J. Alumets, M. Ericsson, J. Fahrenkrug, L. Fahrenkrug, R. Håkanson, P. Hedner, I. Lorén, A. Melander, C. Rerup, and F. Sundler, VIP occurs in intrathyroidal nerves and stimulates thyroid hormone secretion, Nature 287:343 (1980).

60. G. A. Hedge, L. J. Huffman, T. Grunditz, and F. Sundler, Immunocytochemical studies of the peptidergic innervation of thyroid gland in the Brattleboro rat, Endocrinology 115:2071 (1984).

61. T. Grunditz, R. Håkanson, G. Hedge, C. Rerup, F. Sundler, and R. Uddman, Peptide histidine isoleucine amide stimulates thyroid hormone secretion and coexists with vasoactive intestinal polypeptide in intrathyroid nerve fibers from laryngeal ganglia, Endocrinology 118:783 (1986).

62. S. T. Green, J. Singh, and O. H. Petersèn, Control of cyclic nucleotide metabolism by non-cholinergic, non-adrenergic nerves in rat thyroid gland, Nature 296:751 (1982).

63. R. S. Toccafondi, M. L. Brandi, and A. Melander, Vasoactive intestinal peptide stimulation of human thyroid cell function, J Clin Endocrinol & Metab 58:157 (1984).

64. B. Ahrén, R. Håkanson, and C. Rerup, VIP-stimulated thyroid hormone secretion: Effects of other neuropeptides and α- or β-adrenoceptor blockade, Acta Physiol Scand 114:471 (1982).

65. M. L. Brandi, A. Tanini, and R. Toccafondi, Interaction of VIPergic and cholinergic receptors in human thyroid cell, Peptides 8:893 (1987).

66. T. Grunditz, R. Ekman, R. Håkanson, C. Rerup, F. Sundler, F. and Uddman, R., Calcitonin gene-related peptide in thyroid nerve fibers and C cells. Effects on thyroid hormone secretion and response to hypercalcemia, Endocrinology 119:2313 (1986).

67. T. Grunditz, R. Håkanson, F. Sundler, and R. Udd-

man, Neurokinin and galanin in the thyroid gland: Neuronal localization, Endocrinology 121:575 (1987).

68. T. Grunditz, R. Ekman, R. Håkanson, F, Sundler, and R. Uddman, Neuropeptide Y and vasoactive intestinal peptide coexist in rat thyroid nerve fibers emanating from the thyroid ganglion, Regul Pept 23:193 (1988).

69. B. Ahrén, T. Grunditz, R. Ekman, R. Håkanson, F. Sundler, F. and Uddman, R., Neuropeptides in the thyroid gland: Distribution of substance P and gastrin/cholecystokinin and their effects on the secretion of iodothyronine and calcitonin, Endocrinology 113:379 (1983).

70. F. Sundler, and R. Håkanson, Peptide hormone-producing endocrine/paracrine cells in the gastroentero-pancreatic region, in: "Handbook of Chemical Neuroanatomy. Vol 6: The peripheral Nervous System", A. Björklund, T. Hökfelt and C. Owman, eds., Elsevier Sci. Publ., Amsterdam (1988).

71. G. Tramu, A. Pillez, and J. Leonardelli, An efficient method of antibody elution for the successive or simultaneous localiation of two antigens by immunocytochemistry, J Histochem Cytochem 26:322 (1978).

72. J. B. Furness, M. Costa, and J. R. Keast, Choline acetyltransferase- and peptide immunoreactivity of submucous neurons in the small intestine of the guinea-pig, Cell Tissue Res 237:329 (1984).

73. N. Itoh, K. Obata, N. Yanaihara, and H. Okamoto, Human prepro-vasoactive intestinal polypeptide contains a novel PHI-27-like peptide, PHM-27, Nature 304:547 (1983).

74. H. Nawa, T. Hirose, H. Takashima, S. Inayama, and S. Nakanishi, Nucleotide sequences of cloned cDNAs for two types of bovine brain substance P precursor, Nature 306:32 (1983).

75. T. Hökfelt, V. Holets, W. Staines, B. Meister, T. Melander, M. Schalling, M. Schultzberg, J. Freedman, H. Björklund, L. Olson, B. Lindh, L-G. Elfvin, J. M. Lundberg, J. Å. Lindgren, B. Samuelsson, B. Pernow, L. Terenius, C. Post, B. Everitt, and M. Goldstein, Coexistence of neuronal messengers - an overview, in: Coexistence of Neuronal Messengers: A New Principle in Chemical Transmission, T. Hökfelt, K. Fuxe and B. Pernow, eds., Elsevier, Amsterdam (1986).

76. F. Sundler, E. Ekblad, T. Grunditz, R. Håkanson, A. Luts, and R. Uddman, NPY in peripheral non-adrenergic neurons, in: "Nobel Symposium XIV: Neuro-

peptide Y", V. Mutt, T. Hökfelt and K. Fuxe, eds., Raven Press, USA, in press (1989).

77. R. Håkanson, and F. Sundler, The design of the neuroendocrine system: a unifying concept and its consequences, Trends Pharmacol Sci 4:41 (1983).

78. T. Hökfelt, G. Fried, S. Hansen, V. Holets, J. M. Lundberg, and L. Skirboll, Neurons with multiple messengers - distribution and possible functional significance, Progr Brain Res, 65:115 (1986)

79. R. A. Rush, and L. B. Geffen, Dopamine-β-hydroxylase in health and disease, CRC Crit Rev Clin Lab Sci (1980).

80. L. Edvinsson, E. Ekblad, R. Håkanson, and C. Wahlestedt, Neuropeptide Y potentiates the effect of various vasoconstrictor agents on rabbit blood vessels, Br J Pharmacol 83:519 (1984).

81. E. Ekblad, L. Edvinsson, C. Wahlestedt, R. Uddman, R. Håkanson, and F. Sundler, Neuropeptide Y coexists and co-operates with noradrenaline in perivascular nerve fibers, Regul Pept 8:225 (1984)

82. F. Sundler, R. Håkanson, E. Ekblad, R. Uddman, and C. Wahlestedt, Neuropeptide Y in the peripheral adrenergic and enteric nervous systems, Int Rev Cytol 102:243 (1986).

83. C. Wahlestedt, L. Edvinsson, E. Ekblad, and R. Håkanson, Neuropeptide Y potentiates noradrenaline-evoked vasoconstriction: mode of action. J Pharm Exp Ther 234:735 (1985).

84. T. M. Jessell, L. L. Iversen, and A. C. Cuello, Capsaicin-induced depletion of substance P from primary sensory neurones, Brain Res 152:183 (1978).

85. R. Gamse, P. Holzer, and F. Lembeck, Decrease of substance P in primary afferent neurones and impairment of neurogenic plasma extravasation by capsaicin, Br J Pharmacol 68:207 (1980).

86. A. Saria, R. Gamse, J. M. Lundberg, T. Hökfelt, E. Thedorsson-Norheim, J. Petermann, and J. A. Fischer, Co-existence of tachykinins and calcitonin gene-related peptide in sensory nerves in relation to neurogenic inflammation, in: "Tachykinin Antagonists", Fernström Symp Series, R. Håkanson and F. Sundler, eds., Elsevier, Amsterdam (1985).

87. F. Sundler, E. Brodin, E. Ekblad, R. Håkanson, and R. Uddman, Sensory nerve fibers: Distribution of substance P, neurokinin A and calcitonin gene-related peptide, in: "Tachykinin Antagonists", Fernström Symp Series, R. Håkanson and F. Sundler, eds., Elsevier, Amsterdam (1985).

88. F. MÜller, R. O'Rahilly, and J. A. Tucker, The human larynx at the end of the embryonic period proper. I. The laryngeal and infrahyoid muscles and their innervation, Acta Otolaryngol (Stockh) 91:323 (1981).
89. P. E. Sawchenko, and L. W. Swanson, A method for tracing biochemically defined pathways in the central nervous system using combined fluorescence retrograde transport and immunohistochemical techniques, Brain Res 210:31 (1981).
90. G. Skagerberg, A. Björklund, and O. Lindvall, Further studies on the use of the fluorescent retrograde tracer True Blue in combination with monoamine histochemistry, J Neurosci Methods 14:25 (1985).
91. J. C. Helke, and K. M. Hill, Immunohistochemical study of neuropeptides in vagal and glossopharyngeal afferent neurons in the rat, Neurosci 26:539 (1988).
92. D. M. Katz, and H. J. Karten, Substance P in the vagal sensory ganglia: Localization in cell bodies and pericellular arborizations, J Comp Neurol 193:549 (1980).
93. G. Skofitsch, and D. M. Jabobowitz, Galanin-like immunoreactivity in capsaicin sensitive sensory neurons and ganglia, Brain Res Bull 15:191 (1985).
94. S. D. Brain, T. J. Williams, J. R. Tippins, H. R. Morris, and I. MacIntyre, Calcitonin gene-related peptide is a potent vasodilator, Nature 313:54 (1985).
95. L. Huffman, and G. A. Hedge, Effects of vasoactive intestinal peptide on thyroid blood flow and circulating thyroid hormone levels in the rat, Endocrinology, 82:7, (1986).
96. L. Huffman, and G. A. Hedge, Neuropeptide control of thyroid blood flow and hormone secretion, Life Sci 39:2143 (1986).
97. M. Kalisnik, O. Vraspir-Porenta, T. Kham-Lindtner, M. Logonder-Mlinsek, Z. Pajer, D. Stiblar-Martincic, R. Zorc-Pleskovic, and M. Trobina, The interdependence of the follicular, parafollicular, and mast cells in the mammalian thyroid gland: A review and a synthesis, Am J Anat 183:148 (1988).
98. S. Van Noorden, J. M. Polak, and A. G. E. Pearse, Single cellular origin of somatostatin and calcitonin in the rat thyroid gland, Histochemistry 53:243 (1977).

99. Y. Kameda, H. Oyama, M. Endoh, and M. Horino, Somatostatin immunoreactive C cells in thyroid glands from various mammalian species, Anat Rec 204:161. (1982).
100. T. Grunditz, P. Persson, R. Håkanson, A. Absood, G. Böttcher, C. Rerup, and F. Sundler, Helodermin-like peptides in thyroid C cells. Stimulation of thyroid hormone secretion and suppression of calcium incorporation in bone, Proc. Nat. Acad. Sci. USA, in press (1989).
101. F. Sundler, J. Christophe, P. Robberecht, N. Yanaihara, C. Yanaihara, T. Grunditz, and R. Håkanson, Is helodermin produced by medullary thyroid carcinoma cells and normal C cells? Immunocytochemical evidence, Regul Pept 20:83 (1988).
102. M. Hoshino, C. Yanaihara, Y-M. Hong, S. Kishida, Y. Katsumaru, A. Vandermeers, M. Vandermeers-Piret, P. Robberecht, J. Christophe, and N. Yanaihara, Primary structure of helodermin, a VIP-secretin-like peptide isolated from Gila monster venom, FEBS Lett 178:233 (1984).
103. P. Robberecht, J. De Graef, M-C. Woussen-Colle, M-C. Vandermeers-Piret, A. Vandermeers, P. De Neef, A. Cauvin, C. Yanaihara, N. Yanaihara, J. Christophe, Immunoreactive helodermin-like peptides in the rat: a new class of mammalian neuropeptides related to secretin and VIP, Biochem Biophys Res Commun 130:333 (1985).
104. S. Naruse, A. Yasui, S. Kishida, M. Kadowaki, M. Hoshino, T. Ozaki, P. Robberecht, J. Christophe, C. Yanaihara, and N. Yanaihara, Helodermin has a VIP-like effect upon canine blood flow, Peptides 7:237 (1986).
105. T. Grunditz, R. Håkanson, C Rerup, and F. Sundler, Helodermin-stimulated thyroid hormone secretion: Effects of other C cell peptides and α- and β-adrenoceptor blockade, in preparation (1989).

RECEPTORS OF THE THYROID: THE THYROTROPIN RECEPTOR IS ONLY THE FIRST VIOLINIST OF A SYMPHONY ORCHESTRA

Leonard D. Kohn, Motoyasu Saji, Takashi Akamizu, Shoichiro Ikuyama, Osamu Isozaki, Aimee D. Kohn, Pilar Santisteban, John Y. Chan, Shashikumar Bellur, Carlo M. Rotella, Francisco V. Alvarez, and Salvatore M. Aloj

Section on Cell Regulation
Laboratory of Biochemistry and Metabolism
National Institute of Diabetes, Digestive, and Kidney Diseases
National Institutes of Health
Bethesda, MD 20892

INTRODUCTION

The primary role of the thyroid is to produce thyroid hormones; the primary regulator of the thyroid, both its function and growth, is the pituitary glycoprotein hormone, thyrotropin (TSH). Studies of the mechanism by which thyrotropin regulates thyroid cells have been a dominant part of thyroid research for the past several decades because autoantibodies to the TSH receptor have been implicated in the hyperfunction and goiter of autoimmune Graves' disease. Understanding why the TSH receptor, but not receptors for other glycoprotein hormones, is an autoantigen is a major medical concern. Equally of concern has been the mechanism by which the TSH receptor achieves its functional response and the relationship of TSH and its receptor to thyroid growth.

The TSH receptor was one of the first receptors found to be coupled to the cAMP signal transduction system (1). It was presumed that the increased cAMP levels resultant from the TSH-receptor interaction (Fig. 1) induced all functions attributed to TSH: iodide uptake, iodide transport into the follicular lumen, thyroglobulin synthesis, iodination of thyroglobulin, and, ultimately, thyroid hormone formation, degradation, and secretion (2). Initially it was also assumed that the TSH receptor and cyclase complex were one and the same (2).

Today it is evident that both initial assumptions were incorrect. Now it is important to understand how the TSH receptor couples to a cyclase complex which is a distinct molecular grouping of catalytic and regulatory subunits (3). In retrospect, it was also naive to presume the cAMP second message coordinately regulated all steps involved in thyroid hormone formation. Independent regulation of the ability to scavenge iodide and store it, as opposed to the need to secrete thyroid hormone, must exist; otherwise we would be hyperthyroid each time iodized salt or fish were on our dinner plates. Today we realize that multiple signals exist and that each signal, cAMP included, must have some means of being custom tailored to express different responses under different circumstances. This is intuitive clinically in the absence of a linear correlation between hyperfunction and goiter in Graves' disease. The issues now are not whether but how?

It is no surprise that in addition to the TSH receptor, thyroid cells have receptors for a multiplicity of other hormones, growth factors, neurogenic agents, toxins, and bioactive compounds. It should also be no surprise to realize that these other ligands can modulate TSH-induced signal systems and thereby customize the TSH response. The activity of these hormones can in some cases replace TSH, in other cases be absolute requirements for TSH receptor expression, and, in still other situations, result in responses greater than the sum of the parts. As will be shown, they can act transcriptionally or posttranscriptionally, in parallel or in sequence.

The present report will try to show how TSH and its

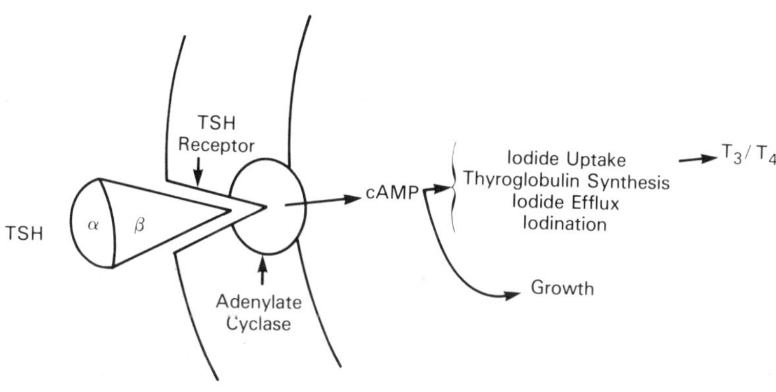

Figure 1. An early concept of the TSH receptor wherein the receptor and adenylate cyclase complex are presumed to be a single molecular entity and the cAMP signal induces all bioactivites of TSH: iodide uptake, thyroglobulin synthesis, iodide efflux into the follicular lumen, iodination and thyroid cell growth.

receptor have moved from the status of conductor to first violinist of a symphony orchestra. It will examine the interrelatedness of several hormone receptors and signals to show how this better relates to the function and growth of the thyroid cell. It will not attempt to be an anthology of all receptors on the thyroid cell nor even a discourse on every possible interrelationship. Finally, it will report on the current studies of the cloning of the TSH receptor. These studies will ultimately be necessary to understand how the TSH receptor is coupled to different signal systems, to understand the function of the first violinist in the orchestra in molecular terms, and to explain, diagnose, and better treat those discordant symphonic events we know as thyroid disease states, from autoimmune Graves' to thyroid cancer.

INSULIN AND IGF-I RECEPTORS ON THE THYROID HAVE A KEY ROLE IN TSH RECEPTOR REGULATED GROWTH AND FUNCTION

Insulin and IGF-I receptors are required for TSH dependent growth of thyroid cells

The development of the FRTL and FRTL-5 thyroid cell lines (4, 5) stands as a key to our current recognition of the importance of insulin and IGF-I receptors to expression of TSH receptor activity. Rat FRTL or FRTL-5 thyroid cells are, as noted in Dr. Taylor's presentation earlier, dependent on TSH for growth; however, TSH-dependent growth requires the presence of insulin and serum factors, which we now know include insulin-like growth factor-I. The work described earlier by Dr Taylor indicated that there is a receptor for both insulin and IGF-I (6). The work to be described below shows that both receptors are critical to thyroid function as well as growth, that both are critical to the expression of signals generated by the TSH receptor, that both, as a result, allow the TSH receptor to be custom tailored to elicit different responses from the same signal, and that the two receptors can be very individual in their effects. These studies have helped change the status of the TSH receptor from the only player to that of an important player in the symphony.

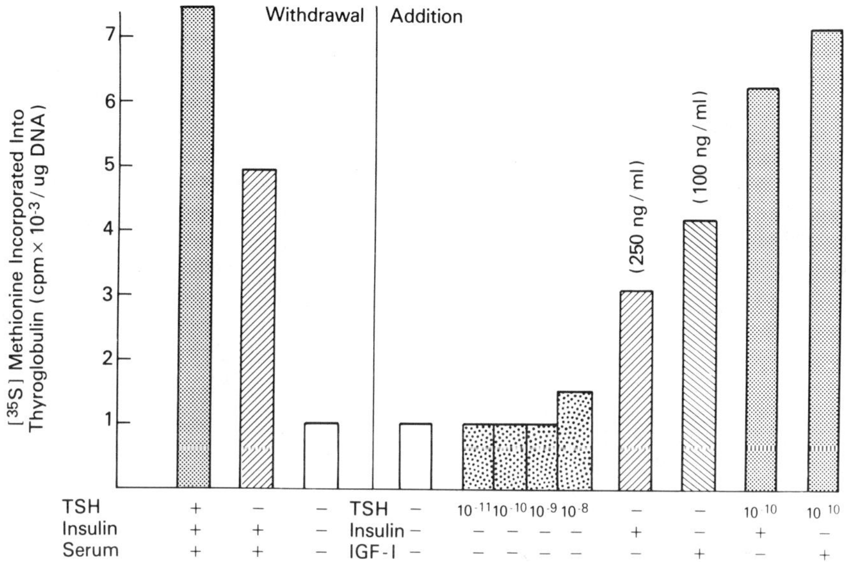

Figure 2. (Left) Effect on thyroglobulin synthesis by FRTL-5 rat thyroid cells of withdrawing, for a three day period, TSH or TSH plus insulin and serum from the medium in which cells are maintained. (Right) Effect of readding TSH at the noted concentrations, insulin (250 ng/ml), or IGF-I (100 ng/ml) to FRTL-5 thyroid cells maintained for 4 days in medium with no added TSH and no insulin (4H) and with only 0.2% serum; [^{35}S]methionine incorporation into immunoprecipitable thyroglobulin was measured 72 hours later.

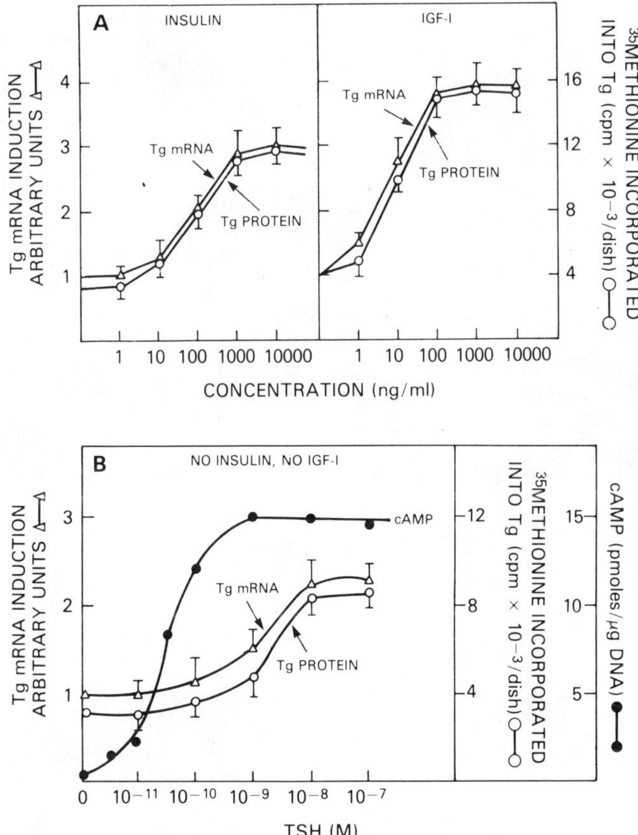

Figure 3 (A) The ability of insulin and IGF-I to increase the synthesis of thyroglobulin reflects an action by these to hormones to increase thyroglobulin mRNA levels. (B) TSH at physiological concentrations does not increase thyroglobulin synthesis or mRNA levels despite its ability to increase cAMP levels. In both experiments FRTL-5 thyroid cells were maintained for 3 days in medium with no added TSH and no insulin as well as with only 0.2% serum. After 36 hours, the thyroglobulin synthesis was measured by exposing one set of duplicate plates to [^{35}S]methionine and isolating the immunoprecipitable thyroglobulin (7). A second set of duplicate plates was used to isolate RNA and, after blotting and hybridization with both a Tg and beta actin cDNA probe, the amount of Tg mRNA was measured by densitometry and expressed in arbitrary units using the no hormone treatment cells as the control, setting them at unity, and comparing the increases in Tg mRNA with beta actin mRNA levels which do not change with insulin, IGF-I or TSH treatment. The cAMP levels were measured in a third duplicate set of plates as described (9).

Coordinate and dependent regulation of thyroglobulin biosynthesis by insulin, IGF-I, and TSH

In examining thyroglobulin synthesis in rat FRTL-5 thyroid cells (7), it was presumed that withdrawal of TSH from the medium, which also contains insulin and 5% calf serum, would eliminate thyroglobulin synthesis, since evidence had accumulated that TSH regulated thyroglobulin gene expression via its cAMP signal (8). Surprisingly, however, thyroglobulin synthesis, measured as $[^{35}S]$methionine incorporation into protein immunoprecipitable by rat antithyroglobulin, decreased less than two-fold and was still a major synthesized protein (Fig. 2A). To reduce thyroglobulin synthesis to low levels required removal of the insulin and serum (Fig. 2A).

In the absence of insulin and serum, the readdition of $1x10^{-10}$ M TSH, a physiologic concentration able to maximally elevate cAMP levels in rat FRTL-5 thyroid cells (9), had no affect on thyroglobulin synthesis (Fig. 2B). In contrast, return of either insulin or IGF-I, alone, to the cells resulted in a 2 to 3 fold increase in thyroglobulin synthesis (Fig. 2B), indicating that these hormones had a major role in thyroglobulin synthesis independent of TSH and its cAMP signal. Further, it was evident that the ability of physiologic levels of TSH to increase thyroglobulin synthesis returned when added with insulin or IGF-I (Fig. 2B). Finally, it was evident that insulin and IGF-I were not additive in their functional expression with TSH (7), unlike the case for growth (6, 9, 10). Thus, in the case of thyroglobulin synthesis, insulin added together with IGF-I was less effective with TSH than was IGF-I plus TSH (7); in the case of growth (6, 9, 10), the three ligands were additive in their activities.

The ability of insulin and IGF-I to increase thyroglobulin synthesis was associated with their ability to increase thyroglobulin mRNA levels (Fig. 3A). Conversely, the inability of physiologic levels of TSH to increase thyroglobulin synthesis in the absence of insulin or IGF-I was associated with its inability to increase to increase thyroglobulin mRNA levels (Fig. 3B). The cAMP signal, though coupled, was clearly not recognized in the absence of insulin and IGF-I (Fig. 3B).

The action of insulin and IGF-I was, like TSH and cAMP, at a transcriptional level (Fig. 4). Similarly the

Effect of Insulin, IGF-I, and TSH On Transcription of Thyroglobulin in RNA from Isolated Nucleii

Hormone Addition	[^{32}P] RNA Input	[^{32}P] RNA Hybridized To: pUC8 Control cDNA	pRTH27 TG cDNA	pA14 Actin cDNA	Transcription: TG Gene	Actin Gene
	(cpm)		(cpm)		(ppm)	
Basal	390,000	50	300	110	640	150
+ Insulin	390,000	55	580	120	1350	170
+ IGF-I	390,000	45	590	110	1400	170
+ TSH (10^{-10})	390,000	50	300	110	640	150
(10^{-8})	390,000	45	500	110	1170	170
+ Insulin + TSH (10^{-10})	390,000	60	870	120	2080	150
+ IGF-I + TSH (10^{-10})	390,000	40	910	105	2230	170

Figure 4. Nuclear run on experiment measuring ability of the noted hormones to increase transcription. Data are obtained as described (7) after UTP labeled nuclear RNA was hybridized to the noted cDNA probes. Nuclei were isolated from cells treated with the noted hormones after 4 days of maintenance in medium with no insulin, no TSH, and with only 0.2% serum.

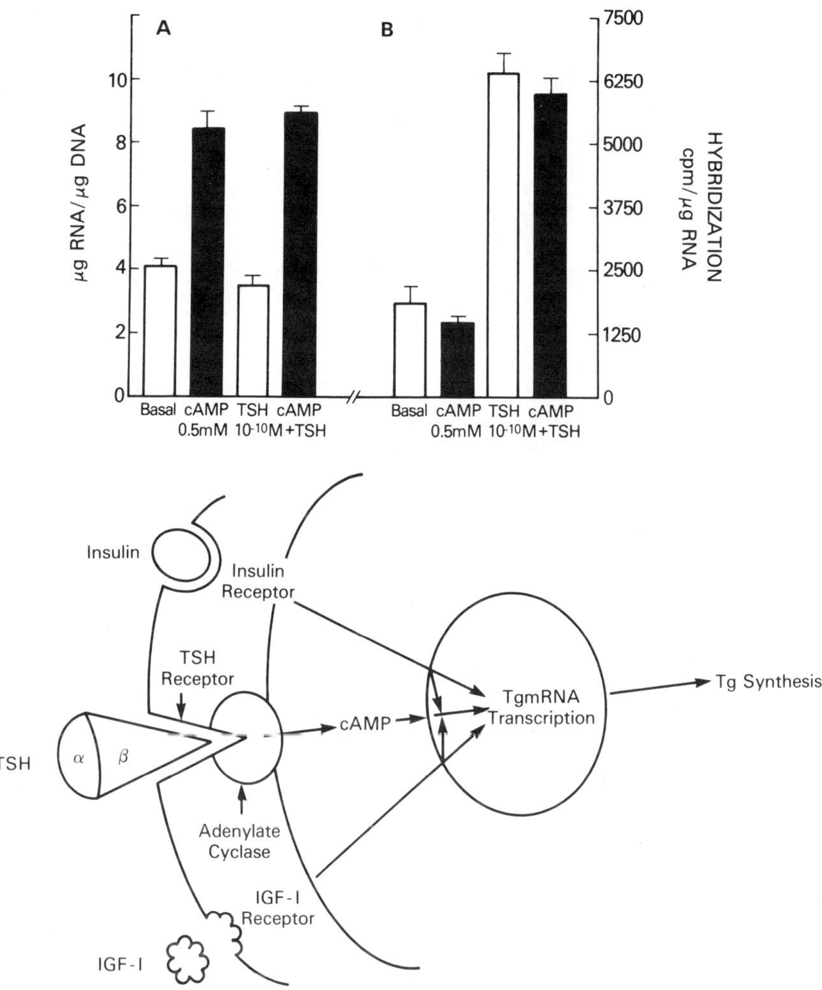

Figure 5 (Top) The effect of TSH and 8-Br cAMP on total poly A+ RNA per microgram DNA (A) and on poly A+ thyroglobulin RNA (B). FRTL-5 thyroid cells were maintained with no insulin, no TSH, no cortisone and with only 1% albumin rather than serum for 7 days before treatment with the noted concentrations of TSH or cAMP analog for 48 hours. Total poly A+ RNA was quantitated assuming absorbance (A)=1cm/0.1% = 25; thyroglobulin poly A+ RNA was measured by hybridization after Northern analysis. The values represent the mean ± SEM from a single experiment which is typical of 3 performed. (Bottom) Model of thyroglobulin synthesis wherein it is induced independently by TSH, insulin, and IGF-I acting at a transcriptional level and wherein the TSH action requires insulin and IGF-I at physiologic concentrations.

additive action of TSH and its cAMP signal was at the transcriptional level (Fig. 4). Of interest, however, was the further observation that TSH and cAMP did not have identical actions in the absence of insulin and IGF-I when transcriptional activity of the ligand and its signal were compared in nuclear "run on" assays. Thus, TSH treatment of thyroid cells maintained with no insulin or IGF-I increased thyroglobulin transcripts but did not increase total transcripts. In contrast, cAMP treatment of cells resulted in increased thyroglobulin and total RNA transcription. This is reflected in their effects on cytoplasmic mRNA levels. Thus, when cells are cultured with no TSH, no insulin, no hydrocortisone, and with only 0.2% serum or 1% bovine serum albumin for 7 days, then treated with 1x10-10M TSH or 0.5mM 8-Br cAMP for 2 days (Fig. 5A), the cAMP but not the TSH increases total poly A+ RNA when compared per microgram DNA. In contrast, TSH but not the cAMP analog increases thyroglobulin mRNA per microgram poly A+ RNA.

Interpretation of this last experiment is complex and requires one to consider that TSH may be initiating specific transcription while "supressing" the cAMP signal for increased total transcription. Thus, the cAMP signal generated by TSH was not mimicking the cAMP analog. One possible explanation for this phenomenon, and the importance of the hydrocortisone depletion, will be apparent below in experiments concerned with actinomycin D "superinduction" of malic enzyme mRNA levels and iodide uptake, both TSH receptor, cAMP- signalled activities. Nevertheless it is clear that the cAMP signal of TSH is modulated by insulin and IGF-I at a transcriptional level, that physiologic expression of TSH receptor action involving its cAMP signal can require insulin or IGF-I, and that insulin and IGF-I have both a coordinate regulatory action with TSH, in this case, as well as an absolute permissive action: they are required for physiologic expression of the TSH receptor cAMP signal. Insulin and IGF-I and their receptors thus have the potential to customize the TSH receptor signal response and this can act be done at a transcriptional level (Fig. 5B).

Numerous questions can be raised as a result of these observations. Are insulin and IGF-I important to the expression of every cAMP signaled, TSH receptor regulated function, i. e. is this a general metabolic phenomenon or a truly customizing mechanism? Are insulin and IGF-I identical in their action in all situations, as is apparent in the case of thyroglobulin, or is their differential action a means of further customizing a TSH regulated response? Is the customizing action of insulin or IGF-I on TSH receptor expression restricted to the cAMP signal system? Do other hormones act in a similar way to modulate and customize TSH receptor signal expression?

Insulin and IGF-I do not similarly modulate all TSH receptor- regulated, cAMP-signalled responses

Iodide uptake, peroxidase activity and mRNA levels, HMG-CoA reductase activity and mRNA levels, and malic enzyme activity and mRNA levels are all increased by TSH and are all cAMP signalled functions.

Like thyroglobulin, TSH elevated iodide uptake requires insulin or IGF-I(Table 1); unlike thyroglobulin neither insulin nor IGF-I appear to have significant activities of their own on iodide uptake. TSH and the cAMP signal similarly increase HMG-CoA reductase mRNA levels only in the presence of insulin (Table 1).

Increases in thyroid peroxidase activity and mRNA levels induced by TSH occur whether insulin or IGF-I are present or absent (Fig. 6). Similarly, insulin or IGF-I have no affect on the ability of TSH to increase malic enzyme activity or mRNA levels (Fig. 7). Neither insulin nor IGF-I have any significant action of their own in these last two cases.

It is therefore evident that insulin or IGF-I and their receptors do not regulate every activity mediated by the TSH receptor and its cAMP signal in an identical manner. Further, it is evident that this customizing action of insulin and IGF-I is not restricted to events, peroxidase activation or iodide uptake, related directly to thyroid hormone formation; "housekeeping functions, for example those involving malic enzyme and HMG-CoA reductase, are similarly customized. Further, it is evident that independent actions of insulin or IGF-I can further customize the TSH receptor response. Finally, it is evident that the tailoring activities of the insulin/IGF-I receptors can regulate gene expression.

TABLE 1

Hormones Present in the Media	Iodide Uptake	HMG-CoA Reductase mRNA levels
		% of Maximal
TSH + Insulin	100	100
TSH - Insulin	15	8

FRTL-5 rat thyroid cells were grown to near confluency in complete medium including TSH, insulin, and 5% serum then maintained for 7 days with no TSH, no insulin, and 5%serum and an additional 3 days with no TSH, no insulin, and only 0.2% serum. The noted hormones were added at $1x10^{-10}$M (TSH) or 10 microgram/ml (insulin) concentrations normally present in the complete medium. Cells were evaluated for iodide uptake after 72 hours and for HMG-CoA reductase mRNA levels after 24 hours. The HMG CoA reductase mRNA level was compared to beta actin mRNA levels to normalize them since beta actin does not change as a function of TSH or insulin treatment.

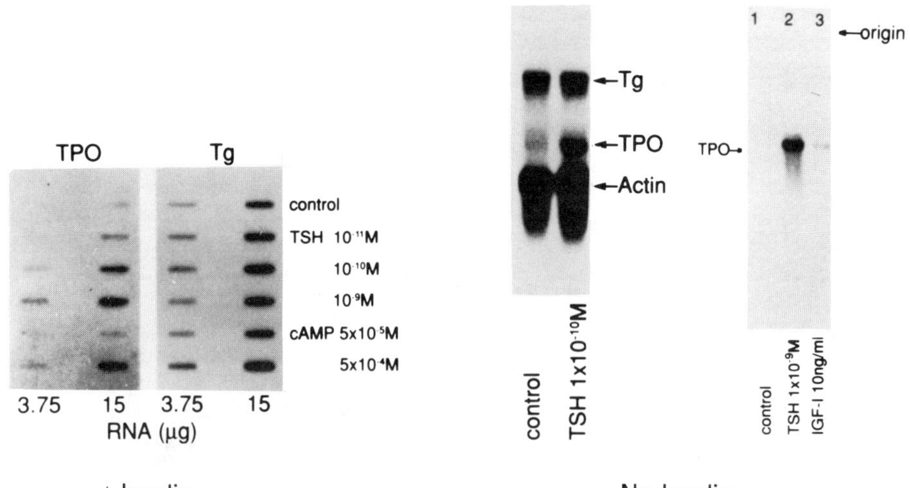

Figure 6. (Left) Ability of TSH and 8-Br cAMP treatment for 24 hours to increase thyroid peroxidase (TPO) or thyroglobulin mRNA levels in cells maintained for 4 days with no TSH but in the presence of 10 micrograms/ml insulin and 5% serum. RNA was isolated from cells and slot blots performed as described (7). The probes were a rat TPO cDNA and a rat Tg cDNA. (Right Panels) Northern analysis measuring the ability of TSH or IGF-I treatment for 24 hours to increase TPO mRNA levels in FRTL-5 thyroid cells maintained for 4 days in medium with no TSH, no insulin and with only 0.2% serum. RNA was isolated from cells and electrophoresed in 1% agarose gels before blotting and hybridization as described (7). In one hybridization a mixture of radiolabeled cDNA probes (TPO, beta actin, and TG) was present; in the other only the radiolabeled TPO probe was added. Washing was performed under stringent conditions as described (7).

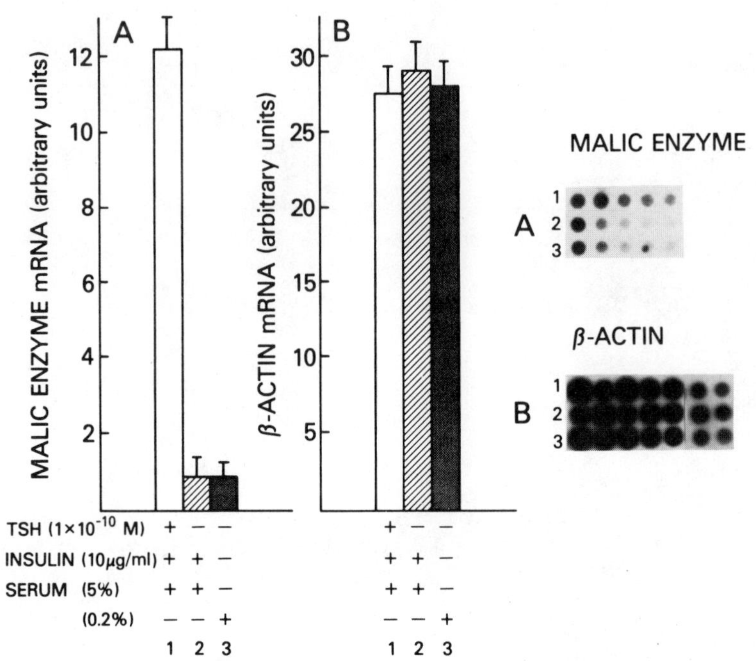

Figure 7. Ability of $1x10^{-10}$M TSH or 10 micrograms/ml insulin with or without serum to increase malic enzyme (A) or beta actin (B) mRNA levels in rat FRTL-5 thyroid cells. Cells were maintained in complete 6H medium including TSH, insulin and 5% serum or were maintained in medium with TSH removed from the complete mixture (20) or with TSH and insulin removed plus only 0.2% rather than 5% serum. RNA was isolated, quantitated by absorbance, blotted at multiple concentrations as noted on right, and hybridized sequentially with the two cDNA probes (right). After autoradiography blots were quantitated by densitometry using arbitrary units (20).

Insulin and IGF-I are not necessarily equivalent in their ability to customize the TSH receptor response nor coordinate in their action with TSH

Insulin, IGF-I and TSH can each independently induce amino acid transport. This is evident in studies of alpha amino isobutyric acid (AIB) transport by FRTL-5 thyroid cells. Thus, as evident in Figure 8, TSH or insulin, given to cells maintained in the absence of TSH, insulin, and in only 0.2% calf serum, can each increase AIB uptake. Further, it is clear that inclusion of insulin in the medium for the 7 day preincubation period in no way alters the ability of TSH to increase AIB uptake (Fig. 8). Similarly, the presence of TSH in the medium during the preincubation period does not affect the ability of insulin to increase AIB uptake (Fig. 8). Each hormone is independent in its action.

These results are different when TSH and IGF-I are similarly compared in AIB uptake studies (Fig. 9). Again, each ligand, TSH or IGF-I, can increase AIB uptake after cells are maintained in medium with no insulin, no TSH, and with only 0.2% serum for a 7 day period (Fig. 9), If, however, IGF-I is included in the medium during the preincubation period, the ability of TSH to increase AIB uptake is lost (Fig. 9); and, if TSH is present, the ability of IGF-I to increase AIB uptake is diminished (Fig. 9). Further evident in this last experiment, the presence of insulin during the preincubation period increases rather than decreases the ability of IGF-I to increase AIB uptake (Fig. 9B). The presence of insulin intensifies, however, the ability of TSH to inhibit the IGF-I-induced increase in AIB uptake (Fig. 9B).

Insulin and IGF-I are thus not necessarily equivalent in their ability to perturb TSH receptor-mediated functions. This allows a further customizing of TSH receptor signalled bioaction.

The nonequivalancy of insulin and IGF-I in their affect on TSH receptor mediated events was also evident when FRTL-5 cell growth was studied. Insulin and IGF-I were each additive with TSH in their ability to increase cell number. The growth of FRTL-5 thyroid cells in culture requires cell attachment; cell attachment is a complex process involving a multiplicity of molecules including surface receptors, proteoglycans, laminin or fibronectin, and collagen (Fig. 10). In studying proteoglycan synthesis, measured by the ability of

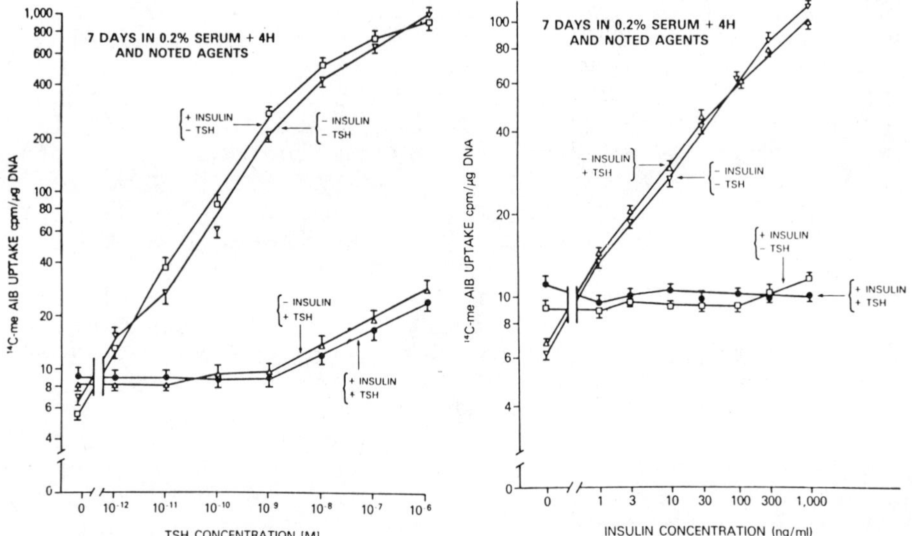

Figure 8. Ability of TSH or insulin to increase aminoisobutyric acid uptake in FRTL-5 rat thyroid cells maintained for 7 days in 0.2% serum, 4H medium, and with or without insulin (left) or with and without TSH (right). In addition , control cells were maintained for the 7 day period with TSH (left) or with insulin (right); the presence of the same ligand during the 7 day preincubation as during the challenge results in a loss of the acute stimulatory effect. After 7 days, the noted concentrations of hormone were added together with radiolabeled aminoisobutyric acid and the amount taken up by the cells measured three hours later using the same procedure described to measure iodide uptake (9).

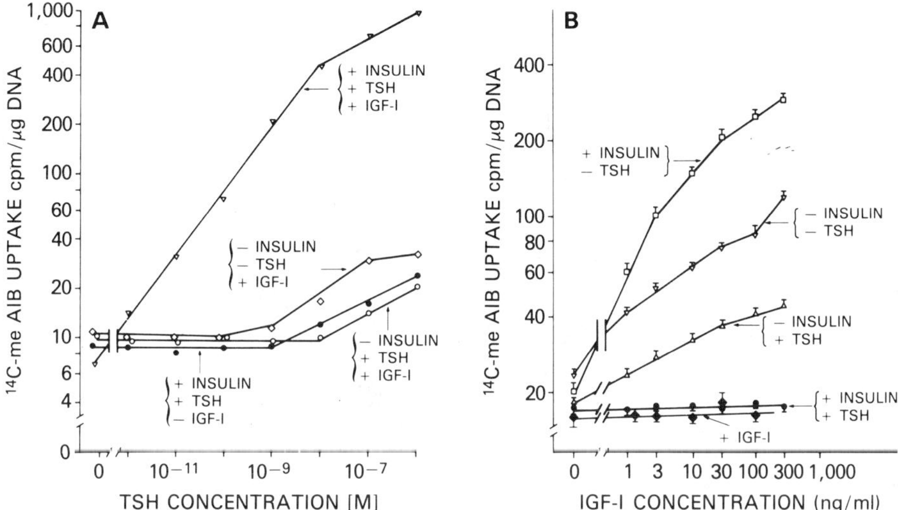

Figure 9. Ability of TSH or IGF-I to increase aminoisobutyric acid uptake in FRTL-5 rat thyroid cells maintained for 7 days in 0.2% serum, 4H medium, and with or without insulin or with and without TSH . In addition, control cells were maintained for the 7 day period with TSH (left) or with IGF-I (right); the presence of the same ligand during the 7 day preincubation as during the challenge results in a loss of the acute stimulatory effect. After 7 days, the noted concentrations of hormone were added together with radiolabeled aminoisobutyric acid and the amount taken up by the cells measured three hours later using the same procedure described to measure iodide uptake (9).

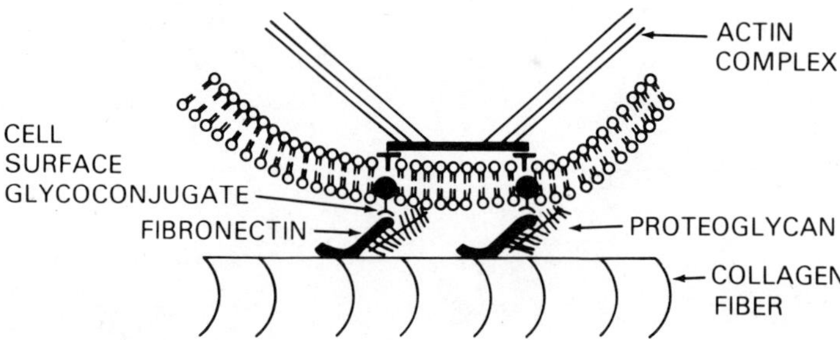

Figure 10. Model of cell attachment to surfaces of other cells or plastic tissue culture dishes wherein attachment requires such factors as collagen, proteoglycans, laminin, or fibronectin. Attachment can be a necessary prelude to growth and function and can influence the activity of a cell by a host of mechanisms related to its association with other cells or connective tissue components.

hormones to increase glucosamine incorporation into glycosaminmoglycans (GAG) in the cells or media, it was noted that the TSH receptor, via its cAMP signal, could increase GAG synthesis (Fig. 11 and References 11, 12); thus TSH, cholera toxin, forskolin, or cAMP analogs were all active in this regard. It was noted however that this action required the presence of insulin (Fig. 11).

When further examined, serum did not significantly add to the insulin action (Fig. 12A, TOP) but could replace insulin as could IGF-I in the ability to express TSH activity. Insulin alone, as well as TSH alone, had minimal activity with respect to increasing GAG synthesis (Fig. 12A TOP). In contrast, however, IGF-I alone was a potent enhancer of GAG synthesis, much superior to insulin (Fig. 12B TOP). Further, IGF-I activity was inhibited slightly by insulin even when IGF-I concentrations were large relative to insulin, indicating that the IGF-I receptor was acting uniquely in this activity (Fig. 12A BOTTOM). This was also evident with mixtures of IGF-I and TSH given to cells maintained with insulin or without insulin; the presence of insulin limited the IGF-I plus TSH response (Fig. 12B BOTTOM).

Once again, the action of IGF-I and insulin appear critical to expression of the action of TSH and are independent in their actions with respect to TSH and its receptor. This is particularly evident when cell attachment is studied (Fig. 13). Thus, plating cells in the absence of TSH and insulin, as well as in low serum (0.2%), results in poor cell attachment. The inclusion in the medium of TSH or insulin alone does not improve cell attachment, whereas the inclusion of IGF-I alone has a salutary effect. TSH plus insulin is better and growth also occurs; TSH, insulin, and IGF-I is best. Insulin and IGF-I and their receptors are thus both critical to TSH dependent growth and cell attachment, they are not identical in their actions, and they are both necessary for the full expression of TSH receptor action.

This interaction between TSH, insulin, and IGF-I receptors with respect to growth extends to their abilities to increase c-myc and c-fos oncogene transcript expression (10). In this action insulin, IGF-I and TSH are almost equally active in increasing oncogene transcript expression and insulin or IGF-I are additive with TSH but not additive with each other (10). The interaction also extends to thymidine incorporation into DNA, a step after oncogene expression but before

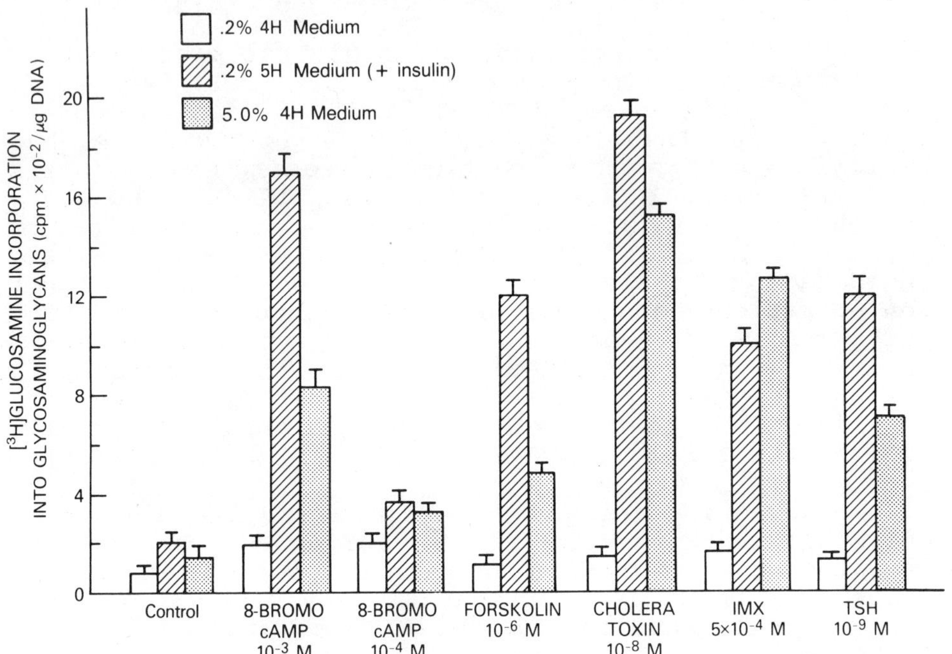

Figure 11. Ability of TSH or the noted cAMP analogs or stimulators - 8 Br cAMP, forskolin, cholera toxin, or isobutylmethylxanthine (IMX) - to increase tritiated glucosamine incorporation into glycosaminoglycans (GAG) associated with the cell pellet of FRTL-5 thyroid cells. Cells were maintained in medium with 0.2% serum and neither TSH nor insulin (4H, open bars), with 0.2% serum plus insulin but no TSH (hatched bars), or in 4H medium containing no insulin or no TSH but including 5% serum (stippled bars). Cells were treated 72 hours with the noted concentrations of ligands in the presence of the tritiated glucosamine before GAG was isolated by a cetylpyridinium precipitation procedure.

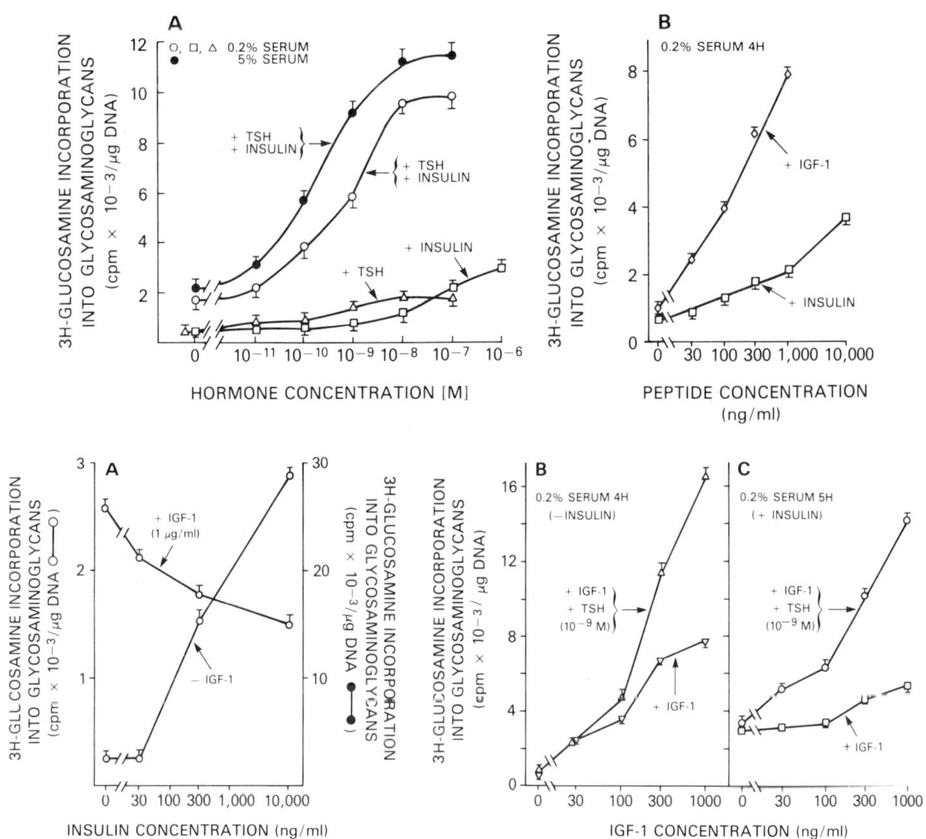

Figure 12 TOP. (A) Ability of TSH or insulin, at the noted concentrations, to increase tritiated glucosamine incorporation into GAG when FRTL-5 cells are maintained (3 days) in 4H medium with no TSH and no insulin and with only 0.2% serum or in the 4H medium with 5% serum. Hormone treatments were for 72 hours; GAG was isolated from cell pellets by a cetylpyridinium precipitation procedure. (B) Ability of insulin or IGF-I to increase tritiated glucosamine incorporation into GAG in FRTL-5 thyroid cells maintained (3 days) with 4H medium and only 0.2% serum. Figure 12 BOTTOM (A) Ability of insulin at the noted concentrations to inhibit the activity of 1 microgram per ml IGF-I in increasing GAG synthesis as measured by tritiated glucosamine incorporation into GAG. (B, C) Ability of TSH and IGF-I together to increase GAG synthesis, measured as glucosamine incorporation, both in the presence (C) and absence (B) of insulin, i.e. in cells maintained in 5H vs. 4H medium plus 0.2% serum.

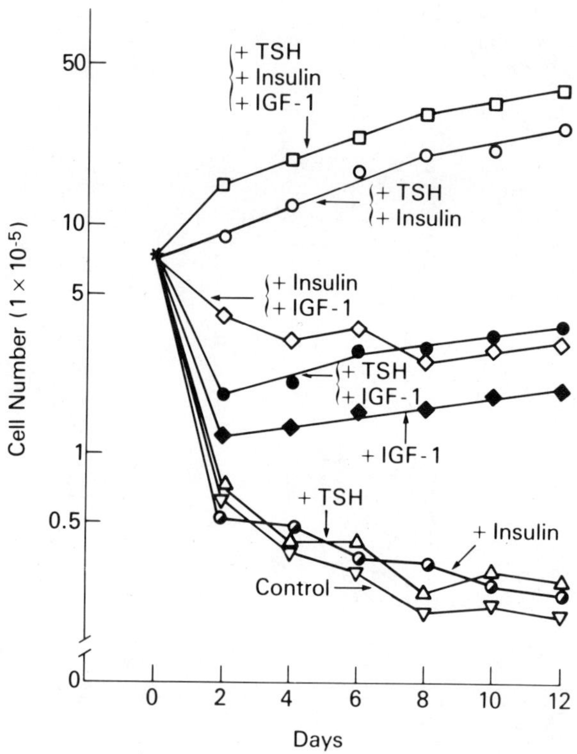

Figure 13. Ability of the noted ligands to cause trypsinized FRTL-5 thyroid cells to attach to plastic dishes and grow as measured by cell number. FRTL-5 cells maintained in complete 6H medium were trypsinized and added to replicate 30 mm tissue culture dishes containing 4H medium, 0.2% serum, and the noted ligands at the following concentrations: TSH, 1×10^{-10} M; insulin, 10 micrograms per ml, IGF-I, 100 ng per ml. At the noted times cells were isolated and counted. Cells were fed fresh medium every third day.

increases in cell number occur. In this case, insulin, IGF-I and TSH are again equally active but insulin or IGF-I cause more than additive increases when mixed together with TSH; insulin and IGF-I are, however, once again not additive with each other (10).

The significance of these interactions between insulin, IGF-I and TSH receptors is thus clear in terms of the interdependent actions of all receptors and ligands for both function and growth. It is also clear that the interaction between insulin, IGF-I and TSH, together with their respective receptors, is very individual to the particular activity examined. Finally, it is clear that insulin and IGF-I receptor modulation of TSH receptor expression is not necessarily equivalent since the two receptors can act individually and independently.

Before leaving the insulin/IGF-I receptor mediated interaction with TSH receptors, one last observation is of interest. In FRTL-5 thyroid cells, the action of TSH to increase mRNA levels of thyroglobulin and HMG-CoA reductase is transcriptional. In contrast, the action of TSH to increase malic enzyme and peroxidase mRNA levels is posttranscriptional in FRTL-5 thyroid cells. It is of interest that the first group is positively regulated by insulin whereas the second is not. These data support the conclusion that insulin and IGF-I can positively regulate TSH receptor-mediated, cAMP-signalled activities at a transcriptional level. Since the role of insulin and IGF-I as positive posttranscriptional regulators of TSH receptor-mediated, cAMP-signalled gene expression remains undefined, it is tempting to speculate the following. An insulin/IGF-I action to increase TSH receptor-mediated, cAMP-signalled gene expression reflects transcriptional rather than posttranscriptional regulation.

RECEPTORS FOR OTHER HORMONES ENLARGE THE ORCHESTRA AND UNCOVER THE COMPLICATED SCORE PLAYED BY THE TSH RECEPTOR

The existence of a multiplicity of receptors for other ligands such as alpha 1 adrenergic receptors, cholinergic receptors, toxin receptors, and other G protein linked receptors will be discussed in detail in separate reports in this meeting. Inhibitory receptors in FRTL-5 thyroid cells, such as adenosine or ATP receptors, have been detailed by two laboratories in recent work (13, 14); these extend observations in the past using other thyroid tissue sources (15). Nevertheless, it seems pertinent to examine one other receptor in further detail since it shows how complex the interrelationships between receptors can become and how the TSH receptor can induce two activities sequentially as the result of inputs from other receptors.

As noted earlier, TSH induced iodide uptake in FRTL-5 thyroid cells when insulin was present but only minimally when it was absent from the medium (Table 1). In these experiments, cells are maintained with no insulin, no TSH, and with only 0.2% serum or with insulin but no TSH and only 0.2% serum. The normal medium for FRTL-5 thyroid cells includes, however, transferrin, hydrocortisone, somatostatin, and glycyl-L-histidyl-L-lysine in addition to insulin and TSH. When cells are maintained in a <u>No Hormone</u> milieu, i.e. without insulin, TSH, hydrocortisone, etc., for 5 days, then exposed to TSH alone, iodide uptake is, surprisingly, even better than when TSH is added to cells maintained in the 5H mixture with all hormone components other than TSH (Fig. 14A). Further, the addition of hydrocortisone is inhibitory (Fig. 14B) and the hydrocortisone affect cannot be explained by a change in cAMP levels (Fig. 14B).

Gordon Tomkins and his coworkers as well as other groups (16, 17), examining the ability of glucocorticoids to increase tyrosine aminotransferase (TAT) activity in liver cells, described a phenomenon known as superinduction (Fig 15). If they used hydrocortisone to increase TAT activity, then, several hours later, gave actinomycin D, they observed a further increase in TAT activity rather than an expected decrease. Studies summarized subsequently by E. B. Thompson (18) argued that the actinomycin D did this because it inhibited the formation of a second factor, also induced by hydrocortisone, which increased TAT mRNA degradation.

TSH induced iodide uptake exhibits the phenomenon of superinduction (Fig. 15 and Reference 19) when actinomycin D is given 24 hours after TSH is added to cells maintained in 5H media. These results suggest that the mechanism predicted by Thompson (18) is also operative in the case of the TSH receptor. Presumably, TSH induces a second factor which increases mRNA degradation and limits the increase in iodide porter mRNA. The second factor acts as a post transcriptional

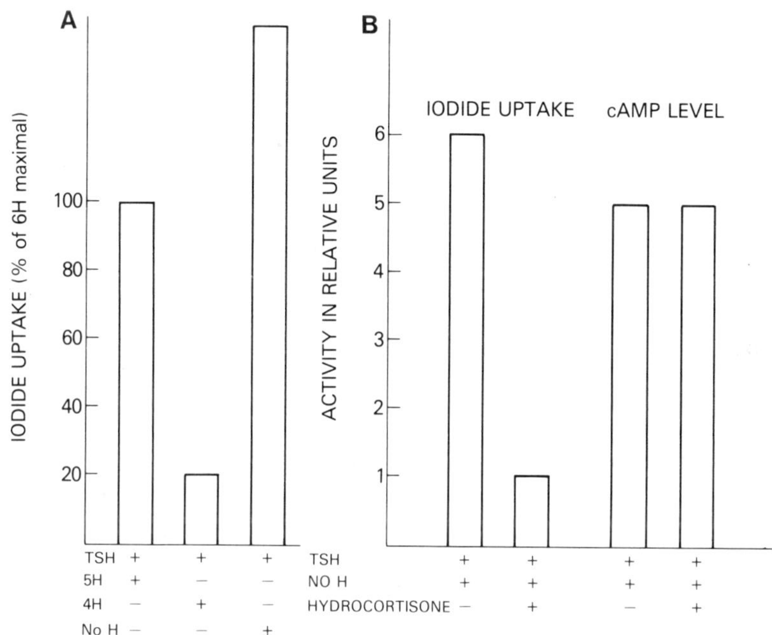

Figure 14. (A) Ability of 1×10^{-10} M TSH to increase iodide uptake into FRTL-5 thyroid cells maintained for 5 days in medium with no TSH (5H) but containing insulin, in medium with no TSH and no insulin (4H), or in medium with none (No H) of the 6 hormone supplement usually added to FRTL-5 thyroid cells: insulin, hydrocortisone, TSH, transferrin, etc. (4, 5). In all cases the medium contained only 0.2% serum. The TSH treatment lasted 3 days; iodide uptake, measured as described (9), was for 30 minutes. (B) Effect of 20 nM hydrocortisone on the ability of TSH to increase iodide uptake or cAMP levels in FRTL-5 cells maintained in No H medium as above and treated with TSH as above. Iodide uptake and cAMP levels were measured as described (9) and are expressed a percent of maximal.

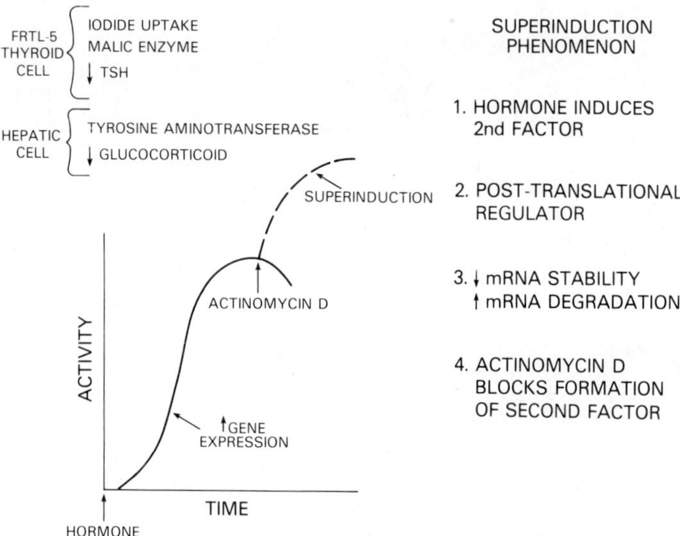

Figure 15. Superinduction model noted when actinomycin D is added to cells several hours (glucocorticoids) or 24 hours (TSH) after initial induction by the two ligands in hepatoma cells and FRTL-5 rat thyroid cells respectively. Superinduction can be measured with tyrosine aminotransferase (TAT) in hepatoma cells (16-18) or iodide uptake (19) and malic enzyme (21) in FRTL-5 thyroid cells. The presumed explanation predicted by E. B. Thompson is noted.

regulator to increase mRNA degradation (Fig. 15).

It is not possible to prove the existence of a factor causing increased mRNA degradation using iodide uptake as a model nor, until recently, was this possible with the glucocorticoid TAT system. In neither case could the degradation of mRNA be directly evaluated. Fortuitously, however, recent studies have noted that TSH induces an increase in malic enzyme mRNA (Fig. 7) and activity levels (20, 21). This increase is cAMP mediated, does not require insulin, is not inhibited by alpha-amanitin, and is not evident in nuclear run on experiments (20, 21). This suggested that TSH, through its cAMP signal, increased malic enzyme mRNA levels by a post transcriptional mechanism. When the ability of TSH to increase malic enzyme mRNA levels was followed as a function of time, it was noted that the initial increase, maximal at 16 hours, was followed by a subsequent decrease to basal levels (Fig. 16). It was further noted that the increase and decrease in malic enzyme mRNA preceded the increase in thymidine incorporation into DNA which is also induced by TSH (Fig. 16).

Cyclohexamide, given 30 minutes before TSH, inhibited the ability of TSH to increase malic enzyme mRNA levels (21); given 24 hours after TSH, cyclohexanmide accelerated the decrease (Fig. 17A). In contrast, actinomycin D, which had no affect on TSH induced increases in malic enzyme mRNA when given 30 minutes before TSH and when malic enzyme mRNA levels were measured for the first 16 hours, markedly attenuated the decrease in malic enzyme mRNA levels when given 24 hours after TSH (Fig 17B).

The action of actinomycin D in this last experiment can be considered another example of superinduction. Further, since the conditions exactly parallel those wherein actinomycin induces superinduction with respect to iodide uptake, the malic enzyme studies would indicate that the mechanism predicted by Thompson (18) is correct. The decrease in malic enzyme mRNA normally evident at 24 hours results from the action of a second factor which increases mRNA degradation. Actinomycin D prevents the formation and action of this second factor.

The sum of the iodide uptake and malic enzyme studies predict, therefore, the following (Fig. 17 BOTTOM). The TSH receptor mediated cAMP signal can increase expression of a particular mRNA by a

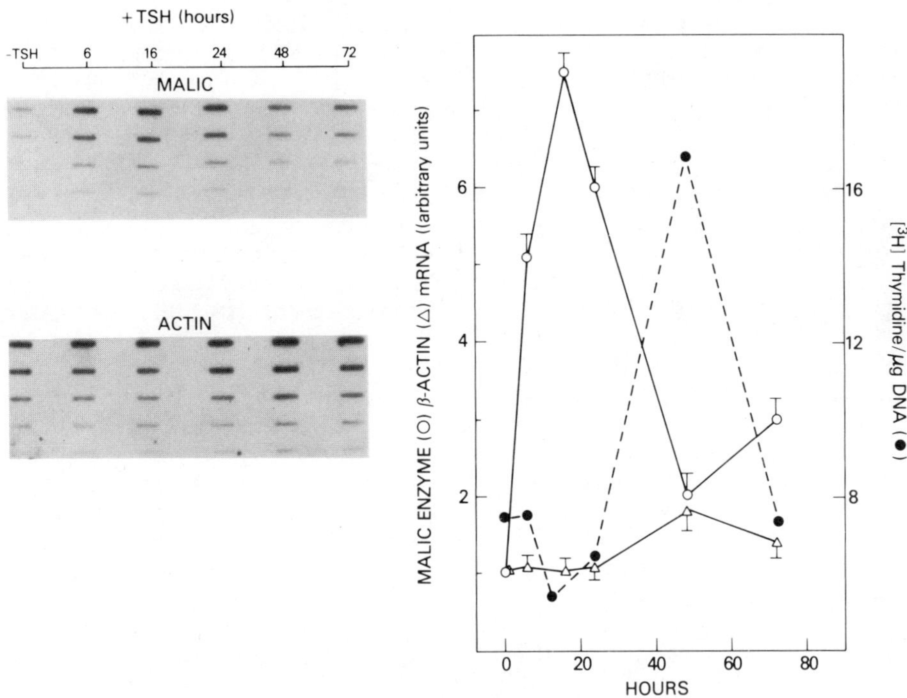

Figure 16. Ability of $1x10^{-10}$ M TSH to increase malic enzyme mRNA levels in FRTL-5 thyroid cells as a function of time, compared to the ability of TSH to increase the rate (measured as a 2 hour pulse) of thymidine incorporation into DNA. FRTL-5 cells were maintained in medium containing 5% serum but with no TSH (5H) for 5 days and then for two additional days in 5H medium with only 0.2% serum before the experiment was started. Fresh medium with or without TSH was added at 72, 48, 24, 16, or 6 hours before harvesting cells and RNA extracted as described (20, 21). Autoradiograms of slot blots containing different dilutions of the RNA extracted and hybridized sequentially with a malic enzyme cDNA probe or a beta actin probe are presented as is the densitometry values, in arbitrary units, of the effect of TSH on the two mRNAs. Densitometry set the control cell values of hybridization to unity for both actin and malic enzyme. The tritiated thymidine incorporation into DNA was measured using duplicate plates; tritiated thymidine was added during the last two hours of the experiment. The incorporation into DNA and measurements of DNA by diphenylamine reagent were otherwise as described (9).

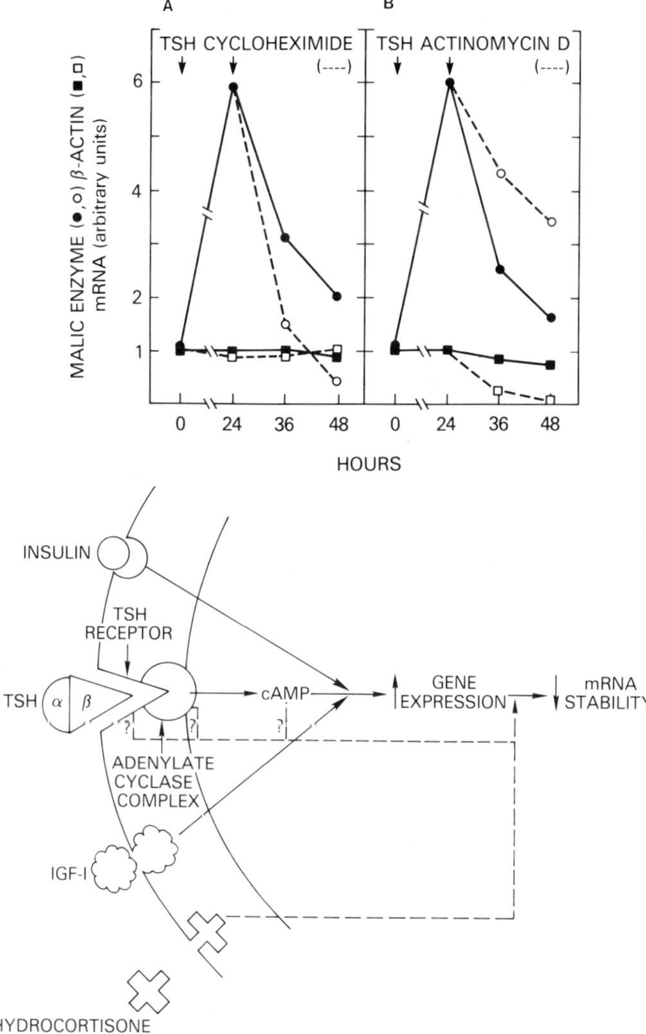

Figure 17(TOP). Effect of cyclohexamide (A) and actinomycin D (B) on TSH induced increases in malic enzyme mRNA levels in FRTL-5 thyroid cells when both antibiotics are added 24 hours after TSH. The experiment was otherwise performed as described in Figure 16.
(BOTTOM) Model wherein TSH regulates expression of a gene by two sequential actions which are sequential in time and regulated by the presence, perhaps, of other hormones and their receptors such as hydrocortisone. The first effect is to increase gene expression at a transcriptional or posttranscriptional locus; the second to decrease or limit gene expression by decreasing mRN stability or increasing degradation.

transcriptional or posttranscriptional mechanism. Insulin and IGF-I play important custom tailoring roles in this situation. In some cases, however, TSH induces a second factor which acts to decrease the expression of the initially increased mRNA. The result is to limit the extent of bioactivity, as in the case of iodide uptake, or even to abolish the increase, as in the case of malic enzyme. The ability of TSH to induce this second factor appears to be regulated by a second hormone; in the case of iodide uptake and malic enzyme, this appears to be hydrocortisone. Obviously, the converse case, that hydrocortisone is the inducer and TSH the permissive agent cannot be excluded. Nevertheless, the complexity of the cross-regulation and the interdependence of the hormones is evident. TSH, as a first violinist, plays a complicated score involving not only other strings but the woodwinds as well.

THE LDL RECEPTOR IN THYROID CELLS: CHOLESTEROL METABOLISM AND TSH RECEPTOR MODULATED GROWTH

In previous considerations, the interrelatedness of hormone receptors and the affects of these relationships on the prime regulatory receptor of the thyroid, the TSH receptor, were addressed. Before proceeding to the structure of the TSH receptor itself, the presence of LDL receptors on thyroid cells must be addressed as well as the relationship between LDL receptors and TSH receptors.

The lipid composition of plasma membrane can dramatically alter its physical properties. For example, FRTL-5 cells cease dividing when exposed to a medium lacking TSH and display major changes in the lipid composition of their plasma membrane resulting in reduction of membrane fluidity (22, 23). The most notable lipid changes involve a more than two fold increase of membrane cholesterol, an increased cholesterol/phospholipid ratio, and an increased ratio of saturated to unsaturated fatty acids. The changes in membrane fluidity and lipid composition can be reversed by TSH or cyclic AMP derivatives.

Altered membrane lipids and membrane fluidity influence the growth of a cell and can affect the expression of receptors and membrane components important for coupling receptors to signal transduction systems. The relationship between cholesterogenesis and cell growth goes further; thus, the pathway of isoprenoid synthesis involves the formation of mevalonate as the product of 3-hydroxy-3-methylglutaryl coenzyme A (HMG-CoA) reductase, the rate limiting enzyme of cholesterol biosynthesis. It has been suggested that mevalonic acid may be the link between cholesterogenesis and cell proliferation since mevalonate is needed to restore proliferation in cells treated with compactin, a competitive inhibitor of HMG-CoA reductase (24, 25).

Since cholesterol metabolism in FRTL-5 cells is a critical TSH receptor-related function which, in turn, can influence the action of a host of other cell receptors and their functions, it is important to understand how TSH regulates cholesterol metabolism in the thyroid cell. FRTL-5 cells possess high affinity LDL receptors which bind, internalize and degrade LDL. When FRTL-5 cells are deprived of TSH, the binding of LDL increases more than two fold. Upon addition of TSH, at a concentration of $1x10^{-10}$ M or greater, LDL binding decreases rapidly and, within 24 hours, reaches the level which is typical of FRTL-5 cells chronically stimulated by TSH.

TSH regulation of LDL receptor activity in FRTL-5 cells could explain why, in the absence of the hormone, these cells accumulate of cholesterol. The relationship between a lower cholesterol uptake and an actively proliferating cell population may relate to the fact that (a) FRTL-5 cells are able to synthesize cholesterol and (b) the pathway of cholesterol biosynthesis and growth intersect. As noted above a key enzyme in cholesterol biosynthesis is HMG-CoA reductase; the key intermediate is the product of this enzyme, mevalonate. Other products of mevalonate such as dolichol or ubiquinone or isopentenyl adenine (26) are required for DNA synthesis and cell duplication. The ability of TSH to downregulate the LDL receptor in FRTL-5 cells would reduce cholesterol uptake but would also act as a signal for the activation of the pathway of endogenous cholesterol synthesis and the synthesis of mevalonate.

Studies of ^{14}C acetate incorporation into cholesterol and other lipids (27) have shown that FRTL-5 cells posses very active cholesterol synthesis, which is unusual amongst mammalian cells. When FRTL-5 cells are made quiescent by withdrawing TSH for seven days and are in a low serum (0.2%) milieu, subsequent addition of TSH to the culture medium increases acetate conversion into cholesterol, up to a maximum of 7-8 fold over the basal level. The effect of TSH on cholesterol synthesis is the result of the induction of greater activity of HMG-CoA reductase and a higher rate of transcription of the HMG-CoA reductase gene (Table 1). Thus, the steady state level of HMG-CoA reductase messenger RNA is increased 7-8 fold by TSH and so is the rate of transcription of the HMG-CoA reductase gene, as assessed by nuclear "run off" assay.

In summary, the LDL and TSH receptors are critically interrelated. This relationship influences the growth, morphology, and, very likely, the function of the cell.

THE TSH RECEPTOR IS NOT A WELL DEFINED ENTITY

The structure of the TSH receptor remains an enigma despite the efforts of a host of laboratories. Binding and purification studies (28-30) have suggested that the thyrotropin (TSH) receptor is composed of both a membrane glycoprotein and membrane ganglioside. The former acts as the high-affinity binding domain on the surface of the cell;. the latter is presumed to couple the binding domain to the adenylate cyclase-G protein signal complex (31, 32) and may modify the affinity as well as specificity of the binding domain. Studies with monoclonal antibodies to the TSH receptor (33-35) support this concept. They also indicate that the TSH receptor is coupled to multiple transducers, for example the phosphoinositide-Ca-arachidonic acid as well as the adenylate cyclase signal system, and that all are necessary for maximal growth and function. It is important to understand the detailed structure of the TSH receptor not only to understand its molecular mechanism of action in coupling signal systems to bioactivity and growth but also to understand the relationship between receptors in thyroid cells.

THE GLYCOPROTEIN COMPONENT OF THE TSH RECEPTOR

From Past Confusion a Picture of This Component Emerges

Purification by standard procedures has uncovered a high molecular weight TSH binding protein of about 300K and a host of smaller species (28-30). One of these was a 15 to 25K glycopeptide, which could be derived by tryptic digestion of either whole cells or solubilized membrane preparations, yet, could still bind TSH (36, 37). Cross-linking and immunoprecipitation studies using monoclonal antibodies to the TSH receptor (38) suggested, however, that a major TSH binding component might be about 70-80K but that there were also 45-55K and 20-30K forms or fragments, particularly if care was not taken to prevent protease digestion. Other higher molecular weight forms, for example 90K, 115-120K, or 140K, also were evident. The same multiplicity of TSH binding proteins was evident when methionine-radiolabeled, solubilized, membrane preparations from rat FRTL-5 thyroid cells were subjected to affinity chromatography on TSH-Sepharose then immunoprecipitated with monoclonal antibodies to the TSH receptor. Of particular note, however, was the observation that the pattern of bands was different if the experiment used cells treated with TSH as opposed to cells not exposed to TSH (35, 39, 40).

Although these last results could be interpreted to reflect the rapid synthesis and breakdown (turnover) of the TSH receptor when cells were exposed to TSH, it was not clear which might be the biosynthetic product, which the processed form, which the aggregate, which the subunit, which the degraded form or even which was the artifact. Further alternative explanations could not be excluded; for example, the bands might represent different TSH receptors which couple to different transduction signals.

Nevertheless, the sum of these studies suggested that the TSH-binding high affinity receptor component had to, in the final analysis, satisfy several structural constraints. First it had to be a glycoprotein. Second it had to have a 15-25K glycopeptide within its structure which could still bind TSH after protease digestion and had to be on the outside of the cell, possibly within a 45-55K larger component able to be released into the medium from cultured thyroid cells under different conditions. This last constraint implied the receptor might have only a single transmembrane domain. Third, any model would have to account for the multiplicity of other TSH-binding proteins as related or processed forms.

Cloning Studies Identify a Graves' Autoantigen which may be Related to the TSH Receptor Membrane Glycoprotein Component

In collaboration with the group from the National Institute of Dental Research interested in the basis of autoimmune phenomena, we immunoscreened a human thyroid carcinoma lambda gt11 expression library with an IgG preparation from a patient with active Graves' disease (41). The IgG preparation was highly positive in assays measuring thyroid stimulating antibodies (TSAbs), thyrotropin binding inhibiting antibodies (TBIAbs) and thyroid growth promoting antibodies (TGPAbs). Although the IgG preparation contained no detectable microsomal or thyroglobulin antibodies, it was presumed that the IgG preparation would react to a multiplicity of autoantigens other than the TSH receptor.

In a separate approach (42) we immunoscreened a FRTL-5 rat thyroid cell lambda gt11 expression library with a polyclonal rabbit antibody developed against FRTL-5 thyroid cell TSH receptor preparations purified by affinity chromatography on TSH-Sepharose and reactive with monoclonal TSH receptor antibody-Sepharose (35, 39, 40). This rabbit antibody immunoprecipitated the same multiplicity of TSH-binding proteins as did the monoclonal antibodies to the TSH receptor and as were evident in purification studies. It could, however, inhibit TSH-induced increases in cAMP levels and thymidine incorporation into DNA (growth) in FRTL-5 cells, indicating that it did indeed contain antibodies directed against the functional TSH receptor. The rat FRTL-5 thyroid cell is a continuously cultured thyroid cell line which maintains most properties of thyroid cells in vivo (5, 9); there was no possibility, therefore, that this cDNA library was contaminated by the presence of other tissues, including lymphocytes.

Immunoscreening with the Graves' autoantibody identified 25 different human cDNA clones. Immunoscreening with the rabbit antibody to the TSH receptor preparation resulted in a single rat cDNA clone. The latter cDNA clone was identical in size, 1.25 Kb, and restriction mapping to one of the 25 human cDNA clones; each exhibited cross-hybridization with the other indicating they were identical or near identical. These results suggested the cDNA coded for an autoantigen related to the TSH receptor.

The cDNA from both clones identified a 2 Kb mRNA in thyroid tissues or cells from a multiplicity of species (Fig. 18) and was present in human IM9 lymphocytes and adipocyte preparations which have TSH receptor activity. THE 2 Kb mRNA was not present in human or rat tissues such brain, liver, kidney or muscle. The presence or

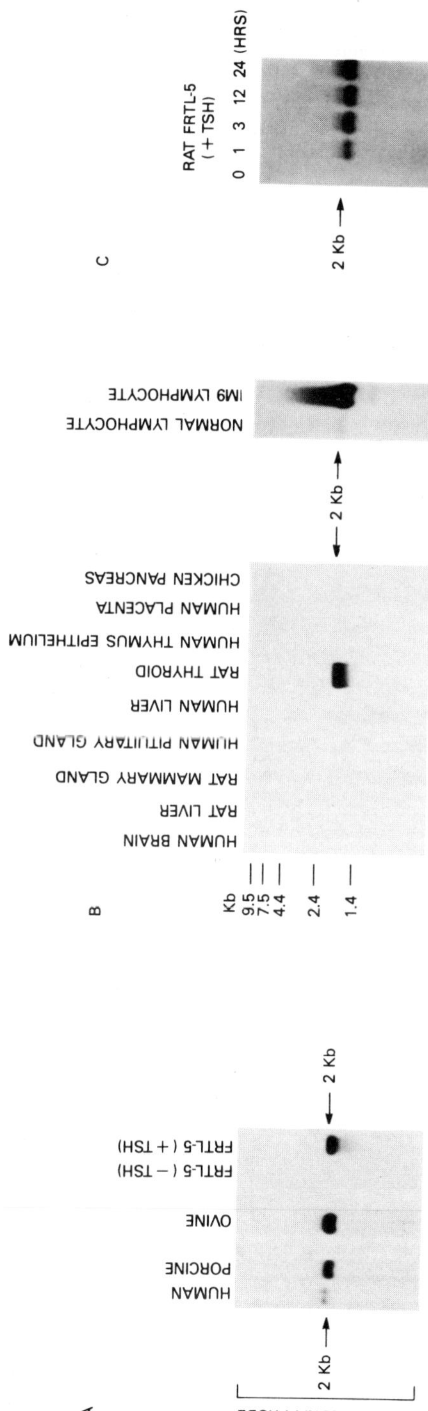

Figure 18. Northern blot analysis of poly A+ mRNA isolated from different thyroid tissues or cells, IM9 and normal lymphocytes, and the other tissues noted using a 1.25 Kb insert derived from the 3' portion of the cDNA of Figure 19. Five micrograms of poly A+ mRNA was applied and resolved on 1% formaldehyde denaturing gels. The same blots were rehybridized with a beta-actin probe to ensure that negative blots did not result from degradation of the mRNA. In (C) the time dependent ability of TSH to increase mRNA identified by this cDNA is noted.

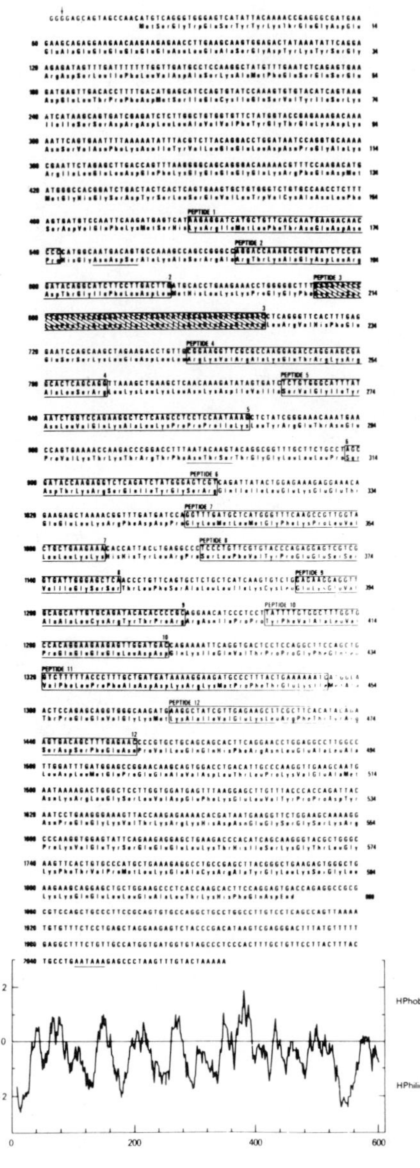

Figure 19. The complete nucleotide and deduced amino acid sequence of a cDNA from the human thyroid carcinoma library (41). The polyadenylation signal AATAAA is underlined. Two potential glycosylation sites are also underlined. A substitution of T for G (arrow) in the sequence of the comparable cDNA from a human Graves' thyroid library defines an in-frame stop codon and the full length sequence. The blocks denote sequences which were used to synthesize peptides for use in the studies of Figure 22.

absence of demonstrable mRNA in poly A+ RNA preparations thus appeared to correlate with the presence or absence of TSH receptor expression in tissues, since studies had established that TSH receptors existed in the adipocytes (43) and IM9 lymphocytes (44), as well as thyroid. Nevertheless, it was evident that the level of expression in different tissues did not relate to functional expression of TSH receptor. This is obvious in the fact that the IM9 lymphocyte transcript was detectable in total RNA preparations whereas in thyroid cells poly A+ RNA is required for Northern analysis. If this were the TSH receptor glycoprotein component, it seemed, therefore, to be similar to the insulin receptor in IM9 lymphocytes in that there is a high level of receptor expression which does not correlate with the function we ordinarily ascribe to the receptor.

Full length clones of each cDNA were isolated and completely sequenced from both the human and rat FRTL-5 cell thyroid libraries. The sequence of the human thyroid carcinoma cDNA clone, together with its predicted amino acid sequence, is presented in Figure 19. Several important features can be discerned. First, there are two potential N-linked glycosylation sites (Asn-X-Ser/Thr, underlined). Second although a hydrophobicity plot of the sequence reveals multiple hydrophobic areas (Fig. 19), only one is compatible with a membrane spanning domain, residues 374-390 (Fig. 19). Third, the clone appears to be full length with a start codon surrounded by a nucleotide sequence in good agreement with consensus start sequences (45), an in-frame stop codon 15 bases upstream (arrow) of this ATG, and a poly A tail 18 bases downstream of a polyadenylation signal (underlined). The clone has an open reading frame of 1827 nucleotides which encodes a protein of 69,812 daltons.

The protein product of the full length clone, obtained after in vitro transcription/translation experiments was an autoantigen in that it reacted with the sera of a multiplicity of Graves' patients, not simply the screening antisera, but not with normal sera similarly diluted (Fig. 20A and reference 41).

The radiolabeled in vitro transcription/translation product was also able to bind to Sepharose-TSH; this binding was inhibited by free TSH but not by free insulin, ACTH, prolactin, cholera toxin, or even hCG (Fig. 20B). The radiolabeled protein could also be immunoprecipitated by a monoclonal antibody to the human

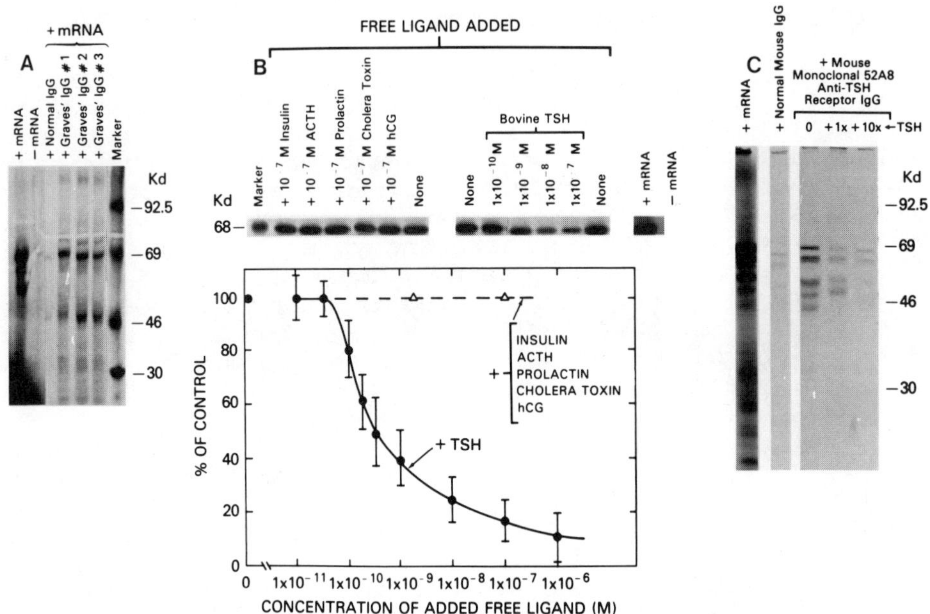

Figure 20. Ability of [^{35}S]methionine -labeled in-vitro translation product of the full length sense transcript from Figure 19 (41) to react with (A) IgG preparations from normals or from patients with Graves' disease, (B) with Sepharose coupled TSH in the presence or absence of the noted concentrations of free hormone or (C) with a monoclonal antibody, 52A8, directed against the TSH receptor (33-35). In each panel there is a minus (-) mRNA control to ensure the specificity of the translation reaction. The ability of free TSH to inhibit the interaction of the radiolabeled translation product with TSH-Sepharose is plotted as % of control, the interaction in the absence of free TSH; these data are derived from densitometry readings of the autoradiograms. The points are the mean of three separate experiments; the bars represent the standard error of the mean. The ability of the [^{35}S]methionine-labeled in-vitro translation product of the full length sense transcript from Figure 19 (41) to react with Sepharose coupled monoclonal antibody 52A8 directed at the TSH receptor was measured both in the absence and presence of free TSH. This antibody is a "mixed" antibody, one which can both stimulate cAMP levels in FRTL-5 thyroid cells and inhibit TSH binding. It is a competitive agonist of TSH.

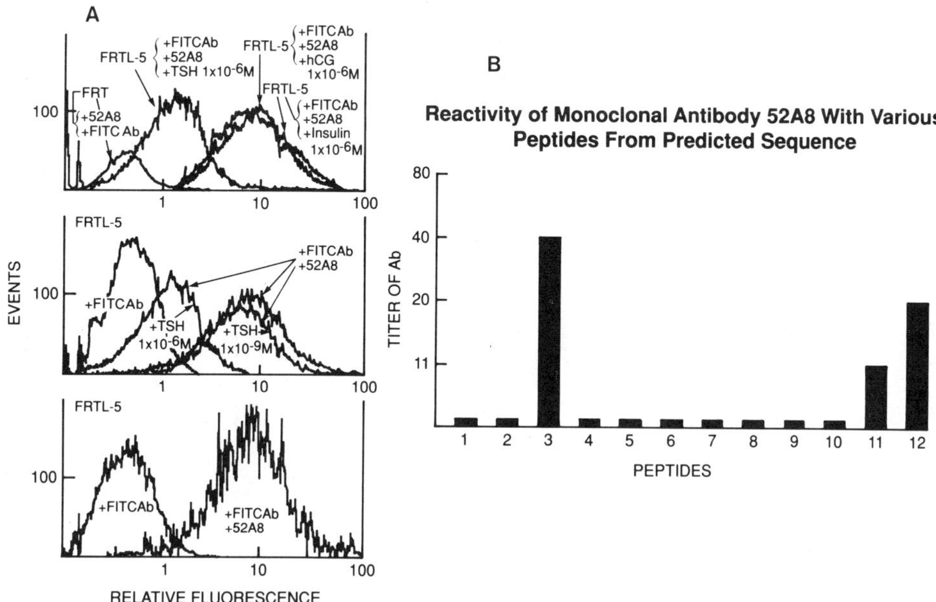

Figure 21A. Ability of the 52A8 monoclonal antibody to the TSH receptor to interact with FRTL-5 thyroid cells in the presence or absence of TSH, insulin, or chorionic gonadotropin (hCG) as measured by fluorescence activated cell sorting (FACS). The bottom panel demonstrates the specificity of the reaction in that the reactivity requires the presence of 52A8 and does not occur with the fluorescein isothiocyanate coupled (FITC) second antibody. The middle panel shows that the TSH inhibition is concentration dependent. The top panel shows that insulin or hCG do not duplicate the TSH inhibition at a high concentration of ligand. Also evident is the absence of the 52A8 reaction with FRT cells which do not have a surface expressed glycoprotein component of the TSH receptor.
Figure 21B. The ability of synthetic peptides matching the different portions of the predicted sequence in Figure 19 (see blocks) to react with monoclonal antibody 52A8 as measured in a solid phase radioimmunoassay.

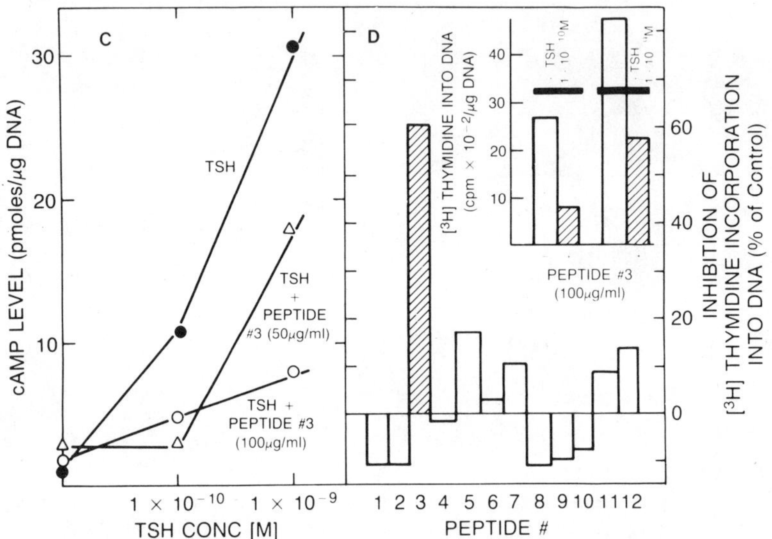

Figure 22. (C) Ability of peptide 3 to inhibit TSH-stimulated cAMP elevations in FRTL-5 thyroid cells. Experiments were performed as described in reference 9. Other peptides tested at the same concentrations had no affect (data not shown). (D) Ability of the different peptides, 100 micrograms/ml, to inhibit 1 x 10^{-10} M TSH stimulated tritiated thymidine incorporation into the DNA of FRTL-5 thyroid cells, an assay which has been shown to measure growth under these conditions (9). The insert tests peptide 3 at different TSH concentrations.

TSH receptor, 52A8; immunoprecipitation by 52A8 was again inhibited by free TSH (Fig. 20C) but not by the ligands above at a 10-fold higher concentration. In all cases (Fig. 20), the largest in vitro transcription/translation product has a molecular weight of approximately 70 Kd, close to the predicted molecular weight of the protein, 69,812. The lower molecular weight transcripts were incomplete translation products since they exhibited similar peptide maps. It is notable that a major protein immunoprecipitated by the autoantibody preparations is around 55K despite its relatively low abundance in the total translated mixture.

Monoclonal antibody 52A8, made against the human TSH receptor (33-35, 46, 47), has been termed a "mixed" antibody since it can be both a competitive antagonist, inhibiting TSH binding, and also a competitive agonist of TSH, stimulating adenylate cyclase and growth activities in FRTL-5 rat thyroid cells. These, as noted earlier, are a strain of continuously cultured cells which maintain many of the functional properties of the thyroid in vitro, including TSH regulation of growth and function. The 52A8 antibody binds to rat FRTL-5 thyroid cells; this binding can be inhibited by TSH but not by the same concentrations of insulin or hCG (Fig. 21A). Twelve peptides representative of different portions of the amino acid sequence predicted were synthesized (Fig. 19) and tested for reactivity with monoclonal 52A8 (Fig. 21B). Peptide 3, residues 212 through 228, was able to inhibit the ability of TSH to increase cAMP levels in FRTL-5 thyroid cells as well as the ability of TSH to increase tritiated thymidine incorporation into FRTL-5 cell DNA (Figs. 22C and 22D, respectively). In both cases, the peptide activity was concentration dependent.

Using 3T3 cells and mouse L cells transfections were performed involving (a) a dextran-DEAE procedure, (b) measurements of transient expression of TSH receptor expression by radiolabeled TSH binding 48 hours later, and (c) "sense" and "antisense" constructs of the full length clone with an SV 40 promotor. Increased expression of TSH-binding could be detected (Table 2) and an affinity as high as 10^{-9} M could be measured in cells transfected with the sense but not the antisense construct. In no case, however, was there an associated ability for TSH to increase cAMP levels when tested 15 min to 3 hours after exposure to TSH ($1x10^{-10}$ or $1x10^{-9}$ M). The TSH binding did, however, appear to be specific (Fig. 23) in that TSH binding was not inhibited by

TABLE 2

Radioiodinated TSH binding to cells transfected with sense (pSVL-FS2) and antisense (pSVL-FA) constructs of the full length clone whose sequence is presented in Figure 19.

CELLS	CONSTRUCT	Kd	SITES/CELL
L-Cells	pSVL-FS2	5×10^{-9} M	920
L-Cells	pSVL-FA	-	<50
3T3 Cells	pSVL-FS2	3×10^{-9} M	330
3T3 Cells	pSVL-FA	-	<50

pSVL (Pharmacia) was digested with Sma1 and dephosphorylated with alkaline phosphatase. Full length insert (41) was purified from agarose gel and filled in with dNTPs to create blunt ends. Vector and insert were ligated and transformed into HB101. Positive clones were selected by ampicillin resistance. Transfection used a dextran-DEAE procedure. After addition of heparin and washing, cells were cultured for 48 hours. TSH binding was measured as described (48).

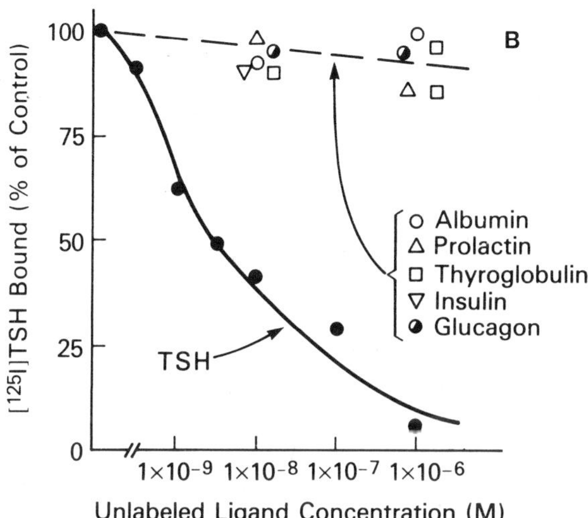

Figure 23. Ability of TSH to bind to 3T3 cells transiently transfected with the full length sense construct (pSVL-FS2), measured 48 hours later with radioiodinated TSH, using whole cells, and using the procedure described in reference 48. The radioiodinated TSH binding was measured in the presence of the noted concentration of unlabeled ligand. The transfection used a Dextran-DEAE procedure.

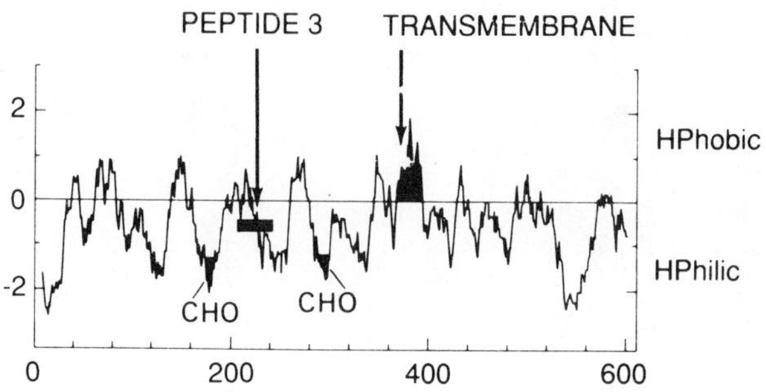

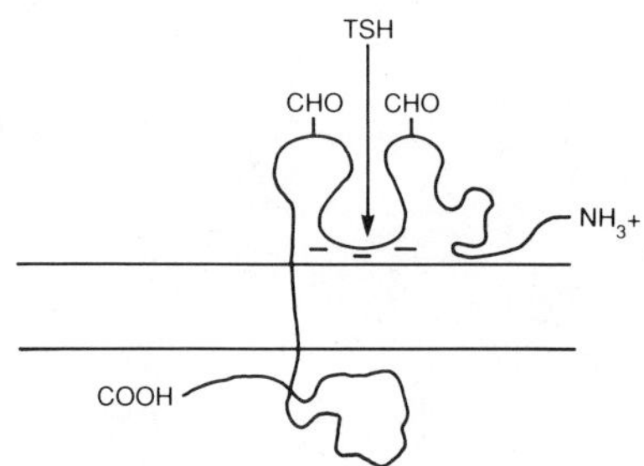

Figure 24. Model of TSH-binding transmembrane glycoprotein predicted from the data in Figure 19 and 22. The hydrophobicity plot (41) at the top is derived from the data of Figure 19. The two glycosylation sites (CHO) are noted as is the transmembrane domain. The region of peptide 3 which interacts with TSH and monoclonal antibodies to the TSH receptor is noted. The model at the bottom places this in the context of the lipid bilayer. A receptor with a single transmembrane domain is predicted; the TSH binding site, which is negatively charged, is between the glycosylation sites.

prolactin, albumin, thyroglobulin, insulin, or glucagon.

In sum, then the cloning studies identified a cDNA clone which coded for a thyroid autoantigen which was able to bind TSH and monoclonal antibodies to the TSH receptor. The autoantigen had two potential glycosylation sites and a single transmembrane domain. Between the two potential glycosylation sites was a peptide which binds a monoclonal antibody to the TSH receptor and inhibits TSH-stimulated growth and function. Modeling these characteristics (Fig. 24) results in a membrane-spanning TSH-binding glycoprotein which has many structural characteristics predicted for the TSH receptor from the early purification studies (28-30). Thus, it has a TSH-binding peptide which lies between two glycosylation sites that could define the 15-25K glycopeptide seen in purification studies; the carbohydrate would possibly protect it from trypsin digestion. There would be a 45-55 K domain external to the membrane, releasable from cells into the medium, and able to bind TSH. TSH binding is notoriously salt sensitive (28-30); the negative charge on the peptide would be compatible with this. Further the negative charge is in line with predictions from ganglioside studies (28-30) which suggest that the TSH-binding domain in the receptor is negatively charged to complement the positive charge on TSH. Its size, 70K, is compatible with a major TSH-binding protein seen in minutes when FRTL-5 thyroid cells are pulsed with radiolabeled methionine (35, 39, 40). The 50-55K form of the protein which is particularly reactive with Graves' autoantibody preparations (49) may be a processed form; multimers could account for the larger forms, i. e. the 280K, 140 K, and even 115-120K (70+50) seen in x-linking, lectin purification, and solubilization studies. Microsequencing should be able to help with at least a negative or positive answer. Because the 70 K form is a biosynthetic precursor it may be present as a non- or poorly glycosylated form which is not evident in lectin purification studies (50).

Supporting the view that this clone might code for a portion of the TSH receptor, the clone produced a TSH binding protein which could be expressed on the surface of cells and could exhibit specific properties of TSH-binding compatible with its identification as TSH receptor. The absence of coupling to the adenylate cyclase could reflect a requirement for a coupling component such as the thyroid specific ganglioside component of the TSH receptor or a missing subunit. This would be consistent with the lack of a primary sequence containing multiple hydrophobic stretches having sequence relationships to G-protein binding domains in the adrenergic receptor. It would be inconsistent with the preliminary report concerning the structure of the hCG receptor as defined in cloning studies (D. L. Segaloff, et. al., Serono Symposium on Glycoprotein Hormones). That structure has a G protein binding domaine. As a result, at this time, alternative explanations for these data must be considered, for example, there is more than one TSH-binding component or receptor in cells and these may be important in expression of autoimmune thyroid disease.

Provocative results have been obtained using a baculovirus expression system (51). Recombinant Autograhpha californica nuclear polyhedrosis virus containing the thyroid cDNA was produced by standard methods. Insect cells transfected with the recombinant virus produced a 70K protein in large amounts; the protein reacted on Western blots with antibodies produced against the peptides synthesized on the basis of the predicted amino acid sequence (Fig. 19). These data supported the conclusion that the predicted sequence is correct. Surprisingly, however, immunofluorescence and fractionation data indicate that the 70K protein is predominantly present in the nuclei of the infected insect cells and has undergone little or no glycosylation. At this point it is not clear what these data mean. Do they represent evidence of complex processing in the insect virus system which is a reflection of the protein in mammalian cells; could the receptor act as a transgenic agent like other receptors? Much remains to be done to complete our understanding and reconcile these results with results of the transfection experiments in mammalian cells.

Regulation of Transcript Expression

In FRTL-5 rat thyroid cells, TSH increases the synthesis and degradation of the TSH-binding glycoprotein defined by the clone in Figure 19, as evidenced by [S^{35}]methionine incorporation into protein immunoprecipitable by a monoclonal antibody to the TSH receptor (35, 39, 40). The 2 Kb mRNA identified by the cDNA described in this report is present in cells grown in the absence of TSH; however, its expression is increased by treatment of FRTL-5 cells with TSH (52). The time course of expression of the mRNA is rapid, consistent with the time course of the

TABLE 3

Effect of TSH and Insulin-like growth factor-I on the transcription in rat FRTL-5 thyroid cells of the TSH-binding protein defined by the ability of its nuclear transcript to bind to its cDNA by comparison to nuclear transcripts for thyroglobulin, beta-actin, and malic enzyme binding to their cDNAs.

	TIME (HOURS) AFTER TSH ADDITION			
	0	6	16	24
TSHBP/ACTIN	1	0.8	1.3	1.2
THYROGLOBULIN/ACTIN	1	1.2	2.4	3.2
MALIC ENZYME/ACTIN	1	0.6	0.9	1.0

FRTL-5 thyroid cells were maintained in 5H medium (no TSH) for 5 days in 5% serum and 2 additional days in 0.2% serum. Nucleii were isolated at the times indicated after the addition of TSH ($1x10^{-10}$M) and incubated in the presence of [^{32}P]UTP for 30 min at 24 C. RNA was purified, denatured, and hybridized with excess amounts of the noted probes which had been immobilized on Nitrocellulose filters. Filters containing a PUC-19 plasmid were included as a control; filters were incubated simultaneously with the radiolabeled nuclear RNA and radioactivity measured to determine the ratios.

immunoprecipitation data using the monoclonal antibody to the TSH receptor and methionine-labeled cells. Of interest, insulin-like growth factor-I (IGF-I) also can increase gene expression (52) and the effect of TSH and IGF-I is additive. The action of TSH appears to be post-transcriptional (Table 3) in contrast to its action on thyroglobulin gene expression.

Chromosome Localization

Using somatic cell human-hamster hybrids (53), 6 loci were identified on 5 different human chromosomes, namely 22q11-13, Xq, 1q, 8, and 10. The presumptive functional chromosome, 22q11-13, is associated with the Sis proto-oncogene. In mice (54), the gene is mapped to a single locus on chromosome 15, also appears to be associated with the sis proto-oncogene, and is on the same chromosome as the thyroglobulin and c-myc genes. Human chromosome 22 does not contain the thyroglobulin or c-myc genes. Southern blotting of EcoRI digested mouse genomic DNA, using the full length cDNA as probe, revealed 3 hybridizing bands of 14, 1.8, and 7.6 Kb from 5' to 3', respectively. Restriction enzyme mapping of the genomic clones suggest the mouse gene is 20-22 Kb.

These results are intriguing with respect to the possibility that the clone is a component of the TSH receptor and/or a very important TSH-binding autoantigen in Graves' disease. First, recent work (55) in patients with Graves' disease and exophthalmos suggests there is a significant increased frequency of P blood group by comparison to patients with Graves' disease who do not have exophthalmos. P blood group antigen is associated with the P1 antigen and in particular to the alpha-4-Gal transferase converting paragloboside to the P1 antigen. This antigen has been reported to be on human chromosome 22. Current studies (W. O. McBride and P. Kendall Taylor, and their collaborators, personal communication) indicate that it maps to the same locus 22q11-13, is also associated with the sis proto-oncogene, and is probably near but not identical to the gene coding for the cDNA described in these studies. Paragloboside and the P1 antigen are glycolipids which can be viewed as structural analogs of gangliosides. This association and these data are very exciting in that they offer the first clue, at a molecular level, as to the relation of Graves', its ophthalmopathy, and the TSH-binding membrane glycoprotein identified by the cDNA in these studies. The TSH binding component of the TSH receptor, rather than the receptor domain important in adenylate cyclase stimulation has been linked to exophthalmos in vitro (29).

Second, the identification of genomic material on the X chromosome is obviously provocative with respect to the dramatically increased frequency of Graves' in females. Whether this is more than fortuitous will, however, require much more understanding of the genomic significance of these multiple gene copies.

THE GLYCOLIPID COMPONENT OF THE TSH RECEPTOR IN FRTL-5 CELLS

When FRTL-5 thyroid cells were radiolabeled with radioactive N-acetyl glucosamine and detergent solubilized membrane preparations from the cells were subjected to sequential purification by TSH-affinity and monoclonal TSH receptor antibody-affinity chromatography, it was noted that preparations of the carbohydrate-labeled glycoprotein component of the receptor could be immunoprecipitated by monoclonal thyroid stimulating antibodies (TSAbs) such as 22A8 and 307H6 (35, 39). This was initially surprising since previous data indicated these TSAbs interacted preferentially with the ganglioside rather than the glycoprotein component of the TSH receptor (28-30, 33-35) in studies wherein the two components were purified separately then reacted with the antibodies. The answer to this dilemma emerged from the following experiment (35, 39, 40).

The carbohydrate radiolabeled preparations of TSH receptor immunoprecipitated by the two types of monoclonal antibodies to the TSH receptor, TSAbs and TBIAbs, were Folch extracted and shown to contain a carbohydrate-radiolabeled ganglioside as well as a carbohydrate-labeled glycoprotein (35, 39, 40). It is notable that this ganglioside has migratory characteristics on thin layer plates of GM_2 or GM_3 and that a ganglioside with similar migratory properties was identified as the "unique" thyroid ganglioside with high affinity to TSH (28-30, 33-35, 39, 40). This ganglioside purifies as a disialoganglioside and is fucosidase sensitive. In sum. FRTL-5 thyroid cells do have complex gangliosides, one of which reacts with monoclonal TSAbs; this ganglioside appears to exist as a tight complex with the glycoprotein component of the TSH receptor.

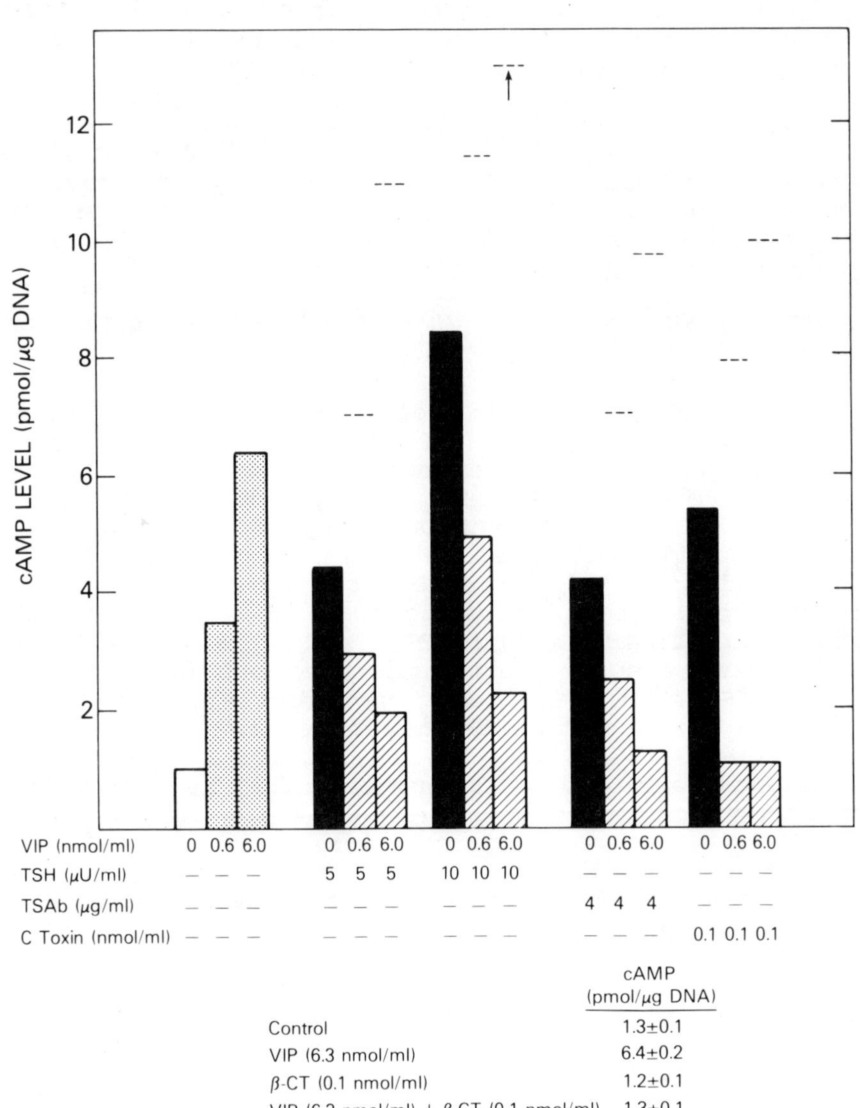

	cAMP (pmol/μg DNA)
Control	1.3±0.1
VIP (6.3 nmol/ml)	6.4±0.2
β-CT (0.1 nmol/ml)	1.2±0.1
VIP (6.3 nmol/ml) + β-CT (0.1 nmol/ml)	1.3±0.1

Figure 25. Ability of TSH, vasointestinal peptide, a human thyroid stimulating antibody and cholera toxin to increase cAMP levels in human thyroid cells in culture when tested at the noted concentrations and either alone or together. The assays were performed as described (31). The dashed lines represent the simple additive effects of the mixture of the ligands predicted from their agonist action when present alone in the incubation mixture.

<u>The ganglioside is related to other hormone receptors on thyroid cells and to coupling to the adenylate cyclase complex</u>

TSH, cholera toxin, and thyroid stimulating autoantibodies (TSAbs) are all able to increase cAMP levels in rat FRTL-5 thyroid cells and in primary cultures of human thyroid cells (31 and Fig. 25). Vasointestinal peptide (VIP) is also able to increase cAMP levels in human thyroid cells (Fig. 25). When, however, VIP is mixed with the TSH, cholera toxin or TSAbs, the ability of the agonists to increase cAMP levels is attenuated (Fig. 25). The agonist action of VIP was also attenuated by the beta subunit of cholera toxin (Fig. 25). These last data suggested (31) that a ganglioside must play an important role in the ability of VIP to couple its receptor to the cyclase complex. Thus, the beta subunit of cholera toxin is the binding subunit whose receptor is considered to be the ganglioside GM_1. Given the data from monoclonal and purification studies indicating a ganglioside was a critical TSH receptor component interacting with TSAbs, it seems reasonable to presume, as predicted (28-38), that a ganglioside will play a critical role in the TSH receptor coupling to the adenylate cyclase complex (Fig. 26).

<u>The ganglioside is a critical cell component interacting with G regulatory subunits of the adenylate cyclase complex</u>

Two studies (57, 58) have now shown that TSH interactions with thyroid cells can block the ability of pertussis toxin to ADP-ribosylate a G protein of the G_i type. These studies have both linked this action to activation of the thyroid adenylate cyclase complex.

A third recent study (32) has shown that under conditions where fucosyl GM_1 can increase FRTL-5 thyroid cell cAMP levels, pertussis toxin can inhibit the ganglioside action.

The sum of these studies continues to support the view that a ganglioside is a critical component of the TSH receptor and is very important in the coupling mechanism allowing the receptor to increase adenylate cyclase activity. The data further indicate the ganglioside acts as an intermediate between the binding

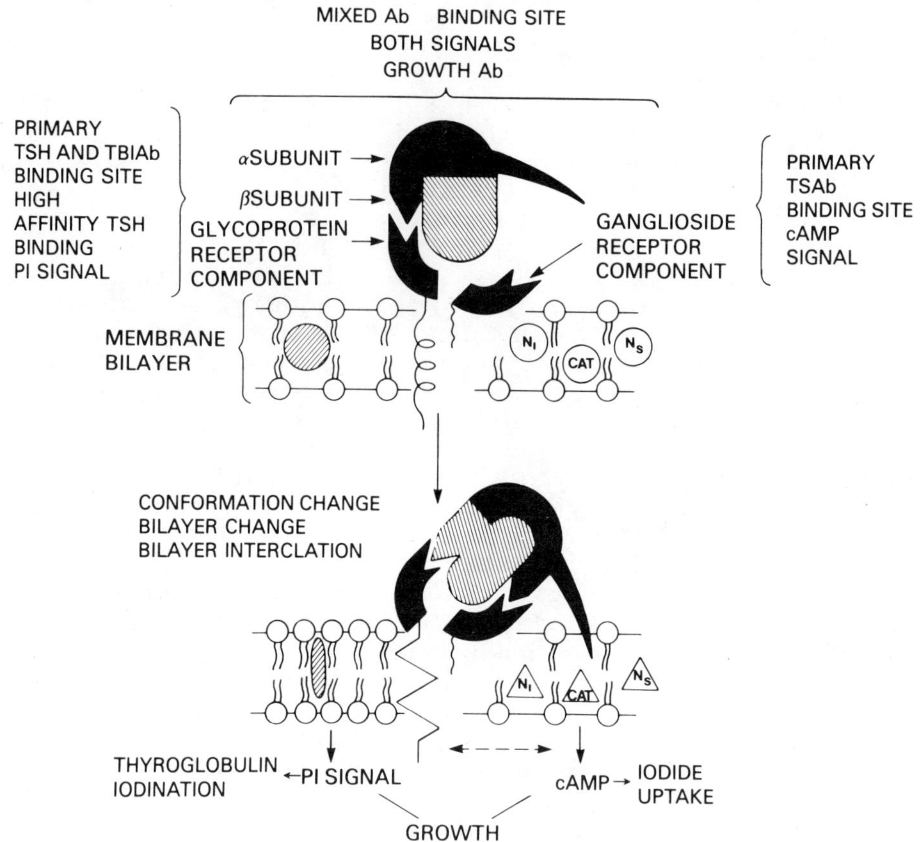

Figure 26. Proposed model of TSH receptor involving a high affinity TSH binding site whose prime membrane component is a glycoprotein and a coupling site to the adenylate cyclase complex involving a ganglioside. The ganglioside can modify the affinity and specificity of the glycoprotein receptor component. The glycoprotein receptor component can activate the Ca/phosphoinositide/arachidonic acid signal system which is important to iodide efflux and iodination of thyroglobulin. The site of interaction proposed for major groups of monoclonal antibodies to the TSH receptor is noted. TSH receptor action involves conformational changes in the hormone, alterations in the membrane bilayer, and intercalation of the alpha subunit of TSH into the bilayer where it is proposed a vasopressin-like peptide sequence described to be on the alpha subunit can interact with enzymes important for ADPribosylation action and components of the adenylate cyclase complex.

site on the glycoprotein component of the receptor and a G protein (Fig 26).

SUMMARY

A basic reason for undertaking these studies was to further our knowledge of the structure and function of the TSH receptor as well as its interaction with other receptors on thyroid cells. The multiplicity of observations suggests the approach is bearing fruit, does not provide a simple answer, and can have pitfalls. We hope they may also contribute to understanding the structure and function of autoantigens in Graves'disease and glycoprotein hormone receptors in general. The authors are grateful to their collaborators in the National Dental Institute, particularly Drs. Bellur Prabhakar, Edward Oates, and Abner Notkins, in the National Cancer Institute, Drs. W. O. McBride and M. Lerman for their contributions to the cloning studies.

REFERENCES

1. G. A. Robison, R. W. Butcher and E. W. Sutherland, "Cyclic AMP," Academic Press, New York (1971).
2. J. E. Dumont, The action of thyrotropin on thyroid metabolism, Vitam. Horm. (N. Y.), 29: 287 (1971).
3. E. M. Ross and A. G. Gilman, Biochemical properties of hormone sensitive adenylate cyclase, Ann. Rev. Biochem., 49: 533 (1980).
4. F. S. Ambesi-Impiombato, L. A. M. Parks and H. G. Coon, Culture of hormone dependent epithelial cells from rat thyroids, Proc. Natl. Acad. Sci. USA, 77: 3455 (1980).
5. F. S. Ambesi-Impiombato, Living, fast-growing thyroid cell strain, FRTL-5. US Patent 4,608,341, August 26 (1986).
6. C. M. Rotella, F. V. Alvarez, N. Perrotti, L. D. Kohn and S. Taylor, Characterization of receptors for insulin and IGF-I on FRTL-5 thyroid cells, in: "Control of the Thyroid Gland: Regulation of its Normal Function and Growth," Plenum Publishing Corp., New York (1989).
7. P. Santisteban, L. D. Kohn and R. DiLauro, Thyroglobulin gene expression is regulated by insulin and IGF-I, as well as thyrotropin, in FRTL-5 thyroid cells, J. Biol. Chem., 262: 4048 (1987).

8. G. Van Heuverswyn, C. Streydio, H. Brocas, S. Refetoff, J. Dumont and G. Vassart, Thyrotropin controls transcription of the thyroglobulin gene, Proc. Natl. Acad. Sci. USA, 81: 5941 (1984).
9. L. D. Kohn, W. A. Valente, E. F. Grollman, S. M. Aloj and P. Vitti, Clinical determination and/or quantification of thyrotropin and a variety of thyroid stimulatory or inhibitory factors performed in vitro with an improved thyroid cell line FRTL-5, US Patent 4,609,622, Sept 2 (1986).
10. O. Isozaki and L. D. Kohn, Control of c-fos and c-myc protooncogene induction in rat thyroid cells in culture, Mol. Endo., 1: 839 (1987).
11. Y. Shishiba, M. Yanagashita and V. C. Hascall, Characterization of proteoglycans synthesized by rat thyroid cells in culture and their response to thyroid stimulating hormone, J. Biol. Chem., 263: 1745 (1987).
12. F. V. Alvarez, C. M. Rotella, W. A. Valente, J. Y. Chan, O. Isozaki, R. Toccafondi, A. D. Kohn and L. D. Kohn, Glycosaminoglycan synthesis in thyroid cells: stimulation by throtropin, insulin-like growth factor I, and IgG preparations from Graves' patients with pretibial myxedema, in: "The Thyroid, 1988," S. Nagataki and K. Torizuka, eds., Excerpta Medica Int. Cong. Series 796, Elsevier Science Publishers, Amsterdam (1988).
13. D. Corda, L. Iacovelli, and M. DiGirolamo, Coupling of the alpha 1·adrenergic receptor and thyrotropin receptors to second messenger systems in thyroid cells: role of G proteins, Horizons in Endocrinology, 52: 169 (1988).
14. F. Okajima, K. Sho and Y. Kondo, Inhibition by islet-activating protein, pertussis toxin, of P2-purinergic receptor-mediated iodide efflux and phosphoinositide turnover in FRTL-5 cells, Endocrinology, 123: 1035 (1988).
15. J. E. Fradkin, W. C. Hardy and J. Wolff, Adenosine receptor- mediated accumulation of cAMP in guinea pig thyroid tissue, Endocrinology, 110: 2018 (1982).
16. L. D. Garren, R. D. Howell, G. M. Tomkins and R. M. Crocco, A paradoxical effect of actinomycin D: the mechanism of regulation of enzyme synthesis by hydrocortisone, Proc. Natl. Acad. Sci. USA, 52: 1121 (1964).
17. J. R. Reel and F. T. Kenney, Superinduction of tyrosine aminotransferase in hepatoma cell cultures: differential inhibition of synthesis and turnover by actinomycin D, Proc. Natl. Acad. Sci. USA, 68: 20 (1968).

18. E. B. Thompson, Glucocorticoid induction of tyrosine aminotransferase in cultured cells, in: Glucocorticoid Hormone Action, J. D. Baxter and G. G. Rousseau, eds., Springer-Verlag, Berlin (1979).
19. C. Marcocci, J. L. Cohen and E. F. Grollman, Efeect of actinomycin D on iodide transport in FRTL-5 thyroid cells, Endocrinology, 115: 2123 (1984).
20. A.D. Kohn, J. Y. Chan, D. Grieco, V. Nikodem, S. M. Aloj and L. D. Kohn, Thyrotropin increases malic enzyme mRNA levels in rat FRTL-5 thyroid cells, Mol. Endo., 3: in press (1989).
21. S. M. Aloj, D. Grieco, V. M. Nikodem, J. E. Rall and L. D. Kohn, Thyrotropin regulation of malic enzyme in FRTL-5 rat thyroid cells, J. Biol. Chem., submitted (1989).
22. F. Beguinot, S. Formisano, C. M. Rotella, L. D. Kohn and S. M. Aloj, Structural changes caused by thyrotropin in thyroid cells and in liposomes containing reconstituted thyrotropin receptor, Biochem. Biophys. Res. Commun., 110: 48 (1983)
23. F. Beguinot, L. Beguinot, D. Tramantano, C. Duilio, S. Formisano, M. Bifulco, F. S. Ambesi-Impiombato and S. M. Aloj, Thyrotropin regulation of membrane fluidity in FRTL-5 thyroid cells, J. Biol. Chem., 262: 1575 (1987).
24. I. Kaneko, Y. Hazama-Shimada and A. Endo, Inhibitory effects on lipid metabolism of cultured cells of ML-2363, a potent inhibitor of HMG CoA reductase, Eur. J. Biochem., 87: 313 (1978).
25. M. S. Brown and J. L. Goldstein, Multivalent feedback regulation of HMG CoA reductase: a control mechanism coordinating isoprenoid synthesis and cell growth, J. Lipid Res., 21: 505 (1980).
26. M. D. Siperstein, Role of cholesterogenesis and isoprenoid synthesis in DNA replication and cell growth, J. Lipid Res., 25: 1462 (1984).
27. M. Bifulco, A. Romano, D. Grieco, and S. M. Aloj, TSH regulation of cholesterol mertabolism in thyroid cells: its relation to cell replication, Ann. d'Endocriologie, Masson, Montpelier (1988).
28. L. D. Kohn, Relationships in the structure and function of receptors for glycoprotein hormones, bacterial toxins, and interferon, in: "Receptors and Recognition, Series A," P. Cuatrecassas and M. F. Greaves, eds., Chapman and Hall, London (1978).
29. P. Laccetti, E. F. Grollman, S. M. Aloj, and L. D. Kohn, Ganglioside dependent return of TSH receptor function in a rat thyroid tumor with a TSH receptor defect, Biochem. Biophys. Res. Commun., 110: 772 (1983).

30 L. D. Kohn, S. M. Aloj, D. Tombaccini D, C. M. Rotella, R. Toccafondi, C. Marcocci, D. Corda and E. F. Grollman, The thyrotropin receptor, in: "Biochemical Actions of Hormones," G. Litwak, ed., Marcel Dekker, New York (1985).

31. L. M. Brandi, C. M. Rotella, F. D. Ledley, L. D. Kohn and R. Toccafondi, Interactions among TSH, vasointestinal peptide, monoclonal antibodies to the TSH receptor and cholera toxin in normal human thyroid cell cultures, J. Clin. Endocrinol. Metab., 62: 1199 (1986).

32. S. Kosugi, T. Mori, M. Iwamori, Y. Nagai and H. Imura, Islet cell-activating protein reverses antifucosyl GM1 ganglioside antibody-induced inhibition of adenosine 3',5'-monophosphate production in FRTL-5 rat thyroid cells, Endocrinology, 124: 1230 (1989).

33. L. D. Kohn, E. Yavin, Z. Yavin, P. Laccetti, P. Vitti, E. F. Grollman and W. A. Valente, Autoimmune thyroid disease studied with monoclonal antibodies to the TSH receptor, in: "Monoclonal Antibodies: Probes for the Study of Autoimmunity and Immunodeficiency," B. F. Haynes and G. S. Eisenbarth, eds., Academic Press, New York (1983).

34. L. D. Kohn , D. Tombaccini, M. DeLuca, M. Bifulco, E. F. Grollman and W. A. Valente, Monoclonal antibodies and the thyrotropin receptor, in: " Monoclonal Antibodies to Receptors: Probes for Receptor Structure and Function," M. F. Greaves, ed., Receptors and Recognition, Series B., 17: 201 (1984).

35. L. D. Kohn, F. V. Alvarez, C. Marcocci, A. D. Kohn, A. Chen, W. E. Hoffman, D. Tombaccini, W. A. Valente, M. DeLuca, P. Santisteban, and E. F. Grollman, Monoclonal antibody studies defining the origin and properties of Graves' autoantibodies, Ann. N. Y. Acad. Sci., 475: 157 (1986).

36. R. L. Tate, H. I. Schwartz, J. M. Holmes, L. D Kohn and R. J. Winand, TSH receptors in thyroid plasma membranes: characteristics of TSH binding and solubilization of TSH receptor activity by trypsin digestion, J. Biol. Chem., 250: 6509 (1975).

37. R. J. Winand and L. D. Kohn , TSH effects on thyroid cells in culture: effects of trypsin on the TSH receptor and on TSH mediated cAMP changes, J. Biol. Chem., 250: 6534 (1975).

38. L. D. Kohn, W. A. Valente, P. Lacettei, J. Cohen, S. M. Aloj and E. F. Grollman, Multicomponent structure of the thyrotropin receptor:

relationships to Graves' disease, Life Sciences, 32: 15 (1983).

39. J. Y. Chan, P. Santisteban, M. DeLuca, O. Isozaki, E. F. Grollman, and L. D. Kohn, TSH receptor structure, Acta Endocrinologia (Copenh), Suppl. 281, 115: 166 (1987).

40. J. Y. Chan, M. DeLuca, P. Santisteban, O. Isozaki, S. Shifrin, S. M. Aloj, E. F. Grollman, and L. D. Kohn, Nature of thyroid autoantigens: the TSH receptor, in: "Thyroid autoimmunity," A. Pinchera, S. H. Ingbar and J. M. McKenzie, eds., Plenum Press, New York (1987).

41. J. Y. Chan, M. Lerman, B. S. Prabhakar, O. Isozaki, P. Santisteban, R. C. Kuppers, E. L. Oates, A. L. Notkins and L. D. Kohn, Cloning and characterization of a cDNA that encodes a 70-kDa novel human thyroid autoantigen, J. Biol. Chem., 264: 3651, (1989).

42. L. D. Kohn, O. Isozaki, J. Y. Chan, T. Akamizu, S. Bellur, M. De Luca, P. Santisteban, A. M. Varutti, S. Grimaz, S. Ikuyama, M. Saji, and G. Owens, The thyrotropin receptor in FRTL-5 thyroid cells: a cloning approach, in: "FRTL-5 Today," H. Perrild and F. S. Ambesi-Impiombato, eds., Elsevier Medical Sciences, Amsterdam (1989).

43. B. R. Mullin, G. Lee, F. D. Ledley, R. J. Winand and L. D. Kohn, Thyrotropin interactions with human fat cell membrane preparations and the finding of a soluble TSH binding component, Biochem. Biophys. Res. Commun., 69: 55 (1976).

44. F. Pekonen and B. D. Weintraub, Thyrotropin binding to cultured lymphocytes and thyroid cells, Endocrinology, 103: 1668 (1978).

45. M. Kozak, An analysis of 5'-noncoding sequences from 699 vertebrate mRNAs, Nucleic Acids Res. 15: 8125 (1987).

46. W. A. Valente, P. Vitti, Z. Yavin, E. Yavin, C. M. Rotella, E. F. Grollman, R. S. Toccafondi and L. D. Kohn, Monoclonal antibodies to the thyrotropin receptor: the identification of blocking and stimulating antibodies, Proc. Natl. Acad. Sci. USA, 79: 6680 (1982).

47. W. A. Valente, P. Vitti, C. M. Rotella, M. M. Vaughan, S. M. Aloj, E. F. Grollman, F. S. Ambesi-Impiombato and L. D. Kohn, Antibodies that promote thyroid growth: a distinct population of thyroid-stimulating autoantibodies, N. Engl.J.Med., 309: 1028 (1983).

48. E. F. Grollman, G. Lee, F. S. Ambesi-Impiombato, M.

F. Meldolesi, S. M. Aloj, H. G. Coon, H. R. Kaback and L. D. Kohn, Effects of thyrotropin on thyroid cell membrane: hyperpolarization induced by hormone-receptor interaction, Proc. Natl. Acad. Sci. USA, 74: 2352 (1977).

49. L. Bartalena, G. Fenzi, P. Vitti, D. Tombaccini, A. Antonelli, E. Macchia, L. Chiovato, L. D. Kohn and A. Pinchera, Interaction of the TSH receptor of rat FRTL-5 thyroid cells with TSH and a thyrotropin-stimulating autoantibody from Graves' patients, Biochem. Biophys. Res. Commun., 143: 266 (1986).

50. B. C. Kress and R. G. Spiro, Studies on the glycoprotein nature of the thyrotropin receptor: interaction with lectins and purification of the bovine protein with the use of Bandeiraca (Griffonia) simplicifolia I affinity chromatography, Endocrinology, 118: 974 (1986).

51. G. P. Allaway, B. S. Prabhakar, A. A. Vivino, J. Y. Chan, L. D. Kohn and A. L. Notkins, Characterization of a novel 70 kilodalton thyroid autoantigen produced in the baculovirus expression system. [Abstract], Proceedings 23rd Annual Meeting European Society for Clinical Investigation, Elsevier, Amsterdam (1989).

52. L. D. Kohn, O. Isozaki, J. Y. Chan, T. Akamizu, S. Bellur, P. Santisteban, S. Ikuyama, M. Saji, S. Doi, K. Tahara, S. Kosugi, H. Sabe, and T. Mori, Characterization of the thyrotropin receptor and other Graves' disease autoantigens, in: "Proceedings International Symposium on Glycoprotein Hormones," W. Chin, ed., Plenum Publishing Corp. New York (1989).

53. J. Y. Chan, M. Lerman, W. O. McBride, P. Santisteban, O. Isozaki, A. L. Notkins and L. D. Kohn, Isolation, characterization, and chromosomal localization of a cDNA clone of an autoantigen in Graves' disease also identified by antibodies to the TSH receptor. [Abstract] 62nd Meeting American Thyroid Association, Endocrinology, 120 (Supplement): T16 (1987).

54. J. Y. Chan, P. Santisteban, C. Kozak, R. C. Kuppers and L.D. Kohn, Genomic organization and chromosomal mapping of a mouse lymphocyte gene: its cDNA sequence is homologous to a thyroid autoantigen. [Abstract] 63rd Meeting American Thyroid Association, Endocrinology, 121 (Supplement): T52 (1988).

55. P. Kendall-Taylor, A. Stephenson, A. Stratton, S. S. Papiha, P. Perros and D. F. Roberts, Differentiation of autoimmune opthalmopathy from Graves' hyperthyroidism by analysis of genetic markers. Clinical Endocrinology, 28: 601 (1988).
56. C. M. Rotella, R. Zonefrate, R. Toccafondi, W. A. Valente, and L. D. Kohn, Ability of monoclonal antibodies to the TSH receptor to increase collagen synthesis in human fibroblasts, an assay which appears to measure exophthalmogenic immunoglobulins in Graves' sera, J. Clin. Endocrinol. Metab. 62: 357 (1986).
57. D. Corda, R. D. Sekura and L. D. Kohn, Thyrotropin effect on the availability of Ni Regulatory protein in FRTL-5 thyroid cells to ADPribosylation by pertussis toxin, Eur. J. Biochem., 166: 475 (1987).
58. F. Riberio-Neto, L. Birnbaumer and J. B. Field, Incubation of bovine thyroid slices with TSH is associated with a decrease in the ability of pertussis toxin to ADPribosylate guanine nucleotide regulatory components, Mol. Endo., 1: 482, (1987).

EXCESS IODIDE INHIBITS THE THYROID BY MULTIPLE MECHANISMS

J. Wolff

National Institutes of Health, Bethesda, Maryland

The many nonsubstrate effects of iodide in the thyroid appear to be due to at least four mechanisms: 1) a possible anion effect of iodide for which the supporting data are conflicting; 2) an inhibition of organic iodine formation (the so-called Wolff-Chaikoff effect); 3) the iodination of critical enzymes in the thyroid gland; and 4) the inhibition of cellular processes by iodinated products such as oxidized iodine itself, or an oxidation reaction involving iodine. The separation into these categories is not firm, but circumstantial evidence suggests that the mechanisms are different. In addition, high levels of iodide will saturate the iodide pump (Ki $\approx 3 \times 10^{-5}$M) (1). In this case, however, the amounts of iodide which enter the thyroid cell remain large, despite transport saturation and are replaced by diffused iodide. Hence this subject will not be discussed here.

I. Anion Effects - Inhibitions in the Presence of Thionamides

The "pure iodide effects" are few and deal mainly with hormone secretion from the thyroid but there is disagreement as to whether or not they are really caused by the anion (Table I). For example, hormone secretion in man appears to be reduced by iodide administration in the presence of antithyroid agents but in dogs and rats (2) the antisecretory effect of iodides is prevented by thionamides. Again, changes in vascularity occur early after refeeding of iodide (3) but such effects may be due either to the anion, or to oxidized or organic forms or hormone. It is not possible to study this phenomenon under conditions where the reduced form of iodine is guaranteed, since thionamides will stimulate the thyroid. In general we have excluded long term iodide pretreatments from these discussions because interpretations are ambiguous.

TABLE I

ACUTE INHIBITORY EFFECTS OF IODIDE ANION
(NOT REVERSED BY THIONAMIDES)

REACTION	COMMENTS	REFERENCES
Pyridine Nucleotide Metabolism	Levels and Oxidation State	4,5
Thyroid Hormone Secretion (Man)	Blocked by Thionamides in Animals	6,7
Reduction of Thyroid Vascularity	By Thallium Uptake	8
Inhibition of Organic Iodine Formation	Wolff-Chaikoff Effect	9,10

*References before 1970 in (10)

Even with the iodide effects that are demonstrable in the presence of thionamides it is difficult to be certain that the "block" is complete. A case in point is the dependence of the antisecretory effect of iodide in rat thyroids on the dose of PTU used (2). Thus, either enough iodide gets through the thionamide block or inhibition is a true anion effect. If the former case, then the PTU-resistant inhibitions would somehow have to be more sensitive to the products of oxidized iodine than the thionamide-sensitive pathways discussed below. This seems unlikely but cannot be ruled out. Alternatively, the two classes of inhibitions result from responses to different iodinated products. This will be expanded below.

If there are true iodide anion effects, then there is a possibility that they should be mimicked by other anions that are related to iodide by hydration enthalpy, size and accumulation by the thyroid (1,11). This has been tested in only one case - reduction in the size of thionamide-induced goiter (12,13). We like to view the antigoitrogenic effects of perchlorate, ReO_4^- etc found many years ago as an anion effect. The mechanism is not understood but may involve changes in growth factors (14) and hence have an extrathyroidal component. The mechanisms by which such effects are produced are unknown.

II. Competition for "Active" Iodine-Inhibition of Organic Iodine Synthesis

When one studies thyroidal organic iodine synthesis as a function of iodide concentration, a linear increase occurs over a considerable range of I^- but, instead of saturating toward a plateau when other factors become rate-limiting, organic iodine formation decreases steeply as a function of iodide concentration (10,15). The order of the effect is >1 and the plateau (if any) is converted to a peak. Total synthesis may decrease to below that of the unsupplemented system. This is the so called Wolff-Chaikoff effect (9). It has been a favorite subject for investigators, has been frequently reviewed (10,16,17,18,19), and our concern here is only with the mechanism by which excess iodide produces the effect, not with the pharmacology.

Iodination reactions in biological systems require some form of oxidized iodine such as $I^{\cdot}$, I^o, I_2, I^+, IO^-, etc. One effect of excess iodide is to compete for one or more of these forms and to convert them to species that are poor or inactive in iodination reactions involving the ortho phenolic position of tyrosine. Initial speculations on the mechanism of the iodide effect were based on the assumption that simple equilibria involving I_2 were involved, as e.g. in $I_2 + H_2O \longrightarrow IOH + H^+ + I^-$, or $I_3^- \longrightarrow I_2 + I^-$. However, to account for other determinants, more detailed rate equations for iodination were developed by including phenolic dissociation constants, a rate limiting step for the leaving proton (demonstrated by an isotope effect) etc. For example (20)

$$k_{obs} = \frac{k_b\ K_1\ K\phi\ K_2}{(K_1 + I^-)(K\phi + H^+)(K_2 + I^-)}$$

where K_1 = triiodide equilibrium
K_2 = is the equilibrium constant for iodine addition to the ortho position forming the protonated intermediate
$K\phi$ = phenolic dissociation constant
k_b = the base catalyzed leaving of the <u>ortho</u> proton

While yet more inclusive rate expressions can be devised, the important point is that frequently these reactions are second order in $1/[I^-]$, i.e. $[I^-]^{-2}$, and thus quite sensitive to iodide inhibition. In practice, the order may lie between 1 and 2 and may itself be a function of iodide concentration and thus may change during the reaction. Despite the seductive authority of such equations, they probably do not apply in the thyroid. Oxidized iodine complexed in thyroid peroxidase is the most likely iodinating species and the potentials and other properties of these species differ substantially from the free chemical forms. Moreover, the rates and products of chemical vs peroxidative or in vivo iodinations are quite different (21,22). Iodide nevertheless competes with substrate for the "active" species. Presumably this occurs while the "active iodine" is bound to the peroxidase, and I_2 is the "stable", and rather unreactive, end product of this competitive side reaction. For this reason the iodide effect has been listed as an anion type of effect in Table I.

There are two competing models for the iodide effect on peroxidative iodinations (Fig 1). One is based on one electron reactions leading to free radicals of iodine and tyrosyl, each on a separate site on the peroxidase. The tyrosyl site accepts iodide with lower affinity but production of a second $I^{\cdot}$ leads to I_2 formation rather than MIT. Tyrosine may also occupy the iodide site thus accounting for the experimental formation of bityrosine (22,23). A patient has been described with a peroxidase defect that permits I_2 formation but not MIT (24); this supports such a two site model. However, the one-electron model would require the formation of compound II from compound I (by a one-electron step) and this is not generally seen and there is little evidence for access of two sites to the heme group.

The second model, which is based on two electron oxidation of I^- to I^+ or IO^-, avoids the compound II problem but is less able to account for bityrosine formation and is less explicit as to whether or not the substitution reaction occurs with thyroglobulin on the peroxidase or through a "free" form of the "active" iodine. Moreover, if the coupling reaction is carried out by compound II, a one-electron reagent, (21, 25-27), then both types of reaction may have to occur in thyroid hormone formation. While the spectra of peroxidase permit much elegant analysis, the multiplicity of redox cycles that are possible has prevented definition of the exact iodination pathway. It is clear, however, that compound I oxidizes the iodide whereas compound II is more likely to be involved in catalyzing the coupling reaction (21,22). Both models account adequately for the iodide effect, and in the time frame of such studies it is perhaps not possible to distinguish two rapid, successive one-electron steps from a two-electron step, and different peroxidases may show different propensities to use one- or two-electron oxidations for the same substrate (26); hence lactoperoxidase may not always be a reliable model.

Iodide also catalyzes the coupling reaction (28), and this effect occurs at high concentrations of the anion. Whether this operates through one of the sites on peroxidases or by other means is not known. In addition, iodide may be involved in a number of side reactions associated with this system. Iodide protects the peroxidase against the formation of inactive compound III when excess H_2O_2 is present (27,29), and can slowly reconstitute native enzyme if compound III has been formed. Another "protective" effect of iodide is its participation in the catalatic destruction of H_2O_2 as indicated in

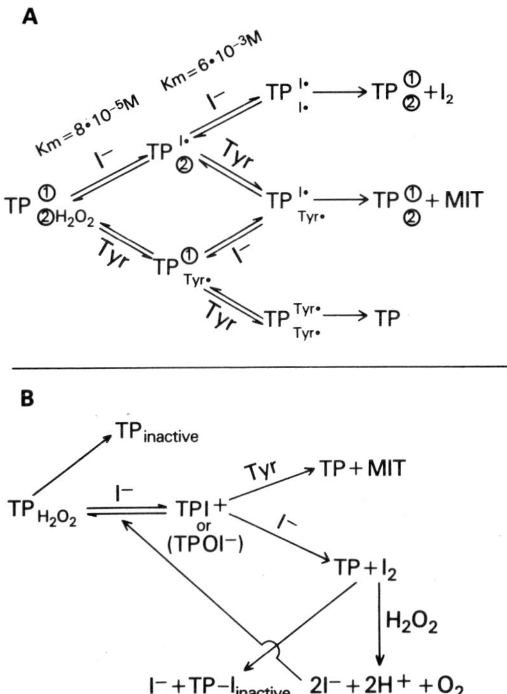

Fig 1. Current models for thyroid peroxidase-catalyzed iodinations. A) free-radical (•) model with two enzyme sites. Site 1 prefers I^- > tyrosine, site 2 prefers tyrosine > I^-; both sites may be occupied by the same ligand but with different affinities. B) Two electron iodination including the futile pathway for H_2O_2 consumption and two possible means for peroxidase inactivation, directly by excess H_2O_2 or indirectly by iodination. (Modified from (18)).

in Fig 1. Since I_2 could be regenerated with the consumption of further H_2O_2, this represents a futile cycle. While it has been shown that H_2O_2 generation is decreased in the presence of excess iodide (30-32), it is not certain whether the catalatic reaction contributes to this potential H_2O_2 deficiency. This reaction may also be related to the prevention of compound III formation mentioned above (27,33).

It is clear, therefore, that iodide can inhibit iodinations through any of the above mechanisms. To what extent iodinations of enzymes or iodinated inhibitors contribute to diminished iodinations in the intact thyroid gland remains to be determined.

III. Inhibitions Requiring Iodide Oxidation - Iodination of Critical Proteins

Initial attempts to explain all the effects of excess iodide on the anion or its competition of "active" iodine could not be sustained. Paradoxically, many of the other inhibitory effects required one or more iodinations, and thionamides prevented many of these inhibitions. Two modes of action can be envisioned: direct iodination and consequent inactivation of selected critical enzymes or cofactors; or the formation of, as yet unknown, iodinated compounds that secondarily inhibit various reactions. A partial list of such effects is presented in Table II. The inhibition of iodide transport probably accounts for the escape from, or adaption to, the acute Wolff-Chaikoff effect (35,36). Interestingly, there is also an effect on organic iodine formation involving oxidized iodine or a product that exists in addition to the iodide mediated competition for "active" iodine that can be demonstrated in isolated or purified systems. A number of the inhibitions requiring oxidized iodine appear to result from effects on adenylate cyclase. Judging from the various stimulators whose effect can be inhibited, the effect does not appear to be on the receptors. There remains, however, some uncertainty as to whether the primary inhibitory effect is on the Gs protein or the catalytic moiety (41,42). cAMP-independent reactions such as Ca^{2+} efflux, membrane potential, and PI turnover are also inhibited. In a number of pathways (secretion, protein synthesis) there is still controversy as to whether or not iodide oxidation is required. Since it is difficult to guarantee that the thionamide block is complete, especially under iodide loads, this question remains difficult to answer. Moreover, some reactions may be inhibited by more than one mechanism.

Under special conditions, when an oxidized form of iodine is allowed to accumulate, (limiting substrate conditions), peroxidase may itself become the substrate for iodination with consequent loss of activity (23,54,55). KI administration has been reported to reduce peroxidase activity in the thyroid by 50% in 2 hours (56), but this is not invariably found (30). It has not been established however, that this occurred by a suicide reaction. It has also been suggested that the inhibition of adenylate cyclase by excess iodide (discussed below) might result from iodination of the catalytic unit (42,57) but this has not been directly demonstrated. Such a proposal would require that the apically located peroxidase/iodine complex can reach the basally located adenylate cyclase. Similarly, Sherwin and Price (58) have suggested that a protein (≈8-10 kDa) believed to be involved in autoregulation may itself be regulated by iodination. The precise function of this protein has not been specified. It has also been shown (59) that membrane tubulin (60) will become iodinated whereas cytoplasmic tubulin will not. However, this is not enhanced by excess iodide. Finally, thyroglobulin hydrolysis can be inhibited by excess iodide in an oxidation-requiring reaction. Whether or not this is by

TABLE II

IODIDE EFFECTS MEDIATED BY IODINATION PRODUCTS

ACTIVITY INHIBITED (References*)	STIMULATORS	COMMENTS
Iodide Transport (34-37)	None or TSH	Probably accounts for escape from Wolff-Chaikoff
(38)		Protein synthesis involved
H_2O_2 Generation (30-32)		Also Catalatic I^- effect
Organic Iodine Synthesis (19,39)	None or TSH	In addition to pure iodide effect
Hormone Secretion (Dog) (19,40,41)	TSH	More sensitive than organic cation Not in man Also on colloid droplets
Adenylate Cyclase (19,41,42)	TSH, PGE, LATS, F^-, Forskolin, Cholera toxin	Catalytic Unit +?Gs ? not receptors Sensitivity varies with stimulator
Glucose Oxidation (19,43)	TSH, PGE, db cAMP	cAMP-mediated
Lactate Production (19,43)	TSH	
Uridine Uptake (19,44)	TSH	Inmase in cmyc mRNA
Thymidine Uptake (44-46)	EGF (insulin)	FRTL-5 cells not thyroid fibroblasts cAMP independent May be stimulated via cyclase inhibition
Protein Synthesis (19,43,47)	TSH	May not require oxidized iodine
Amino Acid Transport (48)	TSH	
Ca2+ Efflux (49)	TSH, db cAMP	
Resting Potential (50)	TSH	
Prostaglandin Synth. and Release (51,52)		Partly due to oxidation?
Phosphatidyl Inositol Turnover (53)	Cholinergic	

*To save space reviews have been cited where possible

iodination rather than by oxidation of -SH groups present in some cathepsins has not been established (61-63). This aspect of iodide inhibition remains largely unsettled but with the greater availability of antibodies to cell constituents, reexamination of the question of the iodination of non-thyroglobulin proteins of the thyroid seems warranted.

IV. Iodinated Inhibitors

It was first suggested in 1954 (64,65) that some of the effects of excess iodide might result from the formation of an inhibitory iodinated compound, and Wollmann & Reed (34) showed conclusively that a brief pre-exposure of thyroids to small amounts of iodide under iodinating conditions markedly decreased the ability of subsequently administered large amounts of iodide to inhibit iodide transport. This has been repeatedly confirmed. Moreover, the inhibition of many other metabolic processes by iodide is prevented by prior or co-administration of thionamides (see Table II) presumably because such drugs prevent the formation of iodinated products. It is implied that iodinated inhibitor compounds are not normally present at inhibitory concentrations. Either the inhibitor had a faster turnover rate than bulk thyroid iodine, or it accumulated only at high iodide loads, i.e. its formation did not compete effectively with protein iodination except at high iodide loads. The low doses effective for Wollmann and Reed (34) suggested that fast formation might be the more important. Once formed, however, excess iodide is no longer required and the inhibition (? inhibitor) persists for many hours (41,42,66).

The nature of the iodinated inhibitor has received intermittent attention. Because thyroid hormones may have direct inhibitory effects on the thyroid gland that are not referrable to pituitary inhibition (19), it has been difficult to rule out rigorously any inhibitory effects of intra-thyroidal T3 or T4. However, T_3 effects differ from KI (19), generally require concentrations higher than attained in the gland, and inhibitions are not produced by T3 under conditions where, e.g., iodoarachidonates (see below) give satisfactory inhibition. Moreover, organic iodine formation shows poor correlation with inhibition of other processes (67).

Lissitzky et al. (68) isolated a number of iodopeptides from mammalian thyroid tissue that could inhibit organic iodine formation in thyroid slices. One peptide had a molecular weight of 3-4 kDa and contained MIT and DIT. Although these peptides were studied further (69), they were never fully identified and the iodopeptide question has not, to our knowledge, been further pursued.

Autoregulation of iodide transport has been shown to involve the participation of a 8-10 kDa protein. Reduction of its level by cycloheximide treatment (58), or during development (70) abolishes the ability to reduce iodide transport in response to iodide excess

Whether an iodinated form of this protein is the transport inhibitor was not directly shown. Moreover, the protein was not involved in iodide-induced inhibition of TSH-stimulated cAMP generation.

None of these derivatives of protein iodination have fulfilled the inhibitory roles proposed for them. However, recent attempts to implicate certain iodinated lipids, though still preliminary, have provided a promising new approach to the postulated iodinated inhibitor and these will be examined in the following sections.

V. Iodine-Lipid Interactions

Iodinated lipids are generally consigned to the waste basket of thyroidology or at best to the "miscellaneous" file destined for oblivion. Nevertheless, there are scattered reports on the iodination of thyroidal lipids that are of chemical interest. The recent chemical characterization of some of the iodinated fatty acids, and the identification of a possible biological role for them, justify a more careful look at this potentially very large class of iodinated compounds. Iodine can interact with lipids in four fundamentally different ways. In two the interaction is non-covalent, while in the two others new covalent bonds are formed. Although the first two may have little to do directly with iodide-induced inhibitions, their understanding is helpful in the overall problem of iodine-lipid interactions. We shall examine these interactions in turn.

A. Electrostatic interactions

Vilkki first demonstrated that iodide ion could be distributed into a nonpolar solvent when that solvent contained certain phospholipids, particularly lecithins (71). This occurred under reducing conditions and no covalent iodine linkages were formed (72). Such interactions can be observed directly by proton magnetic resonance of aqueous suspension of lecithin as a separation of the doublet ascribed to the choline methyl groups. As shown in Fig 2, the separation (by downfield shift of the larger peaks) increases in the same order as in anion preference by the thyroid iodide transport system and Hofmeister effect (11,73). The shift is not dependent on the nature of the cation, but there is some lipid specificity to this interaction since synthetic dioleyl lecithin does not show this anion preference whereas egg lecithin does and thyroid lecithins work the best of the tissues tested. Treatment of these phospholipids with any of the common phospholipases (A, C or D) or by hydrogenation, abolished the binding of iodide (72,74). A structural requirement for an α-acyl, β-nervonyl (24:1) choline phosphatide was suggested but there is very little nervonic acid in thyroid phospholipids (75). However, neutral glycolipids and gangliosides, though not very abundant as a class, contain high percentages of nervonic acid (as well as other monoenoic and long-chain fatty acids) (76-79). Such a phospholipid system could serve as a model for iodide transport in the

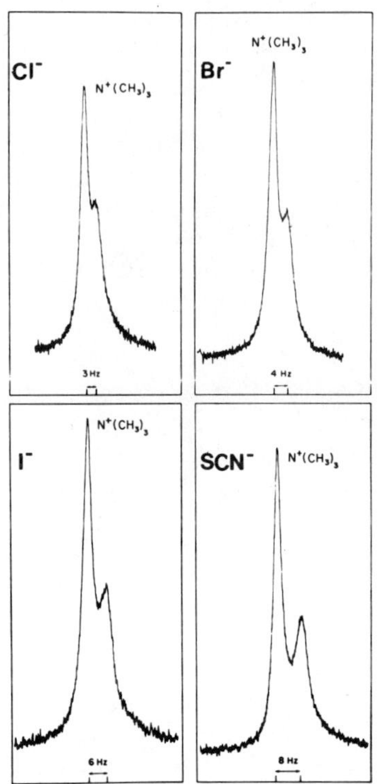

Fig 2. The effect of anions on the polar head group NMR signal in D_2O. The increasing separation of peaks results from a further downfield shift of the downfield peak. 0.1 M sodium salt, 0.044 M egg phosphatidyl choline, 40°C. (Modified from (73)).

thyroid gland (71), and it was later shown (72) that the iodide-lecithin complex was fully reversible and iodide binding to phosphatidyl choline could be competitively displaced by anions related to iodide in a potency series identical to that observed for intact thyroid tissue (Hofmeister series), i.e., the selectivity was of the correct sequence.

Implied in the preference for lecithins was the notion of ion pair formation and from what is known of cation selectivity determinants, a selectivity series for <u>anion</u> preference by the thyroid can be considered diagnostic for an anion exchange mechanism in which the exchanger is a large, weak field cation that allows the hydration enthalpy of the anion to play a decisive role in the selectivity (80,81). That is, electrostatic interactions are relatively weak because of the large radii of the exchanger and are thus less important than the hydration enthalpy as in the relation depicted below (82). If the change in electrostatic energy is $\frac{e^2}{r_c + r_1}$ as the new ion enters the exchanger site, and ΔG_c and ΔG_1 are the changes in the free energies of hydration required to remove water from the contacts between the two ions, then the gain in total free energy is

$$-\frac{e^2}{r_c + r_1} + \Delta G_c + \Delta G_1$$

where, e=electronic charge, r_c=the radius of the cation, r_1=the radius of the entering anion, r_2=the radius of the resident anion. The free energies of hydration of the ions are G_c, G_1 and G_2, respectively. This has to be corrected for removal of the resident counterion (2) by the converse relation:

$$\frac{e^2}{r_c + r_2} - \Delta G_c - \Delta G_2.$$

The net change in free energy of the exchange becomes:

$$\Delta G^\circ_{1/2} = \left(\frac{e^2}{r_c + r_2} - \frac{e^2}{r_c + r_1}\right) - [\Delta G_2 - \Delta G_1].$$

$$\text{and} \quad \Delta G^\circ_{1/2} = - RT \ln K_{1/2}.$$

where $K_{1/2}$ is the selectivity coefficient. The fact that anions such as I^- are large, and hence of weaker field, enhances the hydration effect. Phosphatidyl choline provides such a weak field cation and is thus a reasonable candidate for the exchanger. Whether or not vicinal partial choline charges would enhance selectivity has not been tested. Although there appeared to be some selectivity for thyroid-derived lipid (71,72), other lecithins interact with iodide without being able to bring it into an organic solvent. This discrepancy remains unresolved. Thus, it remains unproved whether such positively charged lipid head groups can account for thyroid anion selectivity or not. Similar arguments may, however, apply to proteins where arginine, or vicinal arginines, may contribute the requisite field properties.

B. "Charge Transfer" Interactions

Everyone who has ever localized lipid spots on thin layer chromatograms with iodine vapor knows that I_2 is soluble in lipids and does not rapidly form C-I bonds under such conditions (i.e., the brown spots don't bleach very rapidly). The color observed is like that seen for I_2 in many solvents that can contribute electrons (e.g. the lone pair of oxygen). With phospholipid liposomes in aqueous media, two new spectral bands appear centering around ≈370 nm and 290 nm; the former is attributed to a blue shifted visible iodine band whereas the ≈290 nm peak is believed to be due to the 1:1 charge transfer complex that is seen only when the phospholipid is present at concentrations above some critical concentration that is well above the critical micelle concentration. The structure of this phase is not known at present. Both peaks show some variation in their maxima but are ascribed to oxygen electrons from the phosphate (83), hence all phospholipids are electron donors. Their potency is, in the order of decreasing affinity constants, sphingomyelin > phosphatidyl choline > phosphatidyl ethanolamine. The NMR spectrum of lecithin with I_2 (in benzene) shows an upfield shift (84), in contrast to what is seen with iodide or other anions (Fig 2). These spectra are seen over a wide range of lecithin concentrations, both below and above a break in the concentration curve that is interpreted as the critical micelle concentration for that particular solvent. Most polar head groups yield the same spectrum (as do brain gangliosides) upon addition of I_2 even when all double bonds are reduced (85). This is ascribed to I_3^- formation by an, as yet, undefined dismutation of I_2. Electron spin resonance studies suggest that the I_3^- formed enters the hydrocarbon region of the micelles (86), and the I_3^- sediments with the ganglioside micelles. Triiodide (or I_5^-, I_7^- etc) is substantially more lipophilic than I^- because of reduced charge density, and I_2 can be shown to be a "carrier" for I^- through artificial membranes; with substoichiometric amounts of I_2 (1% or less) membrane resistance is markedly decreased (87-89). This is completely reversed by reducing agents. A natural example of the use of I_2 for iodide transport appears in the brown algae, especially *Laminaria* (90): iodide is oxidized to I_2, translocated and reduced within the cell. Transport does not occur in the presence of reducing agents. In contrast, *Fucus* species (91,92) transport iodide as the anion.

C. Thyroid Lipids

In order to understand the addition reactions of iodine to thyroid lipids it is important first to understand the substrate available in the gland. Total thyroid lipids have not been frequently analyzed but amount to 14-16 mg/gm wet weight in bovine thyroid tissue (93) (see Table III). Much larger values were reported for rabbit thyroids (94) but a substantial fraction of that lipid was probably due to adipocytes in the thyroid interstitium. Except in cultured cells it is obviously important and difficult to remove all lipid contributions from nonthyroid parenchyma. The absence of polyunsaturated fatty acid may indicate contamination by adipose tissue. The major portion of the total lipid is represented by phospholipids, followed by triglycerides and cholesterol (Table III). While the absolute amounts of lipid may change in stimulated glands, the distribution may remain constant or change (99).

Phospholipids constitute the bulk of thyroid lipids and analysis of polar head groups for various species reveal a striking similarity for all thyroids tested (Table IV). Phosphatidyl choline, phosphatidyl ethanolamine and sphingomyelin make up 85% of the

TABLE III

THYROID LIPIDS FROM VARIOUS SPECIES

	Lipids in Thyroids from					
	Cow[a]	Pig[b]	Man[b]	Sheep(95)	Dog(96)	Man(97)
	mg/g wet weight					
Total Lipids	14			15 (7.3-24)		
Cholesterol	1.4					1.3
Triglyceride	4.1				39%	
Phospholipid	9.2	3.5(M) 8.4(F)	3.6(M) 5.4(F)		58%	5.5
Free Fatty Acid	0.002					

[a])No difference between normal and hypertrophic thyroids (93).
[b])Calculated from lipid P on basis of a mol. wt of 787 (75).

phospholipid. Changes in the functional state of the thyroid tissue did not significantly alter this distribution. Thus dogs on either low or high iodine diets showed no differences in thyroid phospholipid composition (96); normal and hypertrophic bovine thyroids were quite similar (98); and nodular and paranodular tissue of human thyroidectomy material show similar phospholipid patterns (75). On the other hand, in FRTL-5 cells, TSH stimulation led to a change in phospholipid distribution and decreases in the cholesterol/ phospholipid ratios of membranes (99). Moreover, addition of exogenous phospholipids, particularly phosphatidyl inositol, to membranes with the aid of a nonspecific lipid transfer protein causes marked reduction in the activity of TSH-stimulated adenylate cyclase. It was suggested that the locus for this effect was in the coupling of Gs protein and receptor (100).

In addition to high proportions of oleic acid (18:1), the overall phospholipids of thyroids showed significant amounts of unsaturated fatty acids such as linoleic acid (18:2), arachidonic acid (20:4ω6) and docosahexaenoic acid (22:6ω3)(Table V). Individual phospholipids were shown to vary in the contents of unsaturated fatty acids. Thus, phosphatidyl choline was relatively abundant in linoleic acid, and phosphatidyl ethanolamine and especially phosphatidyl inositol were enriched in arachidonic acid containing about twice the fraction of arachidonic acid as do the total phospholipids (101,102). Because of

TABLE IV

DISTRIBUTION OF THYROID PHOSPHOLIPIDS

	Percent of Total Thyroid Phospholipids in					
	Cow	Pig[a]	Man[a]	Dog[b]	Cow(77)	Cow plasma membrane(100)
Phosphatidyl Choline	43	45	41	40	34	40
Phosphatidyl Ethanolamine	28	27	25	25	23	24
Phosphatidyl Serine	5.6	6.8	9.3	18	15	13
Phosphatidyl Inositol	6.5	6.5	4.3			
Sphingomyelin	14	13	14	10	19	23
Cardiolipin	2.8	0.9	2.9	-	3.5	
Phosphatidic Acid	< 1	-	-	3.2		
Lysophosphatidyl Choline	< 1	0.9	1.2	1.7		

[a]Same in nodular and paranodular tissue (75,98).
[b]Same on low and high iodine diets (96).

the great abundance of phosphatidyl choline, the absolute amount of arachidonic acid in phosphatidyl choline is not very different from that in phosphatidyl inositol. As we shall show below, the polyenoic fatty acids are probably the favored substrates for iodination reactions and may thus assume an importance beyond the well known precursor role in prostaglandin, leukotriene etc formation.

D. Covalent Interactions

The chemical halogenation of alkenes and unconjugated polyenoic fatty acids etc. by halogens such as I_2 can be thought of as an addition by electrophilic attack by the positive member of the pair I^+ I^-. The reaction is thought to occur by a carbonium ion intermediate

TABLE V
FATTY ACID COMPOSITION OF THYROID LIPIDS

Fatty Acid	Percent of Total Fatty Acids In:					
	Total Lipid	Triglyceride	Total Phospholipids			
	Cow(93)	Sheep(94)	Man[a]	Pig(102)	Sheep(102)	Rabbit(94)
16:0 Palmitic	22	35	20	20	15	23
16:1 Palmitoleic	1.1	10	tr	1.5	tr	3.8
18:0 Stearic	14	7.3	20	19	23	8.2
18:1 Oleic	34	27	22	37	34	30
18:2 Linoleic	6.8	11	17	12	15	13
18:3 Linolenic	tr	2.2	0.6	1.9	1.0	0.5
20:0 Arachidic	1.7		-	-	-	0.4
20:4(ω6) Arachidonic	7.9		12	7.7	8.8	11
22:0 Behenic	1.4		-			1.9
22:6(ω3)	4.4		3.4			

[a]Normal and nodular tissue did not differ significantly nor did male or female glands (75,98).

on the, as yet, unsubstituted carbon atom which then picks up the negative partner of the ion pair (I^- in this case), from a direction <u>trans</u> to the first iodine. The anion can be the partner of the halogen as in I^+I^- or in halogen halides such as I^+Cl^-, but may be a solvent anion e.g. OH^- when the reaction is carried out in water (the product in that case being an iodohydrin), or the carboxylate ion of a fatty acid to form a lactone, as we shall see below. An alternative proposal has been that a cyclic iodonium is the intermediate, but the pros and cons of these suggestions are beyond the scope of this discussion.

Halogenated lipids and fatty acids are reported in bacteria, fungi, algae, plants and animals including fluorocitrate, ω-fluoro fatty acids from acetic to oleic acid, chlorinated sulfolipids with up

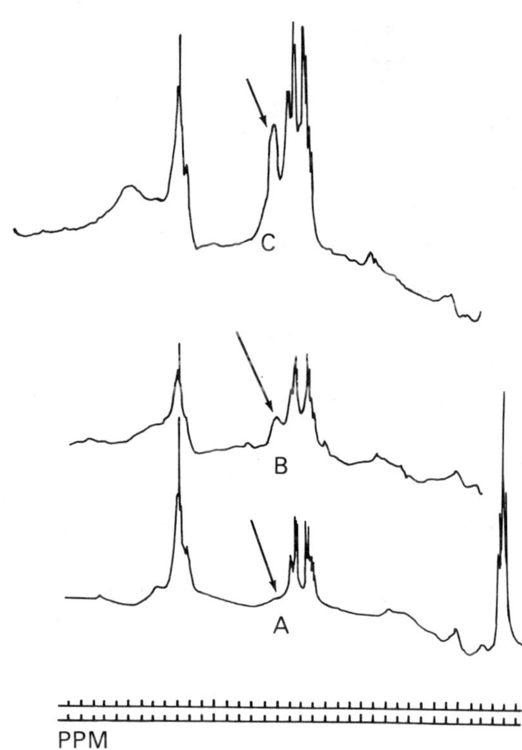

Fig 3. The effect of dietary iodine on the formation of an iodinated lipid in dog thyroid glands. A - low iodine diet; C - high iodine diet; B - I_2 was added to A to show that the lipid was there to be iodinated. The arrows point to the methine iodine peak at 4.5 ppm. (Taken from ref 96).

to 6 Cl/molecule, chlorinated and brominated fatty acids in marine animals. These have been catalogued (103) along with many references to earlier and longer lists of halometabolites. In addition to these naturally occurring halolipids, many investigators have discovered the formation of iodolipids in intact cells exposed to peroxidases, an H_2O_2 source, and I^- for the sake of labeling external proteins (104-108). About a third of the radioiodine incorporated may be present as iodolipids. Most classes of phospholipids are labeled, and it has been shown with phospholipase A_2 that the label resides primarily in the β position of the phospholipid. External iodination of lipid can also occur in isolated hog thyroid cells through the mediation of the cells' own peroxidase that must originally have been associated with the apical membrane when the cell was still polarized (109). Twenty to forty percent of radiodine incorporated at 0.05 μM I^- was present as so-called iodolipids (at the solvent front and extractable into chloroform:methanol). The bulk of this iodolipid formation occurred extracellularly as judged by its sensitivity to exogenous catalase (109).

E. Thyroidal Iodolipids

Anyone who has chromatographed radioiodine-labeled thyroid homogenates will have seen radioactivity near the solvent front in many solvents. Because the radioactivity moves with the mobile phase, it has been assumed to be lipid iodine but this need not always be the case (110). It is, nevertheless, true that iodinated lipids and/or nonpolar substances _can_ be found near the solvent front of chromatographic systems frequently employed for separation of iodoamino acids. Moreover, the formation of iodolipid, can, in special cases, be demonstrated without the use of radioiodine. By nuclear magnetic resonance the presence of an iodinated methine proton peak at 4.5 ppm can be seen (96) (Fig 3). The nature of this material was not further identified.

The formation of covalently linked lipid-like iodine has been studied by a number of investigators both in thyroid slices and _in vivo_. Since peroxidases iodinate lipids of the membrane during attempts to label external proteins (see above), one might suspect that artifacts due to the slice or _in vitro_ techniques might be responsible for much of the iodolipids formed. This is not the case because similar labeling and distribution among phospholipids has been demonstrated in thyroids labeled _in vivo_ (95,98,111,112). Not many detailed time-course studies have been carried out but it is probable that _in vitro_ lipid labeling _is_ faster than _in vivo_ labeling (111,112). All phospholipid, glycolipid and probably triglyceride fractions get labeled to some extent, but both the extent and time courses differ. This is depicted in a graph (Fig 4) drawn from data by Posner and Ordonez (111). It seems probable from the lipid distribution that iodination occurred from internally generated active iodine rather than external sources. The time course for _addition_ of

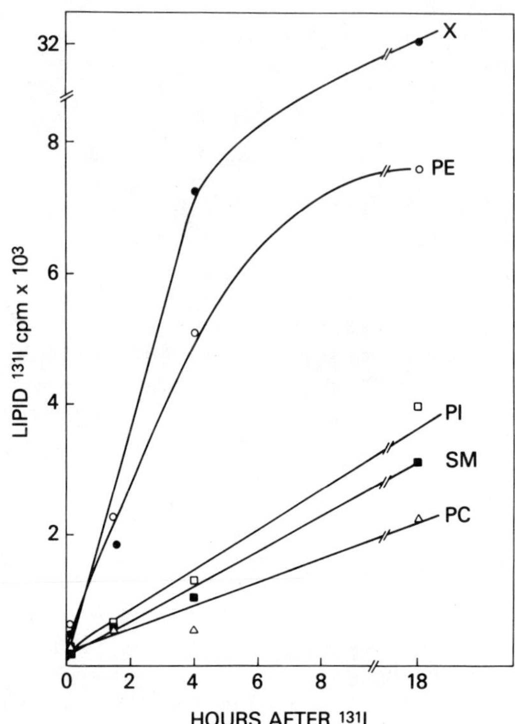

Fig 4. Time course for the labeling with ^{131}I of lipids in rat thyroid glands. PC - phosphatidyl choline; SM -sphingomyelin; PI -phosphatidylinositol; PE - phosphatidyl ethanolamine; X - an unknown iodinated lipid not containing phosphorus (Plotted from data supplied in (111)).

iodine to lipid generally parallels the substitution of iodine in tyrosyl residues (111,112), and shows a high correlation with iodoprotein or T_4 formation (112,113) as depicted in Fig 5. It seems probable that both the aromatic substitution and the addition to double bonds of unsaturated fatty acids compete for the active form of iodine present in thyroid peroxidase. They would thus be similarly sensitive to changes in the availability of the iodinating species and indeed they are: 1) Both are sensitive to PTU and MMI; 2) Both are a function of the degree of differentiation in thyroid carcinomas (112).

Thyroid gangliosides and neutral glyco-sphingolipids, though constituting a small portion of total polar lipids, have received substantial attention because of their potential role in TSH binding

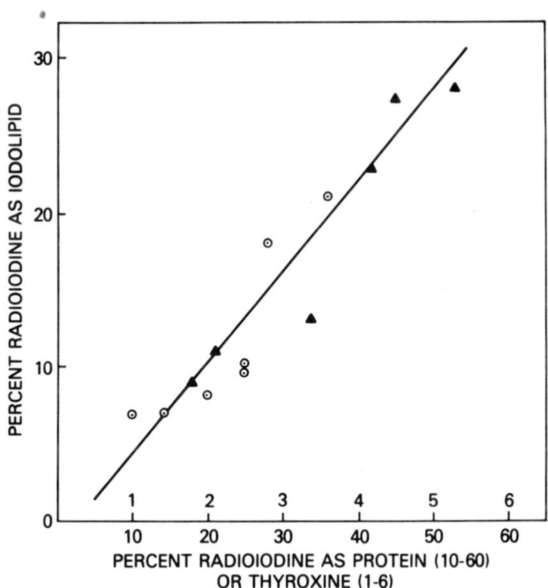

Fig 5. The relation between lipid and protein iodination on thyroxine formation in rat or calf thyroid tissue. Recalculated from refs (112) = ▲, and (113) = ⊙ .

(76,78,97,114,115). These lipids tend to contain a high percentage (≈80%) of saturated fatty acids (mostly C_{16}-C_{18}) and (C_{22}-C_{24}); most of the remainder consists of monounsaturated fatty acids of the same length distribution (76-79) and would thus be expected to be rather poor substrates for iodination. Very recent results in FRTL-5 thyroid cells (E. Grollman - NIH - personal communication) have, however, shown that three iodinated glycosphingolipids can be formed and no other iodinated lipids were seen. One of these appears to be a ceramide with retention times between ceramide trihexoside and globoside. The iodinated fatty acid has not yet been identified.

It has been suggested that the iodine of iodinated phosphatidyl choline and ceramide is a preferred source of iodine for protein iodination (112,116). In support of this it has been shown that covalently ^{125}I-labeled phosphatidyl choline was incorporated into protein of dog thyroid slices preferentially over Na ^{125}I. This process was not blocked by thiosulfate (116). How this scavenging or storage of "active" iodine is accomplished is not clear. The iodohydrins or iodolactones that formed are likely to give up their iodine in alkaline conditions to form epoxides while releasing iodine. Unfortunately, this iodine is thought to take the bond electron with it and appear as iodide (117). However, since peroxidase is involved, and since peroxidative reactions can be reversible, the possibility of preserving "active" iodine has not been ruled out. Transiodination between aromatic residues is a well known process (118), but whether or not iodohydrins or iodoalkanes can participate in such reactions is not known. It is of interest that a plant iodoperoxidase may use an iodinated intermediate for the biosynthesis of ascaridole (119).

F. The Iodinated Fatty Acids

The tremendous versatility of lipids is only slowly being appreciated and the physical basis for much of this is not yet known. One modest example lies in the ability to be halogenated, particularly, iodinated and the large number of novel products that may result.

Early attempts to identify the nature of the products of iodination of lipids in the thyroid gland showed that, in addition to iodination of virtually all lipid classes to a greater or lesser extent, one product was more extensively iodinated and increased progressively as a function of time. A typical time course for iodolipid formation is listed in Fig 4. A number of investigators have pointed out that after exposure of thyroid tissue to radioiodine an abundant labeled compound is formed that does not behave chromatographically like any of the known lipids. Posner & Ordonez (111) described an unknown X that constituted 45% of lipid ^{125}I by 18 h after injection and several groups (95,98,112) found a rapidly and extensively labeled compound, both *in vitro* and *in vivo*, in various species that chromatographed close to but not identical with phosphatidic acid. Finally, Chazenbalk et al. (113) found most of the lipid ^{125}I at 60' in calf thyroid slices in a fraction designated free fatty acids. Since different solvent systems were used, it is not possible to determine any similarities (if any) between these preferentially iodinated fractions. Unknown X, and another unknown that becomes labeled called fraction II (112), contain no phosphorus, are ninhydrin negative, but they may contain a glyco-moiety (orcinol positive) and are resistant to phospholipase A_2 and acid but are alkali labile. Both unknown X and fraction II parallel T_4 formation and are highly correlated. To our knowledge no further studies on these materials have been carried out.

More specific identification of the chemical nature of the iodinated fatty acids was initiated by Boeynaems and coworkers (120-122). Because of the critical role of arachidonic acid in

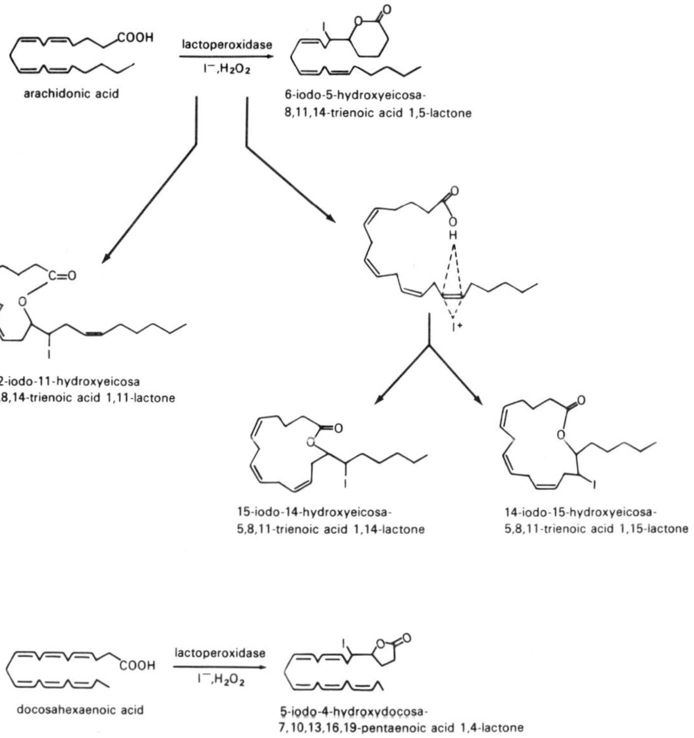

Fig 6. Some iodinated derivatives of polyenoic fatty acids. Details in refs (120-122,124).

transmembrane signalling, these workers studied the iodination of this tetraenoic fatty acid by lactoperoxidase, H_2O_2 and I^- as a model system. The major product found was a 6-iodo-5-hydroxyeicosatrienoic acid as the lactone (Fig 6); this is not unexpected because of the well-known intramolecular iodolactonization of unsaturated acids where the carboxylate is the nucleophile (123). This suggests also that, even though the reaction is peroxidative, it must have some ionic character. Deletion of H_2O_2 or iodide, or addition of catalase, blocks formation of these products. In addition, these authors identified two other lactones of monoiodinated derivatives namely: 15-iodo-14-hydroxy eicosatrienoic acid omega-lactone, and the reverse iodohydrin 14-iodo-15-hydroxyeicosatrienoic acid omega-lactone. Such reactions can also be carried out by eosinophil and myeloperoxidases. All possible monoiodinated derivates (as lactones) have been identified (disregarding any diastereoisomers), as have four different di-iodinated arachidonic acid derivatives (124):

a) 8,15-diiodo-9,14-dihydroxyeicosa - 5,11 dienoic acid;
b) 9,14-diiodo-8,15-dihydroxy..........
c) 8,14-diiodo-9,15-dihydroxy..........
d) 9,15-diiodo-8,14-dihydroxy..........

Clearly, the iodinations are not stereoselective. Other diiodo combinations are possible and the authors conclude that: 1) each of the four double bonds in arachidonic acid is susceptible to iodination; 2) arachidonic acid can be multiply iodinated; 3) the carboxylate moiety does not participate in the formation of all products (i.e. lactonization); hence esters, as in phospholipids or neutral lipids, can also be iodinated in this way. The number of iodo-arachidonic acid derivatives can be calculated to exceed 100 even if we disregard the fact that two chiral centers are created every time an iodohydrin is formed and diastereoisomers are therefore possible. Hence the iodination of this one fatty acid in the thyroid is a tremendous source of compounds of potential biological interest.

Other unsaturated fatty acids can yield an equally complex series of iodinated derivates and Boeynaems et al (122) have shown that docosahexanenoic acid (22:6ω3), which is nearly as abundant in thyroid lipids as is arachidonic acid (Table V), can be iodinated by lactoperoxidase to yield several products among them 5-iodo-4-hydroxy-7,10, 13,16,19 docosapentaenoic acid, γ-lactone (Fig 6). The number of possible iodinated derivatives will, of course, be correspondingly larger than for arachidonic acid. There are many other unsaturated fatty acids and the leukotrienes and retinoids, though conjugated, could provide additional iodinated derivatives.

When thyroid lobes are exposed to arachidonic acid and radioactive iodide _in vitro_, the 6-iodo-5OH derivative (Fig 6) can be readily demonstrated (120). This requires substantial concentrations of both reactants, e.g. 50 μM arachidonic acid and 5 μM KI. At least three other iodinated derivatives are more abundant but have not yet been identified. Methimazole abolished formation of the iodinated arachidonates. Such findings suggest that thyroid peroxidase can perform the same transformations seen with lactoperoxidase, eosinophil peroxidase or myeloperoxidase. Similar findings were obtained when thyroid lobes were exposed to 5 or 25 μM $^{125}I^-$ and increasing concentrations of docosahexaenoic acid. Three peaks of labeled derivatives were found of which one was 5-iodo-4 hydroxy 7,10,13,16,19 docosapentaenoic acid γ-lactone, as also observed after treatment with lactoperoxidase (122). The amount of products was a function of the concentration of both reactants and the reaction was inhibited by methimazole.

It is not clear whether thyroid tissue _not_ supplemented with iodide and arachidonic acid will also produce these iodinated lactones. In favor of such a suggestion are the facts that: 1) stimulation of the thyroid by TSH either increases phospholipase A_2 activity and yields a very rapid release of arachidonic acid especially from PI, or promotes a rapid and transient formation of diacylglyceride by phospholipase C and subsequent arachidonate release _via_ diacylglyceride and monoacyl glyceride lipases (102,125-128). Although stimulators of the phosphatidyl inositol phosphate (IP_3) system have not, apparently, been tested for their effects on phospholipid or arachidonic acid levels, the large concentrations of TSH apparently required suggest that this pathway may be involved. In the presence of indomethacin (to block the metabolism of arachidonic acid) large concentrations of TSH will lead to a doubling of free arachidonic acid levels to 37 nmol/gm tissue (102). 2) Some have found a large proportion of the lipid radioiodine in the free fatty acid or nonphosphatide fraction (113). Since iodoarachidonic acids may exist as free hydroxy acids or as lactones, it is conceivable that unknowns X and II (see above) (which were the most actively labeled) may be the same or related iodofatty acids as seen by Chazenbalk but chromatograph differently as lactones or free acids. 3) Although no studies exist that suggest that small increases in _dietary_ iodine increase thyroidal iodolipids _in vivo_, somewhat larger doses (1 mg I/day) gave clear evidence of leading to a substantial increase in an iodinated lipid (by NMR-see Fig 3) (96). The nature of this material has not been established.

There is thus sufficient reason to suspect that thyroid stimulation on the one hand, and changes in the availability of iodine on the other, _could_ enhance the supply of iodolipids in the gland. Additional evidence by direct chemical or NMR studies should be relatively easy to obtain.

G. Possible Functions of Iodinated Fatty Acids

Although the Boeynaems group (120-122) was unable to detect biological activity in their iodinated arachidonic acid derivatives (particularly 5-hydroxy 6-iodo-eicosatrienoic acid - see Fig 6), inhibition resembling that produced by excess iodide has been found by Pisarev and coworkers (129-132). They have now shown that iodinated arachidonic acid, and in particular 14-iodo-15-hydroxyeicosa-5, 8,11-trienoic acid, either in the free form or as the omega-lactone (see Fig 6), can inhibit various thyroid functions when added to calf thyroid slices in concentrations up to 10^{-4}M. These are listed in Table VI, and include inhibition of iodide "trapping", iodine organification, (the degree of inhibition being inversely proportional to the iodine content of the tissue), uridine incorporation into RNA, amino acid transport and H_2O_2 generation. There was no effect on iodide efflux from the gland. The effects on iodination are similar to those seen with excess iodide even in purified peroxidase systems. It is obvious that these effects are identical to those seen after exposure to excess iodide (Table II) but with the important difference that methimazole could no longer prevent such inhibitions. This

TABLE VI

MIMICRY BY 14-IODO-15-HYDROXY EICOSATRIENOIC ACID ON REACTIONS TYPICALLY INHIBITED BY EXCESS IODIDE
(Taken from Refs 129-133 - compare with Table II)

Iodide-Sensitive Reaction	Concentration [M]	Percent Inhibition	Comment
Iodide Transport (T/M)	10^{-5}	50	Concentration-dependent
Organification	10^{-4}	72	All iodoamino acids and
(Basal)	10^{-5}	40-46	iodolipid decreased (MIT>
(TSH)	10^{-5}	74	DIT>T4)
H_2O_2 Generation	10^{-4}	59	Thyroid peroxidase not affected
cAMP Levels	10^{-4}-10^{-5}	-	Personal communication
	5 μg/ml	32-55	in vivo
α-Aminoisobutyric Acid Transport	10^{-4}-10^{-5}	-	Personal communication
Uridine Uptake	10^{-4}	78	Not influenced by MMI

observation also eliminates the possibility that iodoarachidonic acids could, somehow, serve as a preferred source of iodide or "active" iodine. That is, these compounds were inhibitors in their own right rather than intermediaries in further iodination reactions. Equimolar concentrations of T_3 run in parallel had no inhibitory effects. The group has also established the following potency series: free acid > omega lactone of the same compound > delta lactone of 5-hydroxy-6-iodo-eicosatrienoic acid (132). Arachidonic acid was without effect. The inhibitions are seen within 15 minutes (they appear to be somewhat faster in onset than KI), are dose-dependent and reversible, can be demonstrated also in vivo, and are not sensitive to protein or DNA synthesis inhibitors (129-133). In view of the large numbers of possible iodinated arachidonic acid or docosahexaenoic acid derivatives, it seems highly probable that other derivatives are active and that a more potent inhibitor that is made in the thyroid tissue may eventually be found. Despite many missing pieces to this puzzle, a major regulatory pathway for excess iodide in the thyroid appears thus to have been identified.

VI. Destruction of "Active" Lipids

The fourth way in which excess iodide can impinge on lipids in the thyroid gland is a closely related phenomenon which may stem from similar reactions occurring on biologically active arachidonic acid derivates, i.e., prostaglandins and leukotrienes etc. While it is not yet clear whether or not prostaglandins are normally significant regulators of thyroid function, exogenous PGE_1 binds to thyroid membranes and activates adenylate cyclase (133). Peroxidative conversion of these substances to less active or inactive isomers or oxidation products has been demonstrated in neutrophils and eosinophils (135-137). These conversions are markedly accelerated by iodide and other halides but it is not yet clear whether unstable iodinated intermediates are formed or not. It also remains to be seen whether the oxidation occurs only _via_ double bonds or also _via_ the thioether linkage of the leukotrienes. Some oxidative transformations of arachidonate have been demonstrated in rat thyroids (52). It is, in any case, conceivable that excess iodide may lead to the loss of these substances in the thyroid and thus to modulation of tonic regulation, or to the formation of yet a different class of inhibitors, whether iodinated or oxidized.

VII. Conclusions

It is clear that excess iodide acts at many loci - some stimulated by the cAMP system, some probably via the phosphoinositide/Ca^{2+}/diacyl-glycerol system, and others by neither pathway. Can all these be ascribed to a single mechanism? Probably not. In addition to possible true anion effects, and the direct inhibition of the iodination process, the inhibitions resulting from iodide oxidation may be direct effects on critical enzymes, or may be due to inhibitory compounds derived from unsaturated fatty acids, etc. For years thyroid lipids have been intentionally or unintentionally ignored. It appears now, however, that they deserve more serious attention. Not only could they play a potential role in anion selectivity of the iodide pump, and form charge transfer complexes, but they are subject to covalent modifications that may be important for at least three reasons: a) as substrates for interesting chemical modifications, particularly iodination. With minor lipids taken into account these could number over a thousand possible structures; b) as mediators of thyroid autoregulation and as potential iodine reservoirs; and, c) as possible mediators of thyroid pathology. It is conceivable that some iodinated fatty acids will show preferential inhibition of certain of the reactions listed in Table 2, but this remains to be explored.

Problems that might be amenable to early attack are:
1) The identification of additional active iodinated fatty acids, particularly more potent ones; also structure-function relationships; formation in unfortified thyroid tissue;

formation in unfortified thyroid tissue;
2) Identification of iodinated fatty acids in more complex lipids, and the possibility of changes in function in such combinations;
3) The question of unique functions for unique derivatives;
4) What is the nature of the interaction of iodinated fatty acids with their targets and can this account for the multiplicity of effects -regulatory or pathological?

Thus the major autoregulatory systems operative in the thyroid exist in a paradoxical relation to each other: one depending on the inhibition of iodination reactions, the other upon promotion of iodination of special products. Protection against excess iodide depends, in the first instance, on competition for "active" iodine, and when inhibition of iodination reactions is insufficient, on an alternate substrate for "active" iodine which leads to the formation of inhibitors that interfere with a great many metabolic pathways in the gland. Preliminary evidence suggests that some of these may derive from iodine addition to double bonds of fatty acids.

REFERENCES

1. J. Wolff, Congenital goiter with defective iodide transport, Endocrine Rev. 4:240 (1983).
2. T. Onaya, T. Tomizawa, T. Yamada, and K. Shichijo, Further studies on inhibitory effect of excess iodide on thyroidal hormone release in the rat, Endocrinol. 79:138 (1966).
3. I. Mahmoud, I. Colin, M-C, Many, and J-F, Denef, Direct toxic effect of iodide excess on iodine-deficient thyroid glands, Exp. Molec. Pathol. 44:259 (1986).
4. M.L. Maayan, S.H. Ingbar, Acute depletion of thyroid ATP and pyridine nucleotides following injection of iodine in the rat, Endocrinol. 86:83 (1970).
5. E. Ogata, Y, Yoshitoshi, K, Nishiki, and S. Kobayashi, Dual effect of iodide IV on reduced pyridine nucleotides in rabbit thyroid in situ, Endocrinol. 90:169 (1972).
6. L. Wartofsky, B. Ransil, S.H. Ingbar, Inhibition of iodine of the release of thyroxine from the thyroid gland of patients with thyrotoxicosis, J. Clin. Invest. 49:78 (1970).
7. K. Kasai, H. Suzuki, S-I, Shimoda, Effects of PTU and relatively small doses of iodide on early phase treatment of hyperthyroidism, Acta Endocrinol. 93:315 (1980).
8. J.H. Marigold, A.K. Morgan, D.J. Earle, A.E. Young, and D.N. Croft, Lugol's iodine: its effect on thyroid blood flow in patients with thyrotoxicosis, Br.J.Surg. 72:45 (1985).
9. J. Wolff, I.L. Chaikoff, Plasma inorganic iodide as a homeostatic regulator of thyroid function, J.Biol.Chem. 174:555 (1948).
10. J. Wolff, Iodide goiter and the pharmacologic effects of excess iodide, Am.J.Med. 47:101 (1969).
11. K.D. Collins, M.W. Washabaugh, The Hofmeister effect and the behavior of water at interfaces, Quart. Rev. Biophys. 18:323 (1985).

12. W.D. Alexander, J. Wolff, Antigoitrogenic properties of certain goitrogens, in: "Current Topics in Thyroid Research", C. Cassano, M. Andreoli, eds., Academic Press, New York (1965).
13. W.D. Alexander, J. Wolff, Thyroidal iodide transport VIII: Relation between transport, goitrogenic and antigoitrogenic properties of certain anions, Endocrinol. 78:581 (1966).
14. T. Jolin, G. Morreale de Escobar, and F. Escobar del Rey, 6-Propyl-2-thiouracil vs $KClO_4^-$ -induced goiters, Endocrinol 83:620 (1968).
15. M.E. Morton, I.L. Chaikoff, S. Rosenfeld, Inhibiting effect of inorganic iodide on the formation *in vitro* of thyroxine and diiodotyrosine by surviving thyroid tissue, J.Biol.Chem. 154:381 (1944).
16. S.H. Ingbar, Autoregulation of the thyroid, Mayo Clinic Proc. 47:814 (1972).
17. S. Nagataki, Effect of excess quantities of iodide, in: "Handbook of Physiology", Section 7, vol III, S.R. Geiger, ed., Am Physiol Soc, Washington, D.C. p 329 (1974).
18. J. Wolff, Mechanistic speculations on the iodide effect, in: "Dietary Iodine and Other Aetiological Factors in Hyperthyroidism", MRC Environmental Epidemiol. Unit Scientific Report, No. 9, Southampton p 18 (1987).
19. M.A. Pisarev, Thyroid autoregulation, J. Endocrinol Invest. 8:475 (1985).
20. W.E. Mayberry, J.E. Rall, and D. Bertoli, Kinetics of iodination: I. A comparison of the kinetics of iodination N-acetyl-L-tyrosine and N-acetyl-3 -iodo-L-tyrosine, J.Am.Chem.Soc. 86:5302 (1964).
21. A. Taurog, Thyroid peroxidase-catalyzed iodination of thyroglobulin; inhibition by excess iodide, Arch.Biochem.Biophys. 139:212 (1970).
22. J. Pommier, D. Deme, J. Nunez, Effect of iodide concentration on thyroxine synthesis catalyzed by thyroid peroxidase, Europ.J.Biochem. 37:406 (1975).
23. J. Nunez, J. Pommier, Formation of thyroid hormones, Vitam.Horm. 39:175 (1982).
24. N. Abdelmoumene, J.M. Gavaret, J. Pommier, J. Nunez, A defective thyroid peroxidase in a case of Pendred's syndrome, J.Mol.Med. 3:305 (1978).
25. S. Ohtaki, H. Nakagawa, S. Kimura, I. Yamazaki, Analysis of catalytic intermediates of hog thyroid peroxidase during its iodinating reaction, J.Biol.Chem. 256:805 (1981).
26. M. Nakamura, I. Yamazaki, S. Ohtaki, and S. Nakumura, Characterization of one and two electron oxidations of glutathione coupled with lactoperoxidase and thyroid peroxidase reactions, J.Biol.Chem. 261:13923 (1986).
27. H. Kohler, A. Taurog, H.B. Dunford, Spectral studies with lactoperoxidase and thyroid peroxidase, Arch.Biochem.Biophys. 264:438 (1988).
28. J.L. Michot, J. Osty, and J. Nunez, Regulatory effects of iodide and thiocyanate on tyrosine oxidation catalyzed by thyroid

peroxidase, Eur.J.Biochem. 107:297 (1980).
29. F. Courtin, D. Deme, A. Virion, J.L. Michot, J. Pommier, J. Nunez, The role of lactoperoxidase-H2O2 compounds in the catalysis of thyroglobulin iodination and thyroid hormone synthesis, Eur.J.Biochem. 124:603 (1982).
30. K. Yamamoto, L.J. DeGroot, Function of peroxidase and NADPH cytochrome c reductase during the Wolff-Chaikoff effect, Endocrinol 93:822 (1973).
31. P. Chiraseveenuprapund, I.N. Rosenberg, Effects of H2O2-generating systems on the Wolff-Chaikoff effect, Endocrinol 109:2095 (1981).
32. B. Corvilain, J. Van Sande, J.E. Dumont, Inhibition by iodide of iodide binding to proteins: the Wolff-Chaikoff effect is caused by inhibition of H2O2 generation, Biochem.Biophys.Res.Commun. 154:1287 (1988).
33. R.P. Magnuson, A. Taurog, M.L. Dorris, Mechanism of iodide-dependent catalatic activity of thyroid peroxidase and lactoperoxidase, J.Biol.Chem. 259:197 (1984).
34. S.H. Wollmann, F.E. Reed, Acute effect of organic binding of iodine and the iodide concentrating mechanism of the thyroid gland, Am.J.Physiol. 194:28 (1958).
35. J. Wolff, I.L. Chaikoff, R.C. Goldberg, J.R. Meier, The temporary nature of the inhibitory action of excess iodide on organic iodine synthesis in the normal thyroid, Endocrinol. 45:504 (1949).
36. L.W. Braverman, S.H. Ingbar, Changes in thyroidal function during adaptation to large doses of iodide, J.Clin.Invest. 42:1216 (1963).
37. E.F. Grollman, A. Smolar, A. Ommaya, D. Tombaccini, P. Santisteban, Iodine suppression of iodide uptake in FRTL-5 thyroid cells, Endocrinol. 118:2477 (1986).
38. J.R. Sherwin, W. Tong, The action of iodide and TSH on thyroid cells showing a dual control system for the iodide pump, Endocrinol. 94:1465 (1974).
39. G.D. Chazenbalk, M.A. Pisarev, L. Kraviec, G.J. Juvenal, G. Burton, and R.M. Valsecchi, In vitro inhibitory effects of an iodinated derivative of arachidonic acid on calf thyroid, Acta.Physiol.Pharmacol. Latino Am. 34:367 (1984).
40. G.P. Becks, M.C. Eggo and G.N. Burrow, Regulation of differentiated thyroid function by iodide: preferential inhibitory effect of excess iodide on thyroid hormone secretion, Endocrinol. 120:2569 (1987).
41. J. Van Sande, P. Cochaux, and J.E. Dumont, Further characterization of the iodide inhibitory effect on the cAMP system in dog thyroid slices, Mol.Cell Endocrinol. 40:181 (1985).
42. S. Filletti, B. Rapoport, Evidence that organic iodine attenuates the cAMP response to TSH stimulation by an action at or near the adenylate cyclase catalytic unit, Endocrinol. 113:1608 (1983).
43. J. Wolff, Physiological aspects of iodide excess in relation to radiation protection, J.Mol.Med. 4:151 (1980).

44. N.E. Heldin, F.A. Karlsson, B. Westermark, A growth stimulatory effect of iodide, Endocrinol. 121:757 (1987).
45. R. Gartner, W. Greil, R. Demharter, K. Horn, Involvement of cAMP, I^- and metabolites of arachidonic acid in the regulation of cell proliferation of isolated porcine thyroid follicles, Mol.Cell.Endocrinol. 42:145 (1985).
46. G.P. Becks, M.C. Eggo, G.N. Burrow, Organic Iodine inhibits DNA synthesis and growth in FRTL-5 thyroid cells, Endocrinol. 123:545 (1988).
47. L.J. Valenta, Effect of iodide and TSH on in vitro ^{14}C-amino acid incorporation into rat thyroid protein, Acta Endocrinol. 76:273 (1974).
48. S. Filletti, B. Rapoport, Autoregulation by iodine of thyroid protein synthesis: influence of iodine on amino acid transport in cultured thyroid cells, Endocrinol. 114:1379 (1984).
49. K. Hashizume, M. Kobayashi, T. Onaya, Iodide modulation of Ca^{2+} efflux from mouse thyroid, Endocrinol.Japon. 32:259 (1985).
50. N. Takasu, Y. Handa, A. Kawaoi, Y. Shimizu, T. Yamada, Effects of iodide on thyroid follicle structure and electrophysiological potentials in cultured thyroid cells, Endocrinol. 117:71 (1985).
51. J. M. Boeynaems, N. Galand, J.E. Dumont, Inhibition by iodide of the cholinergic stimulation of prostaglandin synthesis in dog thyroid, Endocrinol. 105:996 (1979).
52. J.M. Boeynaems, D. Pelster, J.A. Oates, W.C. Hubbard, Novel transformations of arachidonic acid by the rat thyroid in vitro, Biochim.Biophys.Acta 665:623 (1981).
53. A. Takeuchi, J. Mockel, Mechanism of increased phosphatidyl inositol turnover in dog thyroid slices in vitro, Ann.d'Endocrinol. 44:54A (1983).
54. B. Rousset, J. Wolff, Lactoperoxidase-tubulin interactions, J.Biol.Chem. 255:2514 (1980).
55. H. Jenzer, U. Burgi, H. Kohler, Irreversible inactivation of lactoperoxidase in the course of iodide oxidation, Biochem.Biophys.Res.Commun. 142:552 (1987).
56. L.J. Valenta, W.C. Florsheim, B.S. Sharma, Acute effects of iodide on the stimulated rat thyroid, Endocrinol. 111:1721 (1982).
57. N.E. Heldin, F.A. Karlsson, B. Westermark, Inhibition of cAMP formation by iodide in suspension cultures of porcine thyroid follicle cells, Mol.Cell.Endocrinol. 41:61 (1985).
58. J.R. Sherwin, D.J. Price, Autoregulation of thyroid iodide transport: evidence for the mediation of protein synthesis -iodide-induced suppression of iodide transport, Endocrinol. 119:2553 (1986).
59. P. Santisteban, A.J. Hargreaves, J. Cano, J. Avila, L. Lamas, Effects of high doses of iodide on thyroid secretion: evidence for the presence of iodinated membrane tubulin, Endocrinol. 117:607 (1985).
60. B. Bhattacharyya, J. Wolff, Membrane-bound tubulin in brain and thyroid tissue, J.Biol.Chem. 250:7639 (1975).

61. N. Bagchi, T. Brown, B. Shivers, R.E. Mack, Effect of inorganic iodide on thyroglobulin hydrolysis in cultured cells, Endocrinol. 100:1002 (1977).
62. C.S. Ahn, I.N. Rosenberg, Proteolytic activity in the rat thyroid gland, Endocrinol. 81:1319 (1967).
63. R.L. Peake, K. Balasubramaniam, W.P. Deiss, Effect of reduced glutathione on the proteolysis of intraparticulate and native thyroglobulin, Biochim.Biophys.Acta 148:689 (1967).
64. W. Vanderlaan, R. Caplan, Observations of a relationship between total thyroid iodine content and the iodide-concentrating mechanism of the thyroid gland in the rat, Endocrinol. 54:437 (1954).
65. N.S. Halmi, R.G. Stuelke, Problems of thyroidal self regulation, Metabolism 5:646 (1956).
66. P. Cochaux, J. Van Sande, S. Swillens, J.E. Dumont, Iodide-induced inhibition of adenylate cyclase activity in horse and dog thyroid, Eur.J. Biochem. 170:435 (1987).
67. E.L. Socolow, D. Dunlap, R.A. Sobel, S.H. Ingbar, A correlative study of the effect of I^- administration on thyroidal I^- transport and organic iodine content, Endocrinol. 83:737 (1968).
68. S. Lissitzky, J. Gregoire, J. Gregoire, N. Limozin, The presence and in vitro activity of free iodinated peptides in the thyroid gland of mammals and man, Gen.Comp.Endocrinol. 1:519 (1961).
69. J.F. Haney, S. Lissitzky, A study of the dialysable iodo-compounds of rat thyroid gland, Gen.Comp.Endocrinol. 3:139 (1963).
70. D.J. Price, J.R. Sherwin, Autoregulation of iodide transport in the rodent: absence of autoregulation in fetal tissue and comparison of material and fetal iodination products, Endocrinol. 119:2547 (1986).
71. P. Vilkki, An iodide complexing phospholipid, Arch.Biochem.Biophys. 97:425 (1962).
72. P.B. Schneider, J. Wolff, Thyroidal Iodide Transport VI. On a possible role for iodide-binding phospholipids, Biochim.Biophys.Acta 94:114 (1965).
73. G.L. Jendrasiak, Halide interaction with phospholipids -proton magnetic resonance studies, Chem.Phys.Lipids 9:133 (1972).
74. P. Vilkki, I. Jaakonmaki, Role of fatty acids in iodide-complexing lecithin, Endocrinol. 78:453 (1966).
75. G.M. Levis, J.N. Karli, B. Malamos, The phospholipids of the thyroid gland, Clin.Chem.Acta 41:335 (1971).
76. G. Van Dessel, A. Lagrou, H.J. Hilderson, W. Dierick, G. Dacremont, Quantitative determination of the neutral glycosyl ceramides in bovine thyroid gland, Biochimie 59:839 (1977).
77. M. Iwamori, K. Sawada, Y. Hara, M. Nishio, T. Fujisawa, H. Imura, Y. Nagai, Neutral glycosphingolipids and gangliosides of bovine thyroid, J.Biochem. (Tokyo) 91:1875 (1982).
78. B. Bouchon, J. Portoukalian, H. Bornet, Major gangliosides in normal and pathological human thyroids, Biochem.Int. 10:531 (1985).

79. G.A.F. Van Dessel, A.R. Lagrou, M. Hilderson, W. Dierick, W. Lauwers, Structure of major gangliosides from bovine thyroid, J.Biol.Chem. 254:9305 (1979).
80. J. Wolff, Iodide transport, anion selectivity and the iodide "trap", in: "Diminished Thyroid Hormone Formation", D. Reinwein, E. Klein, eds., F.K. Schattauer, Stuttgart 3 (1982).
81. E.M. Wright, J.M. Diamond, Anion selectivity in biological systems, Physiol.Rev. 57:109 (1977).
82. D. Reichenberg, Ion exchange selectivity, in: "Ion Exchange -A Series of Advances", Vol 1, J.A. Marinsky, ed., Marcel Dekker, NY 227 (1966).
83. I. Chatterjee, P. Nandy, B.B. Bhowmik, Nature of the interaction of phospholipid liposomes with iodine, Chem.Phys.Lipids 49:57 (1988).
84. G.L. Jendrasiak, NMR study of molecular interactions with phosphatidyl choline, Chem.Phys.Lipids 6:215 (1971).
85. H.C. Yohe, A. Rosenberg, Interaction of triiodide anion with gangliosides in aqueous iodine, Chem.Phys.Lipids 9:279 (1972).
86. G. Jendrasiak, R. Hayes, Spin-label study of the iodine-lecithin interaction, Nature 225:278 (1970).
87. A. Finkelstein, A. Cass, Permeability and electrical properties of thin lipid membranes, J.Gen.Physiol. 52:Suppl 145 (1968).
88. B. Rosenberg, G. Jendrasiak, Semiconductive properties of lipids and their possible relationship to lipid bilayer conductivity, Chem.Phys.Lipids 2:47 (1968).
89. G. Jendrasiak, M. Mangel, Ion-pair movement across bilayer lipid membranes, Nature 234:89 (1971).
90. T.I. Shaw, The mechanism of iodide accumulation by the brown seaweed Lauminaria digitata, Proc.Roy.Soc.B. 150:336 (1959).
91. H. Klemperer, The accumulation of iodide by Fucus ceranoides, Biochem.J. 67:381 (1957).
92. J. Wolff, Thyroid Iodide Transport I. Cardiac Glycosides and the Role of Potassium, Biochim.Biophys.Acta 38:316 (1960).
93. A. Lagrou, W. Dierick, A. Christophe, G. Verdonk, Lipid composition of normal and hypertrophic bovine thyroids, Lipids 9:870 (1974).
94. L.A. Lipshaw, P.P. Foa, The composition and possible physiologic role of the thyroid lipids, Adv.Lipid Res. 12:227 (1974).
95. D.H. Shah, R.C. Shownkeen, V.R. Thakare, Iodinated thyrolipids, Acta Endocrinol. 70:683 (1972).
96. J.L. Rabinowitz, M. Zanger, V. Podolski, Identification by NMR of iodinated lipids in the dog thyroid, Biochem.Biophys.Res.Commun. 68:1161 (1976).
97. L. Svennerholm, Gangliosides of human thyroid gland, BBA 835:231 (1985).
98. G.M. Levis, D.A. Koutras, A. Vagenakis, G. Messaris, C. Miras, B. Malamos, Thyroidal iodinated compounds in nodular goiter, Clin.Chim.Acta 20:127 (1968).
99. F. Beguinot, L. Beguinot, D. Tramontano, C. Duilio, S. Formisano,

M. Bifulco, F.S. Ambesi, S.M. Aloj, TSH regulation of membrane lipid fluidity in the FRTL-5 thyroid cell line, J.Biol.Chem. 262:1575 (1987).

100. H. Depauw, M. De Wolf, G. Van Dessel, H. Hilderson, A. Lagrou, W. Dierick, Modification of TSH-stimulated adenylate cyclase activity of bovine thyroid by manipulation of membrane phospholipid, Biochim.Biophys.Acta 937:359 (1988).

101. T.W. Scott, V. Trikojus, Interactions of phospholipids with thyroglobulin and their influence on the enzyme hydrolysis of this protein, Biochem.Biophys.Acta 215:477 (1970).

102. B. Haye, C. Jacquemin, Incorporation of [^{14}C]arachidonic acid in pig thyroid lipids and prostaglandins, Biochim.Biophys.Acta 487:231 (1977).

103. S.L. Neidleman, J. Geigert, Biohalogenation: principles, basic roles and applications, John Wiley and Sons, NY (1986).

104. A. Bennenson, M. Mersel, A. Pinson, M. Heller, Enzymatic radioiodination of phospholipids catalyzed by lactoperoxidase, Anal.Biochem. 101:507 (1980).

105. T.D. Butters, R.C. Hughes, Surface labeling of human KB cells, Biochem.J. 150:59 (1975).

106. M. Mersel, A. Bennenson, F. Doljanski, Lactoperoxidase-catalyzed iodination of surface membrane lipids, Biochem.Biophys.Res.Commun. 70:1166 (1976).

107. J.F. Poduslo, P.E. Brown, Topographical arrangement of membrane proteins in the intact myelin sheath, J.Biol.Chem. 250:1099 (1975).

108. S.I. Schlager, Specific ^{125}I-iodination of cell surface lipids: plasma membrane alterations induced during humoral immune attack, J. Immunol. 123:2108 (1979).

109. B. Rousset, C. Poncet, J.E. Dumont, R. Mornex, Intracellular and extracellular sites of iodination in dispersed hog thyroid cells, Biochem.J. 192:801 (1980).

110. A. Taurog, W. Tong, I. Chaikoff, An unidentified iodine compound formed by incubation of cell-free preparations of tissue with ^{131}I, J.Biol.Chem. 227:759 (1957).

111. I. Posner, L. Ordonez, Lipid-iodine association in the rat thyroid gland, Biochim.Biophys.Acta 187:588 (1969).

112. D.H. Shah, V.R. Thakare, R.C. Shownkeen, D.N. Pahuja, M.Y. Mandlik, Iodinated thyrolipids: their possible role in hormonogenesis, Acta Endocrinol. 74:461 (1973).

113. G.D. Chazenbalk, M.A. Pisarev, G.J. Juvenal, D.L. Kleiman de Pisarev, H. Mercuri, M. DeTomas, Biosynthesis and regulation of iodolipids in calf thyroid, Acta Endocrinol. 108:72 (1985).

114. B.R. Mullin, T. Pacuszka, G. Lee, L.D. Kohn, R.O. Brady, P.H. Fishman, Thyroid gangliosides with high affinity for TSH, Science 199:77 (1978).

115. G.A.F. Van Dessel, A. Lagrou, H. Hilderson, W. Dierick, W. Lauwers, Structure of the major gangliosides from bovine thyroid, J.Biol.Chem. 254:9305 (1979).

116. J.L. Rabinowitz, C.J. Tavares, Iodinated phospholipids and the in vitro iodination of proteins of dog thyroid gland, Biochem.J. 168:155 (1972).
117. N. Sonntag, Halogenation, dehalogenation, and dehydrohalogenation, in: "Fatty Acids, Part 2", K.S. Markley, ed., Interscience Publ., NY 1073 (1961).
118. B.C. Saunders, B.P. Stark, Studies on peroxidase action XII: transiodination and related processes, Tetrahedron 4:169 (1958).
119. M.A. Johnson, R. Croteau, Biosynthesis of ascaridole: iodide peroxidase-catalyzed synthesis of a monoterpene endoperoxide in soluble extracts of chenopodium ambrosioides, Arch.Biochem.Biophys. 235:254 (1984).
120. J. Boeynaems, W. Hubbard, Transformation of arachidonic acid into an iodolactone by the rat thyroid, J.Biol.Chem. 255:9001 (1980).
121. J. Boeynaems, D. Reagan, W. Hubbard, Lactoperoxidase-catalyzed iodination of arachidonic acid: formation of macrolides, Lipids 16:246 (1981).
122. J. Boeynaems, J. Watson, J. Oates, W. Hubbard, Iodination of docosahexaenoic acid by lactoperoxidase and thyroid gland in vitro: formation of an iodolactone, Lipids 16:323 (1987).
123. P. DeLaMare, Electrophilic Halogenation, Cambridge Univ Press, Cambridge 171 (1976).
124. J. Turk, W. Henderson, S. Klebanoff, W. Hubbard, Iodination of arachidonic acid mediated by eosinophil peroxidase, myeloperoxidase and lactoperoxidase, Biochim.Biophys.Acta 751:189 (1983).
125. B. Haye, S. Champion, C. Jacquemin, Control by TSH of phospholipase A_2 activity: a limiting factor in the biosynthesis of prostaglandins in the thyroid, FEBS Lett. 30:253 (1973).
126. B. Haye, S. Champion, C. Jacquemin, Existence of two pools of prostaglandins during stimulation of the thyroid by TSH, FEBS Lett. 41:89 (1974).
127. Y. Igarashi, Y. Kondo, Acute effects of TSH on phosphatidyl inositol degradation and transient accumulation of diacyl glycerol in isolated thyroid follicles, Biochem.Biophys.Res.Commun. 97:759 (1980).
128. Y. Igarashi, Y. Kondo, Characterization of partial glyceride specific lipases in pig thyroid plasma membranes, Biochem.Biophys.Res.Commun. 97:766 (1980).
129. G. Chazenbalk, M. Pisarev, L. Krawiec, G. Juvenal, G. Burton, R. Valsecchi, In vitro inhibitory effects of an iodinated derivative of arachidonic acid on calf thyroid, Acta Physiol. Pharmacol. Latino Am. 34:367 (1984).
130. M. Pisarev, G. Chazenbalk, L. Krawiec, C. Juvenal, R. Valsecchi, G. Burton, Effects of purified iodolipids on thyroid function in vitro, Proc. 9th Int'l Congress, abstract 225 (1985).
131. L. Krawiec, G. Chazenbalk, S. Puntarulo, G. Burton, A. Boveris, R. Valsecchi, M. Pisarev, The inhibition of $PB^{125}I$ formation in calf thyroid caused by 14-iodo-15-hydroxy-5,8,11-eicosatrienoic

acid is due to decreased H2O2 production, Horm.Metab.Res. 20:86 (1988).

132. G. Chazenbalk, R. Valsecchi, L. Krawiec, G. Burton, G.J. Juvenal, E. Monteagudo, H. Chester, M. Pisarev, Thyroid autoregulation inhibitory effects of iodinated derivatives of arachidonic acid on iodine metabolism, Prostaglandins 36:163 (1988).

133. M. Pisarev, G. Burton, P. Grawitz, G. Chazenbalk, G. Juvenal, D. Kleiman de Pisarev, L. Krawiec, R. Valsecchi, Post-receptor events in growth control, in: "Frontiers in Thyroidology", G. Medeiros-Neto, E. Gaitan, eds., 125 (1986).

134. W.V. Moore, J. Wolff, Binding of prostaglandin E_1 to beef thyroid membranes, J.Biol.Chem. 248:5705 (1973).

135. E.J. Goetzl, The conversion of leukotriene C_4 to isomers of leukotriene B4 by human eosinophil peroxidase, Biochem.Biophys.Res.Commun. 106:270 (1982).

136. W.R. Henderson, A. Jorg, S. Klebanoff, Eosinophil peroxidase-mediated inactivation of leukotrienes B4, C4 and D4, J. Immunol. 128:2609 (1982).

137. J-M. Paredes, S. Weiss, Human neutrophils transform prostaglandins by a myeloperoxidase dependent mechanism, J.Biol.Chem. 257:2738 (1982).

G PROTEIN-LINKED RECEPTORS IN THE THYROID

Daniela Corda, Cinzia Bizzarri, Maria Di Girolamo
Salvatore Valitutti and Alberto Luini

Istituto di Ricerche Biomediche e Farmacologiche "Mario Negri", Consorzio Mario Negri Sud, 66030 S. Maria Imbaro Chieti, Italy

INTRODUCTION

The binding of hormones to membrane receptors results in the activation of intracellular effector(s) such as enzymes or ion channels, which in turn induce a cellular response. In thyroid cells, as in many other cells, growth and differentiation as well as specialized functions such as iodide fluxes and thyroglobulin synthesis are regulated in the above general manner. This chapter is intended to provide an analysis of the types of receptors which in thyroid cells effect this regulation, and of their mechanism of action, with a special emphasis on the role of GTP binding proteins.

It is now accepted that the interaction of a large number of membrane receptors and transducing enzymes is mediated by a family of membrane proteins, the guanine nucleotide binding (G) proteins. G proteins were originally described as the regulatory components of the adenylyl cyclase complex able to couple the inhibitory (Gi) and stimulatory (Gs) receptors to the catalitic subunit of this enzyme[1,2]. Within a few years however it has become evident that these two proteins are members of a large family of membrane proteins that is involved in the modulation not only of the cyclase, but of many other intracellular signalling pathways, including phospholipase C (PLC), phospholipase A2 (PLA2), K^+ channels, Ca^{++} channels. G proteins are distinguishable by their primary sequence, specificity of their coupling to receptors and to transducing enzymes, sensitivity to pertussis and cholera toxins[3,4].

Numerous receptors have been shown to be coupled to G proteins. The primary sequence of several of these receptors has become available and all have been found to share a similar structure consisting of seven transmembrane domains connected by extra and intracellular loops[5-7]. Despite this structural similarity, these receptors are not always characterized by a high homology in their primary sequence[5-7]. Single point mutation, chimeric structures and deletion from the carboxyl-terminus of the cloned receptors have been used to identify the sequences involved in the interaction with agonists and G proteins[5-7]. Rhodopsin, the different classes of adrenergic and muscarinic receptors, the serotonin receptor, belong to this family.

For a more detailed understanding of the above concepts the reader is referred to comprehensive reviews that have recently appeared in the literature[1-7].

Although the structural characteristics of receptors and G proteins are mantained in different cell types, these proteins may use different intracellular mechanism in regulating the function of various tissues.

This chapter will concentrate mainly on the receptors coupled to G proteins that have a role in the regulation of thyroid function, using a continuous line of rat thyroid cells (FRTL5) as a model system. In particular, we will analyze how in these cells TSH, norepinephrine and acetylcholine receptors regulate growth, iodide fluxes and thyroglobulin synthesis by interacting with the adenylyl cyclase, PLC and PLA2.

THE FRTL5 CELL SYSTEM

The FRTL5 cells are a well characterized system which maintains differentiated thyroid function such as the transport of iodide, the synthesis and iodination of thyroglobulin, the release of thyroid hormones[8-14]. These cells are considered a good model for studying mechanisms of cell regulation in general, and of thyroid function in particular.

Similarly to other thyroidal systems, FRTL5 cells depend on the presence of thyrotropin (TSH) for growth and differentiation[8,15-18]. In this system cyclic AMP and its analogues are able to partially mimic the TSH stimulation of growth and of iodide uptake[10,12,17,18]. Other cofactors important for growth regulation are insulin and IGF1[8,19,20]. In FRTL5 cells the TSH effects on growth are distinguishable from those on

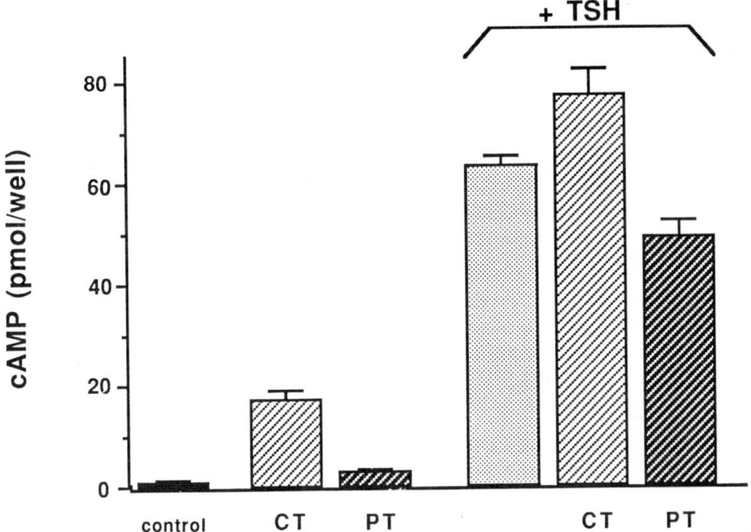

Fig. 1. Levels of cyclic AMP in FRTL5 thyroid cells kept in the absence of TSH for 5-10 days. The FRTL-5 cells used in this and in the following experiments were a continuous line of functioning epithelial cells derived from normal Fisher rat thyroids (obtained from F.S. Ambesi-Impiombato). Their isolation, growth and basic characteristics have been described[8-12]. The cell stimulation and the cyclic AMP evaluation were performed as described[26]. The ligands concentrations were as follows: TSI I and pertussis toxin, 10^{-8}M; Cholera toxin, 10^{-9}M. The results are mean ± S.D. of triplicate determinations, representative of three separate experiments.

thyroglobulin iodination since the sensitivity to the hormone concentration is different in the two cases. TSH maximally stimulates the cyclic AMP dependent phenomena (i.e. growth and protein synthesis) at a concentration thousand fold lower than that required for iodide efflux and thyroglobulin iodination[10,11,14,21-23]. The latter phenomena are independent of cyclic AMP, and involve Ca^{++} and arachidonic acid as probable mediators[21-25]. The role of the adrenergic system in the regulation of these cyclic AMP independent phenomena will be discussed later in this chapter[21-25].

TSH REGULATION OF ADENYLYL CYCLASE

The FRTL5 cells are characterized by a functional adenylyl cyclase sensitive to TSH[10,11,18]. Gi (G inibitory) and Gs (G stimulatory), the two regulatory G proteins coupled

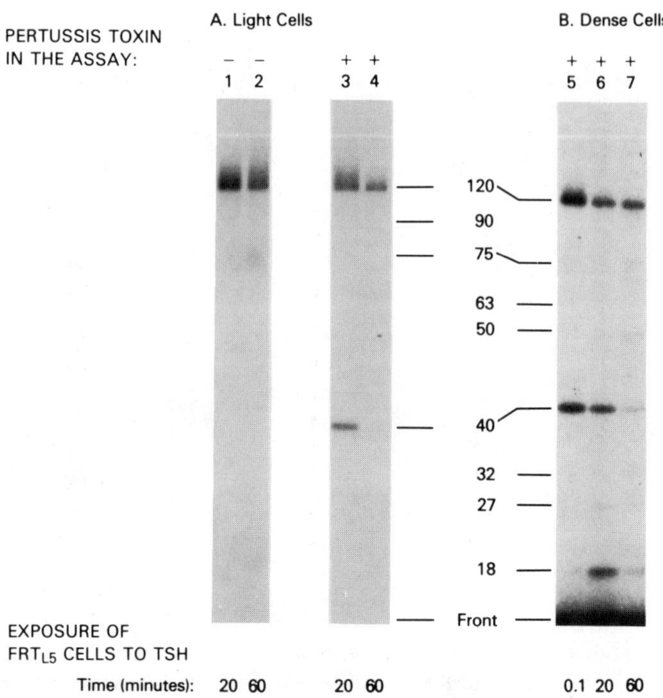

Fig. 2. Autoradiographic analysis of ADP ribosylated proteins in FRTL-5 cell membranes. This figure was taken from ref. 26. The FRTL-5 cells were maintained in 5H medium, i.e. medium without TSH, for 5 days prior to membrane preparation, then incubated with TSH (10^{-8}M) for the indicated time. Pertussis toxin (10^{-7}M) was used in the ADP ribosylation assay, which was carried out as described[26]. The migration of commercial molecular mass markers is indicated.

to the adenylyl cyclase have been evidentiated in this system as the specific substrates of the ADP ribosyl transferase activities of pertussis and cholera toxin, respectively[26].

Fig. 1 shows the effect of TSH, pertussis toxin and cholera toxin on the cyclic AMP levels in FRTL5 cells[26]. Pertussis toxin in this system is able to stimulate the adenylyl cyclase. Its effect is however not additive to the TSH induced increase, suggesting that they may share in part their mode of action (Fig. 1)[26]. Since pertussis toxin is known to act by directly ADP ribosylating the α subunit of Gi, thus functionally inactivating it, we could hypothesize that TSH could use at least in part a mechanism involving the Gi protein. In line with this hypothesis, in a recent study we have demonstrated that TSH modulates the amount of the 40KDa α subunit of the Gi regulatory protein present in FRTL5 cells plasma membranes[26,27]. As shown, FRTL5 cells incubated with TSH for 1 to 60 minutes had a significant decrease in the α subunit of Gi available to pertussis toxin induced ADP ribosylation (Fig. 2)[26,27]. TSH did not change the cholera toxin induced ADP ribosylation of αs, indicating that this effect was specific for αi[26]. Similar data have been recently reported in bovine thyroid slices[28].

These results suggest to us that a) TSH and pertussis toxin could, as noted above, use a partially similar mechanism of adenylyl cyclase activation, namely, that the increase in cyclic AMP levels could result from a decreased inhibition of the catalytic unit of the enzyme rather than from an increased stimulation and b) one of the mechanisms by which TSH could perturb the Gi function could be a decrease in the level of Gi protein present in the plasma membrane. In the bovine thyroid the ADP ribosylation of Gi could be restored by adding detergents to the system. This indicates that this effect could be in part explained by the masking of the Gi protein in the bilayer[28]. Another mechanism that could in theory explain the hormonal regulation of Gi is a TSH dependent ADP ribosylation of αi[22,29]. This could represent a mechanism of competition between the hormone and the toxin for the same site of ADP ribosylation. There are evidences in the literature indicating that TSH increases the ADP ribosylation activity of bovine thyroid membranes, the specific substrate of the TSH induced ADP ribosylation being in that case a peptide of ~40 KDa[30]. From our findings however this does not seem to be the case. It turns out that TSH is able to modulate the ADP-ribosyl transferase activity of FRTL5 cells, but its substrate is a ~27KDa peptide[22,29]. We do not have at this point evidences of any correlation between the 27 and 40 KDa peptides.

Although we could not demonstrate any correlation between the ADP ribosylating activity of TSH and its activation of thyroid function, it is tempting to speculate that the hormonally regulated ADP ribosylation reactions could represent a novel mechanism of cell regulation by hormones, where a peptide relevant for cell function could be activated by this covalent reaction. This mechanism would be very similar to the effect of toxins on the G proteins, which are either activated (Gs) or inactivated (Gi) by an ADP ribosylation.

Adenylyl cyclase, protein synthesis and expression of the norepinephrine receptor

In FRTL5 cells the activation of the adenylyl cyclase by TSH has been related to the synthesis of several proteins[31]. One of the proteins which is under TSH control for its synthesis and expression on the plasma membrane is the $\alpha 1$-adrenergic receptor[32]. FRTL5 cells deprived of TSH for 5-6 days (5H cells) do not fully respond to the

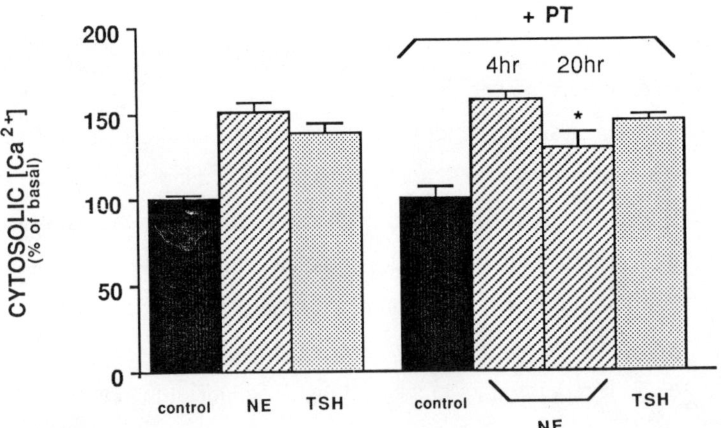

Fig. 3. Cytosolic Ca++ levels in FRTL5 cells loaded with the fluorescence probe Quin2. The basal levels of cytosolic Ca++ were 115±20 nM, the determinations were performed as described[21,38]. Norepinephrine and TSH were used at 10^{-6} M concentration, whereas pertussis toxin was at 10^{-9} M. Data are the mean ± SE of six to eight experiments performed in duplicate. See text for details.

norepinephrine stimulus, at least when PLA2 and PLC activation are used as measure of cell response[22]. The cause of this low sensitivity is the lower number of α1-adrenergic receptors, which are 5 to 10 fold higher in cells kept with TSH when compared to cells deprived of the hormone (5H cells)[32].

Table 1 shows a reduction of almost 90% in the arachidonic acid release upon norepinephrine stimulation in 5H cells. The TSH induced release of arachidonic acid was also markedly reduced in 5H cells (Table 1)[22,23]. We have not investigated further this phenomenon which could be due either to a lower number of TSH receptors, in analogy with what observed in the case of the α1-adrenergic receptors, or to an inefficient coupling of the receptor to the PLA2 in 5H cells[22,23].

The activation of PLC by adrenergic agents was also partially reduced in 5H cells as compared to 6H cells, although to a lesser extent[21,33].

From these data it could be speculated that physiological doses of TSH, by regulating the adenylyl cyclase activity and, as a consequence, the number of α1-adrenergic receptors, also indirectly modulate the adrenergic control of thyroid function.

Table 1. Arachidonic acid release in FRTL-5 cells [a]

	[^{3}H] Arachidonic acid released (percent of basal)	
	6H CELLS	5H CELLS
CONTROL	100 ± 8	100 ± 3
NE (10^{-5} M)	281 ± 8	115 ± 7
TSH (10^{-6} M)	167 ± 21	102 ± 10

[a] The [^{3}H]-arachidonic acid release was measured in FRTL5 cells mantained in the presence of TSH (6H cells) or deprived of it for 5-6 days prior to the experiments (5H cells)[22]. The incubation with TSH and norepinephrine was for 30 min. The experimental procedures have been previously described[21-23]. The results are mean ± SE of three separate experiments performed in duplicate.

TSH, NOREPINEPHRINE AND ACETYLCHOLINE REGULATION OF PHOSPHOLIPASES

The Ca^{++} signal

The role of Ca^{++} in the regulation of thyroid function has been demonstrated in several thyroidal systems[14,21,34,35]. We have shown that TSH increases the cytosolic Ca^{++} levels in FRTL5 cells (Fig. 3)[21]. The dose-effect relationship of this TSH action is well separated from the effect on the cyclic AMP formation since the two dose responses are three orders of magnitude apart (Fig. 4)[21,22]. The Ca^{++} signal is however in a good agreement with the stimulation of iodide efflux, suggesting a regulatory role of Ca^{++} on this phenomenon[14,21]. Similarly, norepinephrine by interacting with an α1-adrenergic receptor increases both cytosolic Ca^{++} levels and the efflux of iodide in FRTL5 cells (Fig. 3 and 5)[14,21-24]. In this system, TSH and norepinephrine also activate PLC and increase the inositol 1,4,5-trisphosphate production[21,33,36,37]. The data so far reported indicate that the increase in cytosolic Ca^{++} is due to the formation of the inositol 1,4,5-trisphosphate, rather than to an opening of a Ca^{++} channel. FRTL5 cells are therefore characterized by a stimulatable PLC coupled to both the adrenergic and TSH receptor[21-23,33,37].

To investigate whether G proteins are involved in the coupling mechanism between

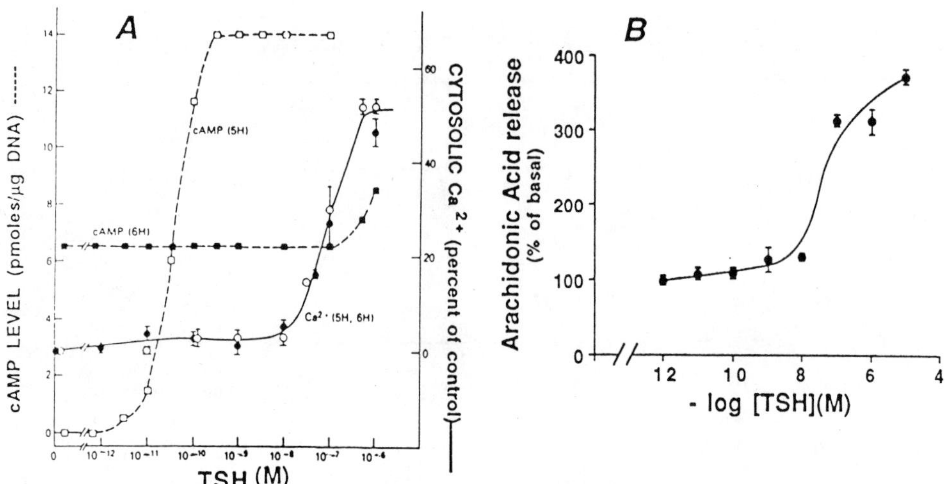

Fig. 4. Dose response curves of the TSH effect on cyclic AMP levels, cytosolic Ca++ (A) and arachidonic acid release (B). Panel A was taken from Ref. 21, panel B from Ref. 22. The experimental procedures were previously described[21,22]. 0.1 μCi [^{3}H]-arachidonic acid/well were used in the overnight cell labelling. Cells were washed twice before adding TSH for 15 min. On the average, about 3000 cpm of [^{3}H]-arachidonic acid were released in the control wells[22].

the α1-adrenergic and TSH receptors and PLC, we have used pertussis toxin. Pretreatment of the FRTL5 cells with this toxin inhibited the efflux of iodide induced by norepinephrine (Fig. 5)[22,38]. These data suggested that the pathway regulated by this receptor could involve a G protein sensitive to pertussis toxin[38]. In contrast, the norepinephrine induced cytosolic Ca^{++} increase, as well as the accumulation of inositol phosphates were only partially affected by the toxin, and the TSH action was not affected by it (Fig. 3)[22,23,33,38]. Since the efflux of iodide and the cytosolic Ca^{++} increase had a different sensitivity to the toxin, it could be hypothesized that a different second messenger, formed via a cascade involving a G protein sensitive to pertussis toxin takes part in the regulation of iodide transport in this cell system[22,23,38]. The activation of PLA2 has a role in this phenomenon, as it will be discussed later[22,24].

Muscarinic regulation of phospholipase C

The cholinergic system has been proposed to intervene in the regulation of thyroid

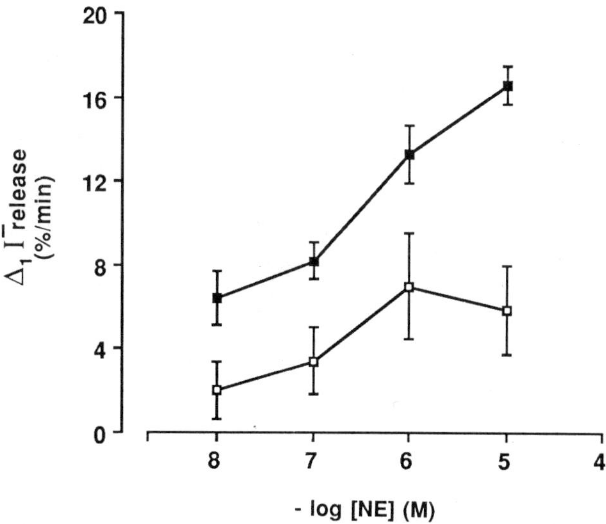

Fig. 5. Dose response curves of the norepinephrine-induced iodide release from FRTL5 cells. The experiments were performed according to the described procedure in control cells (full squares) and in cells preincubated for 4 hr with 10^{-9} M pertussis toxin (open squares)[24,38]. The $\Delta 1 I^-$ release represents the differences in rate of iodide efflux between stimulated and non-stimulated cells [13,24,38]. Data are the mean ± SE of four to six experiments performed in duplicate.

functions[39-41]. In the dog thyroid, which has been one of the systems better characterized from this viewpoint, a cholinergic control of the cytosolic Ca^{++} levels mediated by the activation of PLC has been demonstrated[42,43].

Recently, we have characterized two pharmacologically different muscarinic receptors in FRTL5 cells, which may have a role in the regulation of iodide transport[23,44-47]. The cholinergic agonist carbachol was able to decrease in a dose dependent manner the steady-state iodide content of FRTL5 cells[44,46]. This phenomenon could be related to the activation of either PLC or PLA2 since these are the relevant enzymes in the regulation of iodide transport[22,23].

Unlike in other thyroidal systems, carbachol did not increase the cytosolic Ca^{++} levels in FRTL5 cells, suggesting that PLC is not coupled in a stimulatory manner to the muscarinic receptor (Fig. 6)[45,47]. However this agent was able to reduce the norepinephrine induced increase in cytosolic Ca^{++} (Fig. 6)[45,47]. Carbachol also inhibited

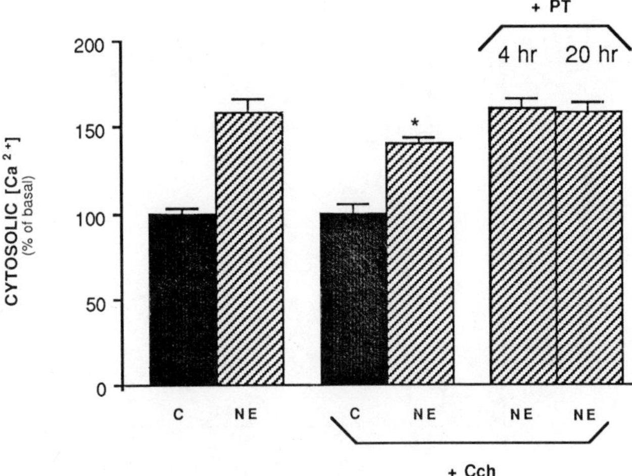

Fig. 6. Effect of carbachol on the cytosolic Ca++ levels in FRTL5 cells. The cytosolic Ca++ levels were meausered with the fluorescent probe Quin2 according to the described procedure[21,45,47]. The concentration of carbachol and norepinephrine were 10^{-6} M and 10^{-5} M, respectively. Pertussis toxin was used at 10^{-8}- 10^{-10} M concentration.

the norepinephrine induced inositol phosphates accumulation, as well as the basal levels of inositol phosphates (Table 2)[47]. The inhibition involved a muscarinic receptor since it was prevented by the muscarinic antagonist atropine[45,47]. We have asked whether this effect of carbachol could be due to a direct modulation of PLC activity or it could be secondary to the muscarinic modulation of a different cytosolic factor and/or second messenger able to decrease the PLC enzymatic activity.

A role of cytosolic Ca++ in the inhibitory regulation of PLC could be excluded since the Ca++ increase induced by the ionophore A23187 did not prevent the carbachol induced inhibition of the inositol phosphate accumulation (Table 2)[47]. A role for cyclic AMP and diacylglycerol could similarly be excluded. These data suggested the possibility of a direct coupling between the muscarinic receptor and PLC[47,48].

The inhibitory effect of carbachol was very sensitive to pertussis toxin pretreatment, indicating that a pertussis toxin sensitive G protein is involved in this inhibitory regulation (Fig. 6)[45,47]. Fig. 7 shows a scheme of the possible mechanisms regulating PLC in FRTL5 cells. Stimulatory and inhibitory receptors coupled to Gp proteins (the G proteins which specifically interact with PLC[49]), either stimulatory (Gps)

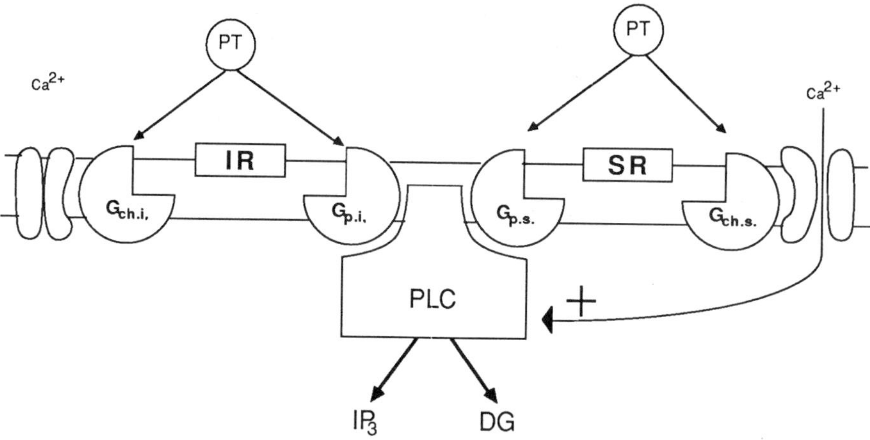

Fig. 7. Possible mechanisms involved in the regulation of PLC activity. IR and SR, inhibitory and stimulatory receptors; Gpi and Gps, inhibitory and stimulatory G proteins; Gchi and Gchs, inhibitory and stimulatory G proteins linked to ionic channels regulation; IP3, inositol 1,4,5-trisphosphate; DG, diacylglycerol. See text for details.

or inhibitory (Gpi), regulate the activity of this enzyme in a manner similar to what has been proposed for the adenylyl cyclase. The possibility that a receptor mediated decrease in cytosolic Ca^{++}, due to the closure of a Ca^{++} channel, inhibits the PLC activity is also illustrated. Such mechanism has been demonstrated in pituitary cells[50].

Recent experiments from our laboratory have shown that the inhibitory effect of carbachol can be observed in FRTL5 cells permeabilized by streptolysin O. In this system norepinephrine increased the inositol 1,4,5-trisphosphate production by 135±17% over the basal. Carbachol inhibited this effect by 50%. Both effects required the presence of GTP.

Taken together these data suggest that a pertussis toxin sensitive G protein provides a direct inhibitory coupling between the muscarinic receptor and PLC (Fig. 7)[45,47,48].

The activation of PLC leads to the formation of another second messenger the diacylglicerol, which is known to directly stimulate protein kinase C. In FRTL5 cells we have used phorbol myristate acetate (PMA), which mimics the stimulation of diacylglicerol on protein kinase C, in order to evaluate the effect of the latter on thyroid functions[51]. Fig. 8 shows that PMA is able to inhibit the iodide efflux induced by norepinephrine[51].

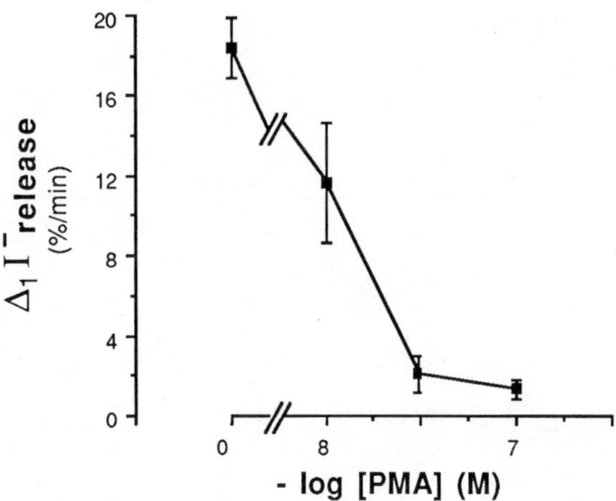

Fig. 8. Effect of phorbol myristate acetate (PMA) on the norepinephrine-stimulated efflux of iodide in FRTL5 cells. See Fig. 5 for details. Data are the mean ± SE of three to six experiments performed in duplicate.

According to our study, this inhibition is due to a direct effect of the protein kinase C on the α1-adrenergic receptor, which is not able to activate PLC and PLA2 in the presence of PMA[51]. This conclusion is supported by the fact that the TSH activation of iodide efflux was not affected by PMA pretreatment, suggesting that the machinery leading to iodide efflux is not a direct substrate for PMA action[51]. In a different cell system it has been demonstrated that the α1-adrenergic receptor is a substrate for protein kinase C induced phosphorylation[52]. In other thyroidal preparations PMA has been shown to exert differential effects on iodide organification, hydrogen peroxide formation and cyclic AMP accumulation, depending on the tissue preparation and on the experimental conditions[53-56]. The role of the protein kinase C pathway in the regulation of thyroidal differentiated functions remains therefore under discussion, whereas its regulation of thyroid cell proliferation is well documented in FRTL5 cells as well as in other thyroid systems[53-58].

The arachidonic acid signal

Arachidonic acid mimics TSH and norepinephrine in stimulating the efflux of iodide

Table 2. Inositol phosphates accumulation in FRTL-5 cells [a]

Addition	Inositol phosphates accumulation (% of basal) Control	Carbachol (10^{-6} M)
NONE	100 ± 5[b]	80 ± 5*
NE (10^{-5} M)	303 ± 29[c]	239 ± 17**
A23187 (10^{-6} M)	105 ± 2	80 ± 7*
NE + A23187	352 ± 40	235 ± 30**

[a] The inositol phosphates accumulation was measured in monolayers of FRTL5 according to the described procedure[33,47]. The incubation with carbachol, A23187 and norepinephrine was for 30 min. The results are mean ± SE of five to ten experiments performed in duplicate. *Significantly different from b ($p < 0,05$) **Significantly different from c ($p < 0,05$) by variance analysis.

from FRTL5 cells[14]. It has been suggested that TSH and adrenergic receptors could use arachidonic acid as a second messenger in the stimulation of thyroid functions[14,22-24]. Both TSH and norepinephrine are able to release arachidonic acid from FRTL5 cells (Fig. 9)[22,23,25]. The dose-response curve of the TSH induced arachidonic acid release is clearly separated from the TSH stimulation of adenylyl cyclase, thus excluding a cyclic AMP mediated phenomenon, whereas it is in a good agreement with the TSH induced increase in cytosolic Ca^{++} levels (Fig. 4)[21,22]. Ca^{++} and arachidonic acid may, in theory, both be formed by the activation of PLC (in this case arachidonic acid would be released by the action of diacylglycerol lipase on the diacylglycerol formed concomitantly with the inositol 1,4,5-trisphosphate). A second possibility is that the two enzymes PLC and PLA2, might form the two second messengers in a indipendent manner. The TSH receptor is coupled to PLC in a pertussis toxin insensitive manner, whereas it is sensitive to the toxin in activating PLA2 (Fig. 9)[22,23]. Although this observation cannot be considered a direct evidence, it suggests that the TSH receptor directly and independently activates PLC and PLA2[22,23].

The situation has been better analyzed in the case of norepinephrine, which has been shown to directly activate PLA2 since a) its effect is insensitive to the diacylglicerol lipase inhibitor RHC 80267 and b) the G protein coupling the α_1-adrenergic receptor to

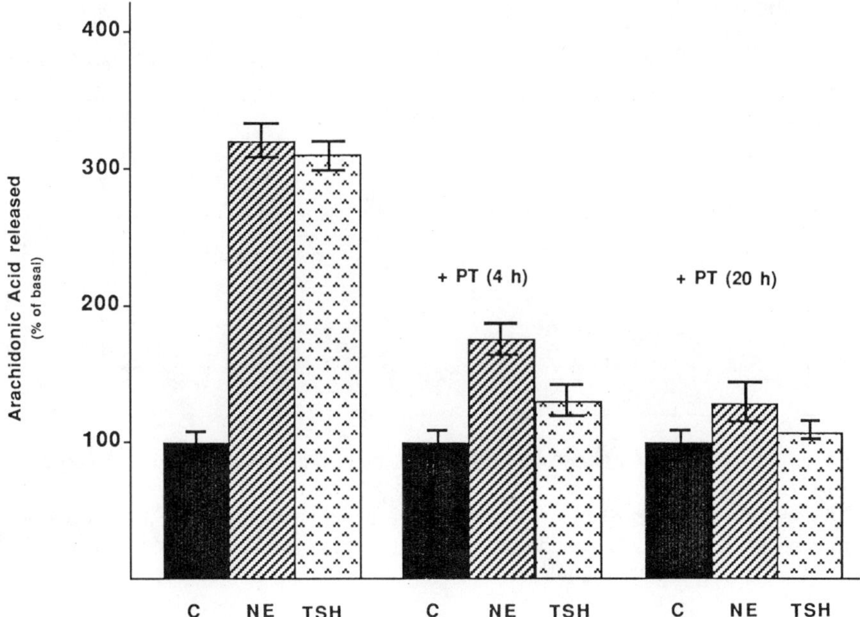

Fig. 9. The effect of pertussis toxin on the TSH and NE stimulated arachidonic acid release from FRTL5 thyroid cells. This figure was taken from Ref. 22. See Fig. 4 for details on the procedure[22]. Pertussis toxin was at a concentration of 10^{-9} M. Norepinephrine and TSH were both added at a 10^{-6} M concentration. The results are mean ± SE of 4 to 6 experiments performed in duplicates.

PLC has a different sensitivity to pertussis toxin from the one coupled to the arachidonic acid release[22,38,59]. Moreover, in permeabilized cells the non-hydrolyzable GTP analog GTPγS was able to induce the release of arachidonic acid in cells treated with neomycin (a specific inhibitor of PLC) demonstrating a) the role of a G protein in the activation of PLA2 and b) the dissociation of the two pathways leading to the Ca^{++} increase (PLC) and to the arachidonic acid release (PLA2)[59].

The TSH and α1-adrenergic receptors modulation of the PLA2 activity have similar sensitivity to pertussis toxin, suggesting the possibility that the same G protein mediates the coupling of these receptors to the enzyme (Fig. 9)[22,23].

In summary, the α1-adrenergic receptor in FRTL5 cells is coupled to PLA2 and PLC via two G proteins which have a different sensitivity to pertussis toxin, whereas the TSH receptor uses a pertussis toxin sensitive G protein in the coupling to the PLA2 activation and a pertussis toxin insensitive pathway in the coupling to PLC[22,23,38].

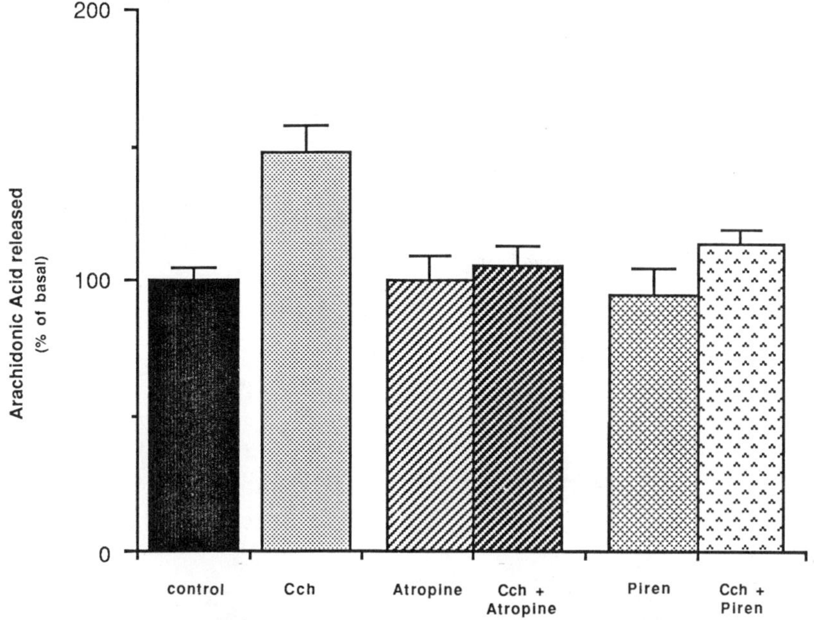

Fig. 10. Effect of carbachol and muscarinic antagonists on the arachidonic acid release from FRTL5 thyroid cells. Carbachol, atropine and pirenzepine were used at a concentration of 10^{-6} M and 10^{-5} M, respectively[44,46]. See Fig. 4 for details on the procedure. Data are the mean ±SE of six to ten experiments performed in duplicate.

Muscarinic activation of phosholipase A2

As mentioned above, the effect of carbachol on the steady-state iodide content of FRTL5 cells could be related to an activation of PLA2[23,44,46]. Carbachol is indeed able to increase the arachidonic acid release in FRTL5 cells in a dose and time dependent manner[23,44,46]. This phenomenon involves a muscarinic receptor of the M1 class since it was inhibited both by the muscarinic antagonist atropine and by the M1 specific antagonist pirenzepine (Fig. 10)[46]. This receptor is therefore different from the muscarinic receptor inhibiting PLC which has been shown to be insensitive to pirenzepine (M2 class)[45,47]. We have mentioned above that G proteins are involved in coupling the α1-adrenergic and TSH receptors to PLA2 activation[22,23,38]. Similarly, the carbachol dependent arachidonic acid release was reduced by ~50% in FRTL5 cells pretreated for 12 hr with pertussis toxin

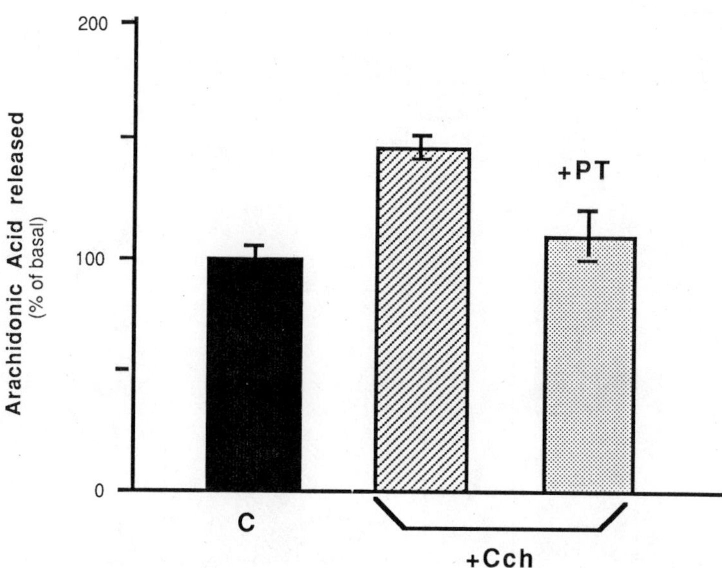

Fig. 11. Effect of pertussis toxin on the carbachol stimulated arachidonic acid release from FRTL5 thyroid cells. The preincubation with pertussis toxin (10^{-9} M) was for 12 hours[44,46]. Carbachol was added at a 10^{-6} M concentration[44,46]. See Fig. 4 for details on the procedure. Data are the mean ± SE of eight experiments performed in duplicate.

(Fig. 11) indicating that a G protein takes part in the coupling between the muscarinic receptor and the PLA2 activation[44,46]. This G protein however has a lower sensitivity to pertussis toxin when compared to the G protein coupled to the α_1-adrenergic and TSH receptors, indicating that in this cell system different G proteins intervene in the activation of PLA2[22,23,38,44,46].

THE FRTL5 CELLS REGULATION

The FRTL5 cells, like most cell types, are exposed to a continuous flow of stimuli leading to their activation or inhibition. Ideally, we would like to know the mechanisms by which the different second messengers generated by the hormonal stimuli interact at the cytosolic level to generate the "perfect" cell functioning.

The following scheme summarizes the intracellular events occurring in FRTL5 cells upon TSH, norepinephrine or carbachol stimulation (Fig. 12). Thyroid hormone formation

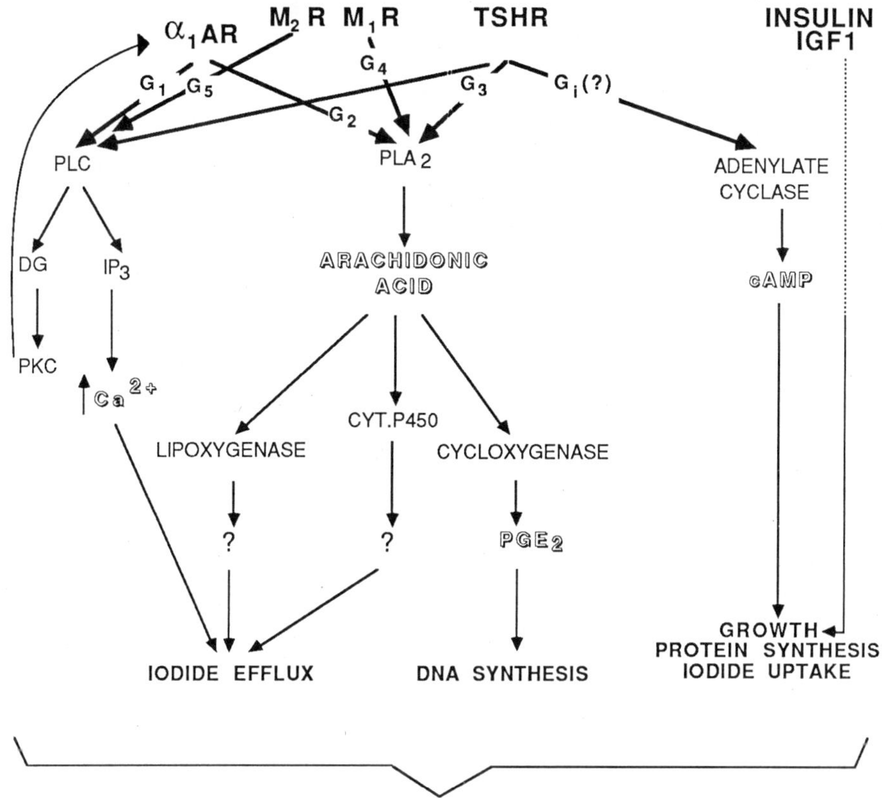

Fig. 12. Biochemical events following the hormonal stimulation of FRTL5 cells. α1AR, TSHR, M1R and M2R indicate the α1-adrenergic, TSH and muscarinic receptors, respectively. The other abbreviations are: G_1, G_2, G_3, G_4, G_5, and Gi different GTP binding proteins; PLC, phospholipase C; PLA_2, phospholipase A_2; DG, diacylglycerol; IP_3, inositol 1,4,5-trisphosphate; cAMP, adenosine 3',5'-cyclic monophosphate; PKC, protein kinase C; CYT.P450, cytochrome P450; PGE2, prostaglandin E_2. See text for details.

requires the synthesis of thyroglobulin and its iodination. Iodide efflux, which precedes iodination, is induced both by TSH and norepinephrine, which act by stimulating PLC and PLA2. Carbachol decreases the activity of PLC. Ca^{++} and the arachidonic acid metabolites are second messengers involved in the iodide efflux regulation. Two G proteins sensitive to pertussis toxin mediate the coupling of the α1-adrenergic receptor to PLC and PLA2.

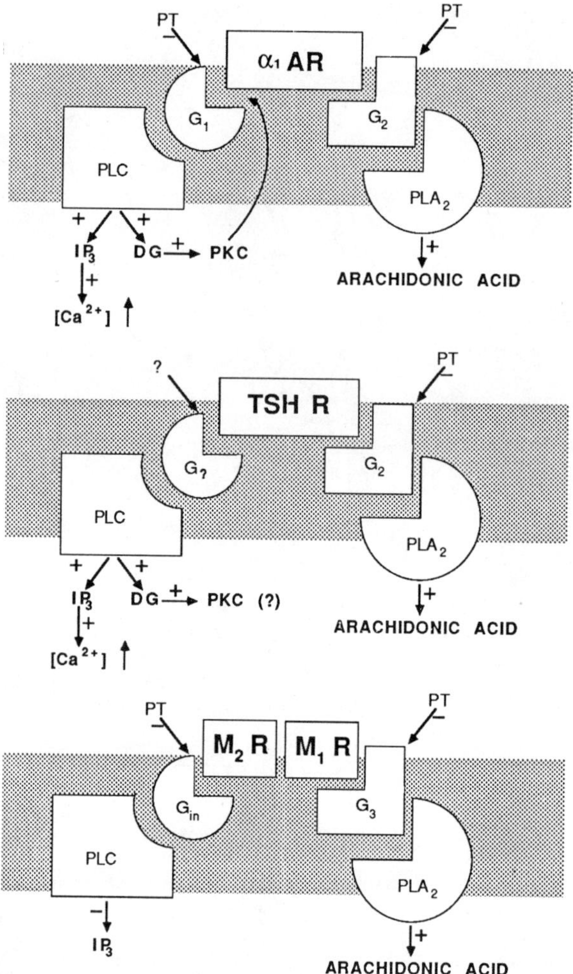

Fig. 13. Scheme of the coupling of the α1-adrenergic, TSH and muscarinic receptors to PLC and PLA2. See legend to Fig. 12 for the abbreviations and text for details.

A G protein sensitive to pertussis toxin couples the TSH receptor to PLA2. G proteins with different sensitivity to pertussis toxin mediate the coupling of the M2 and M1 muscarinic receptors to the inhibition of PLC and to the activation of PLA2, respectively. The adrenergic activation of PLC causes the activation of protein kinase C by diacylglycerol. In FRTL5 cells this represent a negative feedback regulation of the α1-adrenergic receptor which is in this way uncoupled from the transducing enzyme[22,23,51]. Therefore the adrenergic activation of PLC can both switch on (via the inositol 1,4,5-trisphosphate formation) and switch off (via the protein kinase C activation) α1-adrenergic signalling mechanism.

The TSH receptor is coupled to the adenylyl cyclase system. The cyclic AMP produced leads to the regulation of growth, iodide uptake and protein synthesis. Growth is in part regulated also via the PLA2 pathway. Infact, the prostaglandin E2 formed via the α1-adrenergic activation of the cyclooxygenase, is able to increase DNA synthesis (Fig. 12)[59]. It will be interesting to investigate the interplay among the adrenergic, muscarinic and TSH regulation of PLC and PLA2 activity to modulate thyroid functions.

Fig. 13 summarizes our present knowledge of the coupling of the adrenergic, muscarinic and TSH receptors to PLC and PLA2. We can speculate at this point that the number of receptors to be described in FRTL5 could still increase, in particular if we consider the possibility that subclasses of receptors of the same family could define the specificity of the coupling to the different transducing enzymes. For example, the availability of several muscarinic antagonists has made possible the identification of two subclasses of muscarinic receptors. However, recent data from the molecular cloning of five subtypes of muscarinic receptors, suggest that this subclassification could be more complex than what we have considered so far[5]. We could therefore hypothesize that the adrenergic and TSH regulation of these phospholipases could be due to receptors subclasses, similarly to what was observed for the M1 and M2 muscarinic receptors. We are experimentally evaluating this possibility for the α1-adrenergic receptor. As for TSH receptors, unfortunately there are no available tools at this point to distinguish between possible receptors subclasses.

It should be added that in a recent report it has been shown that in FRTL5 cells PLC is regulated also by a purinergic receptor which uses G proteins[60]. The interaction among the purinergic, adrenergic, muscarinic and TSH stimuli is still unclear.

Summary

The FRTL5 cell line has the advantage that its hormonal activation leads to important and measurable thyroid function such as the transport of iodide and the iodination of thyroglobulin. Secondly, the coexistence in the plasma membrane of these cells of several physiologically relevant receptors (TSH, α1-adrenergic, M1 and M2 muscarinic, insulin, IGF1) coupled to at least three transducing enzymes (adenylyl cyclase, PLC, PLA2) gives the possibility to analyze the interaction among second messengers in the cell activation process. This has allowed us and others to show that in the case of the iodide efflux regulation at least two second messengers (Ca^{++} and arachidonic acid) mediate the adrenergic stimulation, whereas the TSH activation of the same phenomenon probably uses other signals in addition to Ca^{++} and arachidonic acid. Growth is mostly regulated by TSH, that activates the adenylyl cyclase by a mechanism that may involve the modulation of the availability of Gi. TSH is also able to regulate an endogenous ADP ribosyl transferase in FRTL5. This could be a novel mechanism of cell regulation by this hormone, but the role of this phenomenon in the physiological action of TSH is still unclear.

Aknowdledgments. This study was partially supported by FIDIA S.p.A., by the Italian Association for Cancer Research and by L' Agenzia per la Promozione e lo Sviluppo del Mezzogiorno (PS.35.93/IND). C.B. and M.D.G. were the recipients of fellowships from the Centro di Formazione e Studi per il Mezzogiorno-Formez (Progetto Speciale "Ricerca Scientifica Applicata nel Mezzogiorno").

REFERENCES

1. M. Schramm, and Z. Selinger, Message transmission: receptor controlled adenylate cyclase system, *Science*, 225: 1350-1356 (1984).
2. A.G. Gilman, G Proteins and dual control of adenylate cyclase, *Cell*, 36: 577-579 (1984).
3. A.G. Gilman, G proteins: transducers of receptor-generated signals, *Ann. Rev. Biochem.*, 56: 615-649 (1987).
4. J.P. Casey, and A.G. Gilman, G protein involvement in receptor-effector coupling, *J.Biol. Chem.*, 263: 2577-2580 (1988).
5. T.I. Bonner, The molecular basis of muscarinic receptor diversity, *TINS*, 12: 148-151 (1989).
6. R.J. Lefkowitz, and M.G. Caron, Adrenergic receptors: models for the study of receptors coupled to guanine nucleotide regulatory proteins, *J. Biol. Chem.*, 263: 4993-4996 (1988).
7. B.K. Kobilka, T.S. Kobilka, K. Daniel, J.W. Regan, M.G. Caron, and R.J. Lefkowitz, Chimeric $\alpha 2$ -, $\beta 2$-adrenergic receptors: delineation of domains involved in effector coupling and ligand binding specificity, *Science*, 240: 1310-1316 (1988).
8. F.S. Ambesi-Impiombato, R. Picone, and D. Tramontano, Influence of hormones and serum on growth and differentiation of the thyroid cell strain, *FRTL*, in: "Cold Spring Harbor Symposia on Quantitative Biology", D.A. Serbasku, G.H. Sato, and A. Pardee, Vol. 9: 483-492, Cold Spring Harbor (1982).

9. F.S. Ambesi-Impiombato, L.A.M. Parks, and H.G. Coon, Culture of hormone-dependent functional epithelial cells from rat thyroids, *Proc. Natl. Acad. Sci. USA*, 77: 3455-3459 (1980).

10. W.A. Valente, P. Vitti, L.D. Kohn, M.L. Brandi, C.M. Rotella, R. Toccafondi, D. Tramontano, S.M. Aloj, and F.S. Ambesi-Impiombato, The relationship of growth and adenylate cyclase activity in cultured thyroid cells: separate bioeffects of thyrotropin, *Endocrinology,* 112: 71-79 (1983).

11. P. Vitti, C.M. Rotella, W.A. Valente, J. Cohen, S.M. Aloj, P. Laccetti, F.S. Ambesi-Impiombato, E.F. Grollman, A. Pinchera, R. Toccafondi, and L.D. Kohn, Characterization of the optimal stimulatory effects of Graves' monoclonal and serum immunoglobulin G on adenosine 3', 5' -monophosphate production in FRTL-5 thyroid cells: a potential clinical assay, *J. Clin. Endocrinol. Metab.,* 57: 782-791 (1983).

12. S.J. Weiss, N.J. Philp, F.S. Ambesi-Impiombato, and E.F. Grollman, Thyrotropin-stimulated iodide transport mediated by adenosine 3', 5'-monophosphate and dependent on protein synthesis, *Endocrinology,* 114: 1099-1107 (1984).

13. S.J. Weiss, N.J. Philp, and E.F. Grollman, Iodide transport in a continuous line of cultured cells from rat thyroid, *Endocrinology,* 114: 1090-1098 (1984).

14. S.J. Weiss, N.J. Philp, and E.F. Grollman, Effect of thyrotropin on iodide efflux in FRTL-5 cells mediated by Ca^{2+}, *Endocrinology,* 114: 1108-1113 (1984).

15. F. Lami, P. Roger, L. Contor, S. Reuse, E. Raspe, J. Van Sande, and J.E. Dumont, Control of thyroid cell proliferation: the example of the dog thyrocyte, in: *Hormones and cell regulation*, J. Nunez, and J.E. Dumont, 153: 169-180. John Libey, London (1987).

16. J.E. Dumont, J.C. Jauniaux, and P.P. Roger, The cyclic AMP-mediated stimulation of cell proliferation, *TIBS* , 14: 67-71 (1989).

17. D. Tramontano, A.C. Moses, B.M. Veneziani, and S.H. Ingbar, Adenosine 3', 5'-monophosphate mediates both the mitogenic effect of thyrotropin and its ability to amplify the response to insulin-like growth factor I in FRTL5 cells, *Endocrinology*, 122: 127-132 (1988).

18. S. Jin, F.J. Hornicek, D. Neylan, M. Zakarija, and J.M. Mc Kenzie, Evidence that adenosine 3'-5' monophosphate mediates stimulation of growth in FRTL5 cells, *Endocrinology,* 119: 802-810 (1986).

19. D. Tramontano, G.W. Cushing, A.C. Moses, and S.H. Ingbar, Insulin-ike growth factor I stimulates the growth of rat thyroid cells in culture and synergizes the growth-promoting effect of thyrotropin and of Graves IgG, *Endocrinology*, 119: 940-942 (1986).

20. O. Isozaki, and L.D. Kohn, Control of c-fos and c-myc proto-oncogene induction in rat thyroid cells in culture, *Mol. Endocrinol.*, 1: 839-848 (1987).

21. D. Corda, C. Marcocci, L.D. Kohn, J. Axelrod, and A. Luini, Association of the changes in cytosolic Ca^{2+} and iodide efflux induced by thyrotropin and by the stimulation of α1-adrenergic receptors in cultured rat thyroid cells, *J. Biol. Chem.*, 260: 9230-9236 (1985).

22. D. Corda, L. Iacovelli, and M. Di Girolamo, Coupling of the α1-adrenergic and thyrotropin receptors to second messenger systems in thyroid cells. Role of G-proteins, in: *"Horizons in Endocrinology"*, M. Maggi and C.A. Johnston, 169-180 Raven Press, New York, (1988).

23. D. Corda, M. Di Girolamo, and C. Bizzarri, Variety of signal transduction pathways in FRTL5 thyroid cells, in: *FRTL5 Today*, F.S. Ambesi-Impiombato and H. Perrild, 95-98 Elsevier, Amsterdam, (1989).

24. C. Marcocci, A. Luini, P. Santisteban, and E.F. Grollman, Norepinephrine and thyrotropin stimulation of iodide efflux in FRTL-5 thyroid cells involves metabolites of arachidonic acid and is associated whith the iodination of thyroglobulin, *Endocrinology,* 120: 1127-1133 (1987).

25. R.M. Burch, A. Luini, D.E. Mais, D. Corda, J.Y.Vanderhoek, L.D. Kohn, and J. Axelrod, α1-Adrenergic stimulation of arachidonic acid release and metabolism in rat thyroid cell line, *J. Biol. Chem.*, 261: 11236-11241 (1986).

26. D. Corda, R.D. Sekura, and L.D. Kohn, Thyrotropin effect on the availability of Ni regulatory protein in FRTL-5 rat thyroid cells to ADP-ribosylation by pertussis toxin, *Eur. J. Biochem.*, 166: 475-481 (1987).

27 L.D. Kohn, S.M. Aloj, D. Tombaccini, C.M. Rotella, R. Toccafondi, C. Marcocci, D. Corda, and E.F. Grollman, The thyrotropin receptor, *Biochemical Action of Hormones,* 12: 457-512 (1985).

28. F. Ribeiro-Neto, L. Birnbaumer, and J.B. Field, Incubation of bovine thyroid slices with thyrotropin is associated with a decrease in the ability of pertussis toxin to adenosine diphosphate ribosylate guanine nucleotide regulatory components, *Mol. Endocrinol.,* 1: 482-490 (1987).

29. D. Corda, L. Iacovelli, and M. Di Girolamo, Thyrotropin regulated ADP ribosyl-transferase activity in thyroid cells, Submitted for publication.

30. P. Vitti, M.J.S. De Wolf, A.M. Acquaviva, M. Epstein, and L.D. Kohn, Thyrotropin stimulation of the ADP-ribosyltransferase activity of bovine thyroid membranes, *Proc. Natl. Acad. Sci. U.S.A.,* 79: 1525-1529 (1982).

31. C. Marcocci, J.L. Cohen, and E.F. Grollman, Effect of actinomycin D on iodide transport in FRTL-5 thyroid cells, *Endocrinology,* 115: 2123-2132 (1984).

32. D. Corda, and L.D. Kohn, Thyrotropin upregulates α1-adrenergic receptors in rat FRTL-5 thyroid cells , *Proc. Natl. Acad. Sci. USA* , 82: 8677-8680 (1985).

33. E. Bone, D.W. Alling, and E.F. Grollman, Norepinephrine and thyroid-stimulating hormone induce inositol phosphate accumulation in FRTL-5 cells, *Endocrinology*, 219: 2193-2200 (1986).

34. H.A. Lippes, and S.W. Spaulding, Peroxide formation and glucose oxidation in calf thyroid slices: regulation by protein kinase-C and cytosolic free calcium, *Endocrinology*, 118: 1306-1311 (1986).

35. K. Haraguchi, C.S.S. Rani, and J.B. Field, Effects of thyrotropin, carbachol, and protein kinase-C stimulators on glucose transport and glucose oxidation by primary cultures of dog thyroid cells, *Endocrinology*, 123: 1288-1295 (1988).

36. N.J. Philp, and E.F. Grollman, Thyrotropin and norepinephrine stimulate the metabolism of phosphoinositides in FRTL-5 thyroid cells, *FEBS Lett.*, 202: 193-196 (1986).

37. J.B. Field, P.A. Ealey, N.J. Marshall, and S. Cockcroft, Thyroid-stimulating hormone stimulates increases in inositol phosphates as well as cyclic AMP in the FRTL-5 rat thyroid cell line, *Biochem J.*, 248: (1987).

38. D. Corda, and L.D. Kohn, Role of pertussis toxin sensitive G proteins in the alph α1-adrenergic receptor but not in the thyrotropin receptor mediated activation of membrane phospholipases and iodide fluxes in FRTL-5 thyroid cells, *Biochem. Biophys. Res. Commun.,* 141: 1000-1006 (1986).

39. K. Yamashita, and J.B. Field, Elevation of cyclic guanosine 3', 5'-monophosphate levels in dog thyroid slices caused by acetylcholine and sodium fluoride, *J. Biol. Chem.*, 247: 7062-7066 (1972).

40. M.L. Maayan, E.M. Volpert, and A. From, Acetylcholine and norepinephrine: compared actions on thyroid metabolism, *Endocrinology*, 112: 1358-1362 (1983).

41. J. Van Sande, J.E. Dumont, A. Melander, and F. Sundler, Presence and influence of

cholinergic nerves in the human thyroid, *J. Clin. Endocrinol. and Metab.*, 51: 500-502 (1980).

42. C.S.S. Rani, A.E. Boyd, and J.B. Field, Effects of acetylcholine, TSH and other stimulators on intracellular calcium concentration in dog thyroid cells, *Biochem. Biophys. Res. Commun.,* 131: 1041-1047 (1985).
43. I. Graff, J. Mockel, E. Laurent, C. Erneux, and J.E. Dumont, Carbachol and sodium fluoride, but not TSH, stimulate the generation of inositol phosphates in the dog thyroid, *FEBS Lett.,* 210: 204-210 (1987).
44. M. Di Girolamo, C. Bizzarri, and D. Corda, A muscarinic receptor is coupled to phospholipase A2 in FRTL5 thyroid cells, in: *FRTL5 Today,* F.S. Ambesi-Impiombato and H. Perrild, Elsevier, Amsterdam, In press.
45. C. Bizzarri, M. Di Girolamo, and D. Corda, Muscarinic inhibition of the norepinephrine induced increase in cytosolic calcium in FRTL5 thyroid cells, in: *FRTL5 Today,* F.S. Ambesi-Impiombato and H. Perrild, Elsevier, Amsterdam, In press.
46. M. Di Girolamo, C. Bizzarri, and D. Corda, Muscarinic regulation of phospholipase A2 in thyroid cells - Role of a G protein, Submitted for publication.
47. C. Bizzarri, M. Di Girolamo and D. Corda, Muscarinic inhibition of phospholipase C activity. A direct mechanism involving a G protein, Submitted for publication.
48. C. Bizzarri, M. Di Girolamo, and D. Corda, Muscarinic inhibition of phospholipase C activity in thyroid cells. Involvement of an inhibitory G protein, (abstracts), Eur. J. Cell Biol., Suppl. Vol. 48, In press.
49. S. Cockcroft, Polyphosphoinositide phosphodiesterase: regulation by a novel guanine nucleotide binding protein, Gp, *TIBS* ,12: 75-78 (1987).
50. L. Vallar, and J. Meldolesi, Mechanisms of signal transduction at the dopamine D2 receptor, *TIPS,* 10: 74-77 (1989).
51. D. Corda, and L.D. Kohn, Phorbol myristate acetate inhibits α1-adrenergically but not thyrotropin-regulated functions in FRTL-5 rat thyroid cells, *Endocrinology*, 120: 1152-1160 (1987).
52. L.M.F. Leeb-Lundberg, S. Cotecchia, J.W. Lomasney, J.F. DeBernardis, R.J. Lefkowitz, and M.G. Caron, Phorbol esters promote α1-adrenergic receptor phosphorylation and receptor uncoupling from inositol phospholipid metabolism, *Proc. Natl. Acad. Sci. USA,* 82: 5651-5655 (1985).
53. C.S.S. Rani, and J.B. Field, Comparison of effects of thyrotropin, phorbol esters, norepinephrine, and carbachol on iodide organification in dog thyroid slices, follicles,

and cultured cells, *Endocrinology*, 122: 1915-1922 (1988).

54. L. Contor, F. Lamy, R. Lecocq, P.P. Roger, and J.E. Dumont, Differential protein phosphorylation in induction of thyroid cell proliferation by thyrotropin, epidermal growth factor, or phorbol ester, *Mol. Cell Biol.*, 8: 2494-2503 (1988).
55. B. Haye, J.L. Aublin, S. Champion, B. Lambert, and C. Jacquemin, Tetradecanoyl phorbol-13-acetate counteracts the responsiveness of cultured thyroid cells to thyrotropin, *Biochem. Pharm.*, 34: 3795-3802 (1985).
56. L.K. Bachrach, M.C. Eggo, W.W. Mak, and G.N. Burrow, Phorbol esters stimulate growth and inhibit differentiation in cultured thyroid cells, *Endocrinology,* 116: 1603-1609 (1985).
57. K. Takada, N. Amino, T. Tetsumoto, and K. Miyai, Phorbol esters have a dual action through protein kinase C in regulation of proliferation of FRTL5 cells, *FEBS Lett.,* 234: 13-16 (1988).
58. A. Lombardi, B.M. Veneziani, D. Tramontano, and S. H. Ingbar, Independent and interactive effects of tetradecanoyl phorbol acetate on growth and differentiated functions of FRTL-5 cells, *Endocrinology*, 123: 1544-1552 (1988).
59. R.M. Burch, A. Luini, and J. Axelrod, Phospholipase A2 and phospholipase C are activated by distinct GTP-binding proteins in response to α1-adrenergic stimulation in FRTL-5 thyroid cells, *Proc. Natl. Acad. Sci. USA,* 83: 7201-7205 (1986).
60. F. Okajima, K. Sho, and Y. Kondo, Inhibition by islet-activating protein, pertussis toxin, of P2-purinergic receptor-mediated iodide efflux and phosphoinositide turnover in FRTL-5 cells, *Endocrinology*, 123: 1035-1043 (1988).

ADP RIBOSYLATION AND G PROTEIN REGULATION IN THE THYROID

James B. Field, Fernando Ribeiro-Neto, Madoka Taguchi
William Deery, CS Sheela Rani and Daniela Pasquali

Diabetes Research Laboratory
St. Lukes Episcopal Hospital
Department of Medicine
Baylor College of Medicine
Houston, TX 77030

Although most of the metabolic effects of TSH on the thyroid reflect its activation of the adenylate cyclase-cAMP system (1), other signalling systems mediate the effect of other agonists such as acetylcholine (2) and phorbol esters (3). Furthermore effects of TSH on desensitization (4) and ^{32}P incorporation into phospholipids (1) are not mediated by cAMP. The phosphatidylinositol 4,5-bisphosphate cascade which increases intracellular Ca^{2+} and activates protein kinase C is present in the thyroid and may be important for the regulation of several metabolic effects (5-9). ADP ribosylation of various proteins is another possible signalling system for cell regulation (10-13). Although this process may involve either poly ADP ribosylation or mono ADP ribosylation, the present discussion will be limited to the latter process.

Vitti et al reported that a 40 KDa protein was ADP ribosylated in bovine thyroid plasma membranes and that such ADP ribosylation was increased by TSH (10). This same substrate was ADP ribosylated by cholera toxin. The effect of TSH was present within 1 minute, was 80% maximal by 2 min and was dependent on the amount of TSH. 1 nM TSH produced an effect which was maximal with 100 nM. Thyroglobulin, insulin, FSH, LH and HCG were ineffective. The TSH stimulation of ADP ribosylation was postulated to be linked to the activation of adenylate cyclase since an inhibitor of the TSH stimulated ADP ribosylation also decreased the hormone's activation of adenylate cyclase. Furthermore TSH stimulation of ADP ribosylation was more rapid and achieved maximal rates faster than its stimulation of adenylate cyclase. Finally when membranes were prepared in hypotonic buffer, NAD increased TSH stimulation of adenylate cyclase.

Filetti and Rapoport also reported that TSH stimulated ADP ribosylation in permeabilized dog thyroid cells as shown in Table 1 (11). The maximum effect was present in 30-60 minutes and required 100 mU/ml hormone. The stimulation involved the ADP ribosyl transferase rather than any change in the substrate pool size or specific activity since it was evident even when a 1000 fold excess of NAD was added. Mono ADP ribosylation rather than poly ADP ribosylation was primarily involved. This effect of TSH was not mediated by cAMP since it was inhibited by dibutyryl cAMP and isobutylmethylxanthine. The stimulation of ADP ribosylation was linked to TSH-induced desensitization (11-13), a process which is independent of cAMP (4) but related to NAD. Thus nicotinamide (50 mM) and N'-methyl nicotinamide inhibited both TSH stimulated ADP ribosylation and desensitization (Table 2). Since N'-methyl nicotinamide cannot be incorporated into an oxidatively functional NAD, the effect of NAD must be other than on electron transport. In addition, nicotinamide accelerated the recovery from TSH-induced desensitization. Arginine and arginine methyl ester which can be ADP ribosylated also inhibited TSH-induced desensitization in thyroid 19 HT cells (12). These compounds decreased cholera toxin mediated ADP ribosylation providing further evidence for the hypothesis that mono ADP ribosylation is important in TSH desensitization. However, this effect of arginine and arginine methyl ester could not be obtained in other types of thyroid cells. Other inhibitors of poly ADP ribose polymerase such as thymidine, 5 bromouridine and pyridoxine also prevented TSH desensitization. In contrast to TSH-induced desensitization, nicotinamide did not prevent homologous desensitization due to prostaglandin E_1 or adenosine.

TABLE 1

Effect of TSH on ADP ribosylation in dog thyroid cells

	Time in minutes		
	0	15	30
	pmol ADP ribose/mg protein		
None	0	0.47 ± 0.08	0.76 ± 0.01
TSH (100 mU/ml)	-	0.75 ± 0.05	1.32 ± 0.29

Reprinted with permission from Filetti, S. and Rapoport, B., J. Clin. Investigation 68:461, 1981

TABLE 2

Effect of nicotinamide and analogues to prevent TSH induced desensitization in human thyroid cells

	pmol cAMP/10^6 cells	
	15 min	6 hours
Control	38 ± 3.5	38 ± 3.5
TSH (100 mU/ml)	830 ± 40	393 ± 12
TSH + nicotinamide	1040 ± 110	1152 ± 128
TSH + N'-methyl nicotinamide	1093 ± 90	1027 ± 100

Reprinted with permission from Filetti, S. et al. **J. Biol. Chem.** 256:1072, 1981.

Despite the reports that TSH stimulated ADP ribosylation in thyroid tissue (10,11,13), other investigators have not observed such an effect (14,15). While Rebois et al found some evidence for endogenous ADP ribosyltransferase activity in membranes from FRTL cells, addition of TSH was without effect (14). In contrast cholera toxin ADP ribosylated 41,45 and 47 KDa polypeptides. The assays were done with 5 mM M_gCl_2 which is essential for cholera toxin ADP ribosylation but inhibits the effect of pertussis toxin (16). Thus it is possible that the incubation conditions would inhibit ADP ribosylation even though during stimulation of adenylate cyclase, cholera toxin, but not TSH, caused ADP ribosylation of specific membrane proteins (14). The failure to detect ADP ribosyl-transferase might reflect the activity of a processing enzyme which released AMP (13). In contrast to the results of Vitti et al (10), Rebois reported that NAD was not necessary for stimulation of adenylate cyclase by TSH (14). Rebeiro-Neto, using conditions that would be optimal for either cholera or pertussis toxin ADP ribosylation found no evidence for endogenous ADP ribosylation in membranes from bovine thyroid slices which had been incubated with or without TSH (15).

However, TSH did have an effect on the subsequent ADP ribosylation of a 40 KDa substrate for pertussis toxin in bovine thyroid and FRTL-5 membranes (15,17). Incubation of bovine thyroid slices with TSH for 2 hours decreased the pertussis toxin mediated ADP ribosylation of a 40 KDa polypeptide in membrane preparations by 40-60% (Fig 1) (15). This was not due to destruction of GTP or

NAD. Inhibition was present as early as 1 minute and persisted for 30 minutes of incubation of the membranes with pertussis toxin (Fig 2). The effect of TSH required at least a 60 min incubation and 10 mU/ml of the hormone (Fig 3). Although these conditions were similar to those necessary for TSH induced desensitization of adenylate cyclase (18) and ADP ribosylation has been implicated in TSH desensitization (11-13), the two effects are probably unrelated. Thus incubation of thyroid slices with pertussis toxin for 6 hours decreased the subsequent pertussis toxin ADP ribosylation of the 40 KDa substrate but did not modify TSH induced desensitization (15). Similar results were obtained using FRTL-5 cells (4). In addition, activation of G_i with α_2 adrenergic stimulation potentiated the TSH-induced desensitization. Furthermore PGE_1, which also causes homologous desensitization of the adenylate cyclase system in bovine thyroid slices (Fig 4) (15), had no effect on the subsequent pertussis toxin mediated ADP ribosylation in bovine thyroid plasma membranes (Fig 5). The effect of TSH to decrease ADP ribosylation of the 40 KDa substrate by pertussis toxin appears to reflect a change in the availability of the substrate since treatment of the membranes with 0.3% Lubrol PX prior to assay of ADP ribosylation abolished the difference between the slices incubated with and without TSH (Fig 6). In contrast to the effects of TSH on the pertussis toxin substrate, the hormone did not alter the ADP ribosylation induced by cholera toxin (15,17). Corda et al reported that incubation of FRTL-5 cells with either TSH or pertussis toxin, but not cholera toxin, decreased pertussis toxin mediated ADP ribosylation of a 40 KDa polypeptide in the membranes of the cells (17). An effect of TSH was present after 20 min incubation of the cells and after 60 min incubation, the pertussis toxin substrate appeared to be completely ADP ribosylated.

TABLE 3

Conditions favoring ADP ribosylation

	Cholera Toxin	Pertussis Toxin
GTP	+++	++++
ATP	0	+++
Mg^{2+}	+++	inhibits
Pi	+++	inhibits
Lubrol extraction	no effect	25-30 fold increase

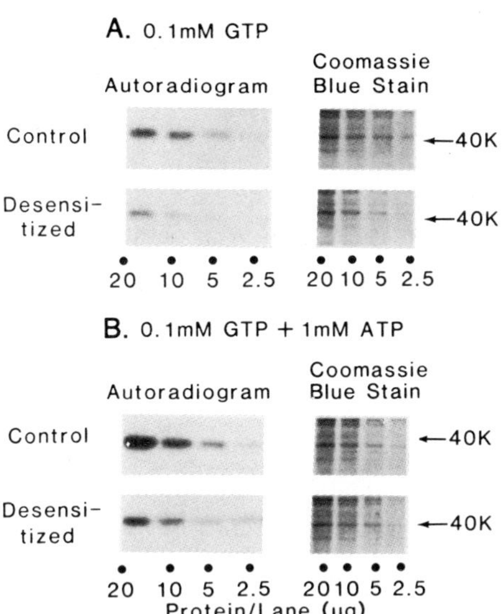

Figure 1. Effect of TSH treatment of bovine thyroid slices on ADP ribosylation of the 40 KDa band in thyroid membranes using different amounts of membrane proteins and nucleotides. The desensitized membranes were prepared from slices which had been previously incubated with TSH for 2 hours. Reprinted with permission from Ribeiro-Neto, F., et al., Mol. Endocrinology 1:482, 1987.

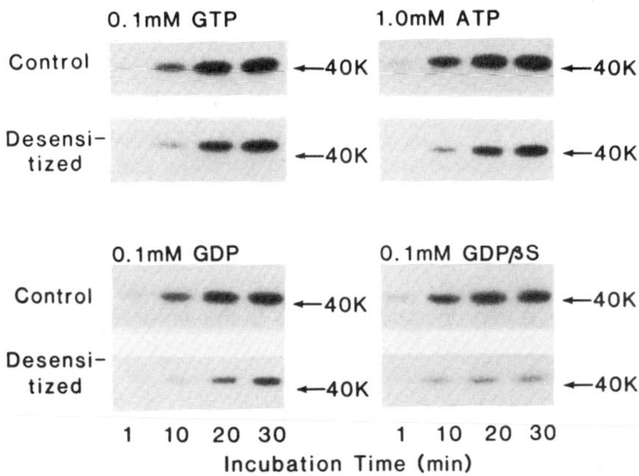

Figure 2. Effect of TSH treatment of bovine thyroid slices on ADP ribosylation of the 40 KDa band in thyroid membranes assayed at various times of incubation and with different nucleotides. Reprinted with permission from Ribeiro-Neto, F. et al., Mol. Endocrinology 1:482, 1987.

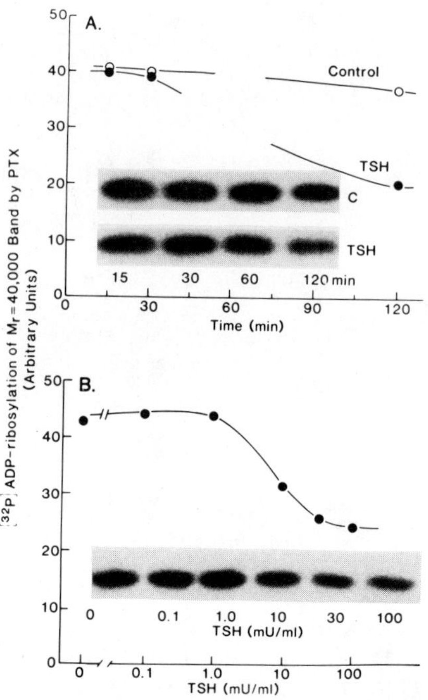

Figure 3. Time and concentration dependence of TSH-induced decreased pertussis toxin catalyzed ADP ribosylation of the 40 KDa bands in bovine thyroid membranes. Reprinted with permission from Ribeiro-Neto, F. et al., Mol. Endocrinology 1:482, 1987.

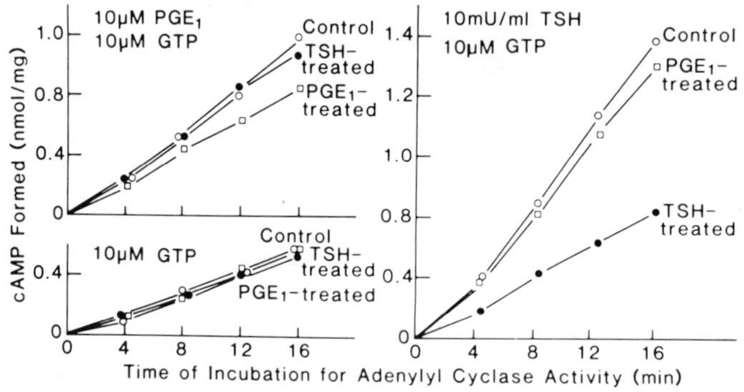

Figure 4. Comparison of the effect of treating bovine thyroid slices with either TSH or PGE_1 on basal, TSH and PGE_1 stimulated adenylate cyclase in plasma membranes. Reprinted with permission from Ribeiro-Neto, F. et al., Mol. Endocrinology 1:482, 1987.

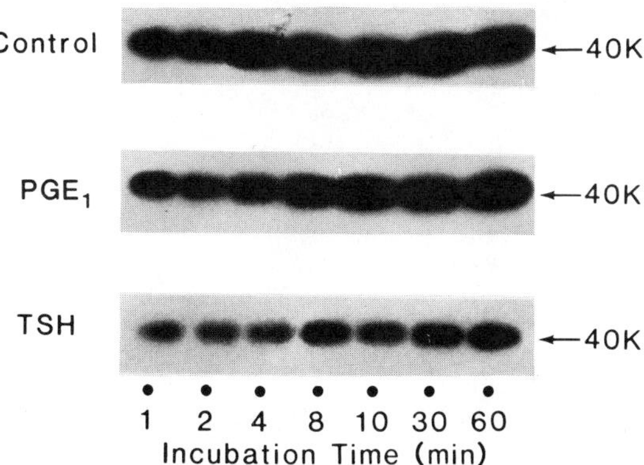

Figure 5. Lack of significant effect of treatment of thyroid slices with PGE_1 on subsequent ADP ribosylation of the 40 KDa band in plasma membranes. Reprinted with permission from Ribeiro-Neto, F. et al., Mol. Endocrinology 1:482, 1987.

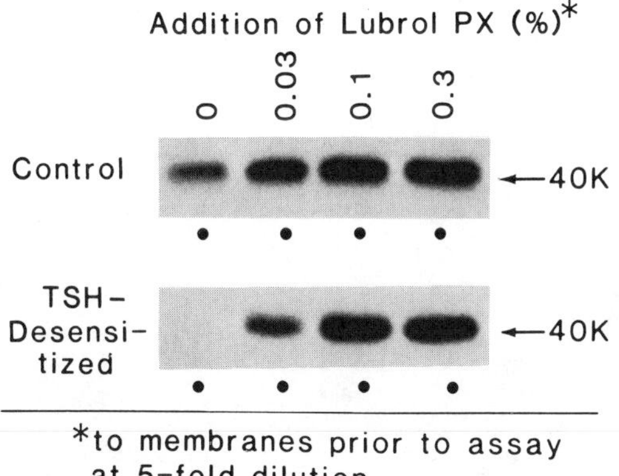

Figure 6. Effect of Lubrol PX extraction of control and desensitized bovine thyroid slices prior to assay of ADP ribosylation of the 40 KDa band in plasma membranes. Reprinted with permission from Ribeiro-Neto, F. et al., Mol. Endocrinology 1:482, 1987.

TABLE 4
Effect of TSH and pertussis toxin on cAMP in FRTL-5 cells

	pmol/well
Control	< 1
TSH 1 nM	63 ± 2
Pertussis Toxin 10 nM	3 ± 0.1
TSH + Pertussis Toxin	49 ± 3

Reprinted with permission from Corda, D. et al. **Eur. J. Biochem.** 166:475, 1987.

Another approach to evaluating the role of ADP ribosylation in thyroid tissue is examination of effects of cholera and pertussis toxins on various parameters of thyroid metabolism. It is recognized that such studies are restricted to those polypeptides which are substrates for the two toxins while ADP ribosylation of other polypeptides might be important. Furthermore, effects of cholera or pertussis toxin could reflect actions other than ADP ribosylation. Substrates for both cholera and pertussis toxin have been repeatedly demonstrated in thyroid tissue (10-17). Despite some variability depending on the type of the thyroid tissue, the substrate for pertussis toxin is approximately 40 KDa while that for cholera toxin has ranged from 42 to 50 KDa. Table 3 indicates that the assay conditions favoring ADP ribosylation of the substrates for the two toxins are quite different.

A role for ADP ribosylation in the TSH activation of adenylate cyclase was proposed by Vitti et al (10) and discussed above. Cholera toxin increases cAMP in thyroid tissue (17,4) and potentiates the effect of TSH via ADP ribosylation of G_s (10). However, incubation with TSH does not alter the ability of cholera toxin to ADP ribosylate G_s or function in an assay for G_s using cyc^- cells (20,21). Effects of pertussis toxin on cAMP have not always been consistent. Corda et al reported that pertussis toxin increased cAMP in FRTL-5 cells and potentiated the effect of forskolin (17). However, the same investigator observed that the toxin decreased the stimulatory effect of TSH on cAMP (Table 4). Opposite results were observed in dog thyroid slices in which the effect of TSH was potentiated by pertussis toxin (Table 5) (22). Furthermore, incubations of dog thyroid slices with pertussis toxin for 15-22 hours reversed the norepinephrine inhibition of TSH stimulated cAMP accumulation but had no effect on the inhibition induced by carbachol or iodide. Such a result is not unexpected since norepinephrine acts via G_i while carbachol and iodide do not. Carbachol inhibition has been attributed to stimulation of phosphodiesterase while the mechanism for iodide inhibition is unknown (22).

TABLE 5

Effect of pertussis toxin on norepinephrine, carbachol and iodide inhibition of TSH stimulation of cAMP in dog thyroid slices

	pmol cAMP/100 mg wet weight
TSH 1 mU/ml	1637 ± 25
TSH + Norepinephrine 10^{-4}M	820 ± 114
TSH + Carbachol 10^{-5}M	1021 ± 16
TSH + IAP 250 ng/ml	2552 ± 473
TSH + IAP + NE	2327 ± 401
TSH + IAP + Carbachol	1302 ± 258

Reprinted with permission from Cochaux, P. et al. FEBS Lett. 179:303, 1985.

Phosphatidylinositol 4,5-bisphosphate hydrolysis with production of inositol trisphosphate (IP_3) and diacylglycerol is another signalling system in the thyroid (5-9). This pathway is probably responsible for increased intracellular Ca^{2+} and activation of protein kinase C which can mediate many of the metabolic events in the thyroid (2,3,23). Although TSH stimulates phosphatidylinositol 4,5-bisphosphate in the thyroid (5-8), its physiologic significance is uncertain since relatively large amounts of the hormone are required and the effect is not very rapid. However, this pathway is probably responsible for many, if not all, of the effects of carbachol on the thyroid such as increased glucose oxidation (24), ^{32}P incorporation into phospholipids (25), iodide organification (2), and increased intracellular Ca^{2+} (26). Phosphatidyl 4,5-bisphosphate hydrolysis is also involved in the α_1 adrenergic stimulation of intracellular Ca^{2+} and iodide efflux (27). While pertussis toxin, but not cholera toxin, pretreatment of normal dog thyroid cells had no effect on TSH stimulation of IP_3 formation, it did inhibit the carbachol effect (Table 6). Pertussis toxin also inhibited the norepinephrine, but not the TSH activation of phospholipase C in FRTL-5 cells (28,29). Such results suggest that two different G proteins are involved in activation of phospholipase C. Similar results were obtained in other tissues in which effects of one agonist but not another were decreased by pertussis toxin (30,31). In FRTL-5 cells pretreatment with pertussis toxin for 4-20 hours inhibited by 67% norepinephrine stimulation of iodide efflux (28) without any effect on basal or TSH stimulated activity. Although pertussis toxin decreased norepinephrine stimulation of phospholipase C and iodide efflux, it had much less effect on intracellular Ca^{2+} (28). The reason for this is not clear especially since Corda et al postulated that iodide efflux mediated by norepinephrine reflected hydrolysis of phosphatidylinositol 4,5-bisphosphate (28). However, Okajima et al postulated that agonists may increase intracellular Ca^{2+} by a mechanism that does not involve hydrolysis of PIP_2 (32). They reported that ATP stimulated IP_3 formation, intracellular Ca^{2+} and iodide efflux in FRTL-5 cells by a P_2-purinergic receptor. Although pertussis toxin inhibited the responses to 1 uM ATP, it had much less of an effect at higher concentrations of the nucleotide. They concluded that ATP stimulated phospholipase C by two different pathways, a pertussis toxin sensitive and a pertussis toxin insensitive one. The G protein involved in activation of phsopholipases A and C by norepinephrine also seem to be distinct since the former is sensitive to pertussis toxin while the latter is not (29).

TABLE 6

Effect of cholera and pertussis toxin on TSH and carbachol stimulation of inositol phosphate accumulation in dog thyroid cells

	% of control values stimulated by	
Pretreatment	TSH (250 mU/ml)	Carbachol 10^{-6}M
None	164 ± 10	204 ± 15
Cholera toxin 10 ug/ml	95 ± 9	147 ± 13
Perussis toxin 100 ng/ml	147 ± 10	154 ± 9

In normal dog thyroid cells, TSH and phorbol esters cause rapid dephosphorylation of 19 and 21 KDa polypeptides which have many characteristics of myosin light chains (33). The effect of TSH was evident within 1 minute and reached a maximum at 15 min. It was obtained with 2.5 mU/ml TSH. Calcium and calmodulin appear-ed to be involved in the stimulation of dephosphorylation by both TSH and phorbol esters (34). The effect of TSH was mediated by cAMP since it was reproduced by dibutyryl cAMP, forskolin, cholera toxin and prostaglandin E_1 (33). Pertussis toxin had no effect on the stimulation induced by TSH or phorbol esters. It is not known what function such dephosphorylation plays in thyroid gland metabolism or whether, except for augmenting cAMP, other G proteins are involved.

In conclusion, evidence has accumulated that ADP ribosylation occurs in the thyroid but the results have been conflicting as to whether the process is stimulated by TSH. TSH-induced desensitization does not seem to involve ADP ribosylation of either the cholera or pertussis G protein substrate. Although these G protein substrates may be involved in other metabolic reactions in the thyroid such as phosphatidylinositol 4,5-bisphosphate hydrolysis and its subsequent consequences, different agonists appear to utilize different G proteins for the same metabolic effect as judged by their sensitivity to pertussis toxin.

ACKNOWLEDGEMENTS

This work was supported by USPHS Grants DK 26088 and DK 27685. We also wish to acknowledge Mary Ann Farabee for her expert secretarial assistance.

REFERENCES

1. J. B. Field, "Mechanism of action of TSH, in the Thyroid," Harper and Row, New York, (1978).
2. C. DeCoster, J. Mockel, J. Van Sande, J. Unger and J. E. Dumont, The role of calcium and guanosine 3':5'-monophosphate in the action of acetylcholine on thyroid metabolism, Eur. J. Biochem. 104:199 (1980).
3. Y. Yoshimura, A. Dekker, M. Ferdows, C.S.S. Rani, and J. B. Field, Effects of phorbol esters on metabolic variables in the thyroid, Endocrinology 119:2018 (1986).
4. H. Hirau, R. P. Magnusson and B. Rapoport, Studies on the mechanism of desensitization of the cyclic AMP response to TSH stimulation in a cloned rat thyroid cell line, Mol. Cell. Endocrinol. 42:21 (1985).
5. E. A. Bone, D. W. Alling, and E. F. Grollman, Norepinephrine and thyroid-stimulating hormone induce inositol phosphate accumulation in FRTL-5 cells, Endocrinology 119:2193 (1986).
6. J. B. Field, P. A. Ealey, N. J. Marshall, and S. Cockcroft, Thyroid stimulating hormone stimulates increases in inositol phosphates as well as cyclic AMP in the FRTL-5 rat thyroid cell line, Biochem. J. 247:519 (1987).
7. E. Laurant, J. Mockel, J. Van Sande, I. Graff and J. E. Dumont, Dual activation by thyrotropin of the phospholipase C and cyclic AMP cascades in human thyroid, Mol. Cell. Endocrinol. 52:273 (1987).
8. M. Taguchi, and J. B. Field, Effects of thyroid-stimulating hormone, carbachol, norepinephrine, and adenosine 3',5'-monophosphate on polyphosphatidylinositol phosphate hydrolysis in dog thyroid slices, Endocrinology 123:2019 (1988).

9. I. Graff, J. Mockel, E. Laurent, C. Erneux, and J. E. Dumont, Carbachol and sodium fluoride, but not TSH stimulate the generation of inositol phosphates in the dog thyroid, FEBS Lett. 210:204, (1987).
10. P. Vitti, M. J. S. DeWolf, A. M. Acquaviva, M. Epstein, and L. D. Kohn, Thyrotropin stimulation of the ADP ribosyltransferase activity of bovine thyroid membranes, Proc. Nat. Acad. Sci. USA 79:1525, (1982).
11. S. Filetti, and B. Rapoport, Hormonal stimulation of eucaryotic cell ADP-ribosylation. Effect of thyrotropin on thyroid cells, J. Clin. Invest. 68:461, (1981).
12. S. Filetti, N. A. Takai, and B. Rapoport, Prevention by nicotinamide of desensitization to thyrotropin stimulation in cultured human thyroid cells, J. Biol.Chem. 256:1072, (1981).
13. M. J. S. DeWolf, P. Vitti, F. S. Ambesi-Impiombaba, and L. D. Kohn, Thyroid membrane ADP ribosyltransferase activity. J. Biol. Chem. 256:12287, (1981).
14. R. V. Rebois, S. K. Beckner, R. O. Brady, and P. H. Fishman, Mechanism of action of glycopeptide hormones and cholera toxin: What is the role of ADP ribosylation? Proc. Natl. Acad. Sci. 80:1275, (1983).
15. F. Ribeiro-Neto, L. Birnbaumer, and J. B. Field, Incubation of bovine thyroid slices with thyrotropin is associated with a decrease in the ability of pertussis toxin to adenosine diphosphate-ribosylate guanine nucleotide regulatory component(s), Mol. Endocrinol. 1:482, (1987).
16. F. Ribeiro-Neto, R. Mattera, D. Grenet, R. D. Sekura, L. Birnbaumer, and J. B. Field, Adenosine diphosphate ribosylation of G proteins by pertussis and cholerat toxin in isolated membranes. Different requirements for and effects of guanine nucleotides and Mg^{2+}, Mol. Endocrinol. 1:472, (1981).
17. D. Corda, R. D. Sekura, and L. D. Kohn, Thyrotropin effect on the availability of Ni regulatory protein in FRTL-5 rat thyroid cells to ADP-ribosylation by pertussis toxin, Eur. J. Biochem. 166:475, (1987).
18. S. J. Shuman, U. Zor, R. Chayoth, and J. B. Field, Exposure of thyroid slices to thyroid-stimulating hormone induces refractoriness of the cyclic AMP system to subsequent hormone stimulation, J. Clin. Invest. 57:1132, (1976).
19. K. Mashiter, G. D. Mashiter, R. L. Hauger, J. B. Field, Effects of cholera and E. coli enterotoxins on cyclic adenosine 3',5'-monophosphate levels and intermediary metabolism in the thyroid, Endocrinology 92: 541, (1973).
20. B. Rapoport, S. Filetti, N. Takai, and P. Seto, Studies on the desensitization of the cyclic AMP response to thyrotropin in thyroid tissue, FEBS Lett. 146:23, (1982).
21. Y. Totsuka, T. B. Nielsen, and J. B. Field, Effect of thyrotropin-induced desensitizsation of bovine thyroid

adenylate cyclase on the nucleotide regulatory protein, Endocrinology 113:1088, (1983).
22. P. Cochaux, J. Van Sande, and J. E. Dumont, Islet-activating protein discriminates between different inhibitors of thyroidal cyclic AMP system, FEBS Lett. 179:303, (1985).
23. K. Haraguchi, C. S. S. Rani, and J. B. Field, Effects of thyrotropin, carbachol, and protein kinase-C stimulators on glucose transport and glucose oxidation by primary cultures of dog thyroid cells, Endocrinology 123:1288, (1988).
24. I. Pastan, B. Herring, P. Johnson, and J. B. Field, In vitro stimulation of glucose oxidation in thyroid by acetylcholine, J. Biol. Chem. 236:340, (1961).
25. M. Altman, H. Oka, and J. B. Field, Effect of TSH, acetylcholine, epinephrine, serotonin and synkavite on ^{32}P incorporation into phospholipids in dog thyroid slices, Biochim. Biophys. Acta. 116:586, (1966).
26. S. C. S. Rani, A. E. Boyd III, and J. B. Field, Effects of acetylcholine, TSH and other stimulators on intracellular calcium concentration in dog thyroid cells, Biochem. Biophys. Res. Commun. 131:1041, (1985).
27. D. Corda, C. Marcocci, L. D. Kohn, J. Axelrod, and A. Luini, Association of the changes in cytosolic Ca^{2+} and iodide efflux induced by thyrotropin and by the stimulation of $_1$-adrenergic receptors in cultured rat thyroid cells, J. Biol. Chem. 260:9230, (1985).
28. D. Corda, and L. D. Kohn, Role of pertussis toxin sensitive G proteins in the alpha$_1$ adrenergic receptor but not in the thyrotropin receptor mediated activation of membrane phospholipases and iodide fluxes in FRTL-5 thyroid cells, Biochem. and Biphys. Res. Commun. 141:1000, (1986).
29. R. M. Burch, A. Luini, and J. Axelrod, Phospholipase A_2 and phosphalipase C are activated by distinct GTP-binding proteins in response to $_1$ adrenergic stimulation in FRTL-5 thyroid cells, Proc. Nat. Acad. Sci. USA 83:7201, (1986).
30. S. Cockroft, and J. Stutchfield, G-proteins, the inositol lipid signalling pathway, and secretion, Phil. Trans. R. Soc. Lond. 320:247, (1988).
31. S. Schnefel, H. Banfic, L. Eckhardt, G. Schultz, and I. Schultz, Acetylcholine and cholecystokinin receptors functionally couple by different G-proteins to phospholipase C in pancreatic acinar cells, FEBS Lett. 230:125, (1988).
32. F. Okajima, K. Sho, and Y. Kondo, Inhibition by islet-activating protein, pertussis toxin, of P_2-purinergic receptor-mediated iodide efflux and phosphoinositde turnover in FRTL-5 cells, Endocrinology 123:1035, (1988).
33. M. Ikeda, W. J. Deery, T. B. Nielsen, M. S. Ferdows, and J. B. Field, Dephosphylation of 21 K and 19 K polypeptides in response to thyroid stimulating hormone in cultured thyroid cells. Endocrinology 119:591, (1986).

34. M. Ikeda, W. J. Deery, M. S. Ferdows, T. B. Nielsen, and J. B. Field, Role of cellular Ca^{2+} in phosphorylation of 21 K and 19 K polypeptides in cultured thyroid cells - effects of phorbol esters, trifluorperazine and TMB-8, Endocrinology 121:175, (1987).

THE INOSITIDE AND ARACHIDONIC ACID SIGNAL SYSTEM

Eduardo G. Lapetina

Division of Cell Biology, Burroughs Wellcome Co.

Research Triangle Park, NC 27709

INTRODUCTION

The concept that inositol phospholipid hydrolysis is a very early event and is responsible for transducing the effect of hormone-receptor stimulation to the cell interior is now widely accepted[1]. The activation of these specific receptors stimulates phospholipase C which degrades membrane-bound phosphatidylinositol 4,5-bisphosphate to produce two second messengers: inositol 1,4,5-trisphosphate, which can liberate Ca^{2+} from intracellular stores[1], and 1,2-diacylglycerol, which activates protein kinase C[2]. The membrane-bound transducer that relates the message from the receptor to the phospholipase C seems to be a specific GTP-binding protein[3,4] that is referred to as Gp, where p stands for phosphoinositide.

In most cases, the same agonists that cause the stimulation of phospholipase C will also induce the activation of phospholipase A_2[5]. This activity hydrolyses the arachidonic acid esterified at the 2-position of phosphatidylcholine, phosphatidylethanolamine, phosphatidylinositol and phosphatidic acid. The liberated arachidonic acid is immediately metabolized by the action of the cyclooxygenase and lipoxygenase activities[6]. The products that are formed have been shown to have important biological roles[6].

It has been proposed that the Ca^{2+} that is mobilized as a consequence of the activation of phospholipase C is needed for the subsequent activation of phospholipase A_2[6]. However, recent information suggests that phospholipase C and phospholipase A_2 can be activated independently[7].

Hydrolysis of Inositol Phospholipids by Phospholipase C

The inositol phospholipids are located within the plasma membrane and they comprise phosphatidylinositol, phosphatidylinositol 4-monophosphate, and phosphatidylinositol 4,5-bisphosphate[1]. These phospholipids can be metabolized by specific kinase phosphomonoesterases and phosphodiesterases[1]. Phosphatidylinositol can be phosphorylated by phosphatidylinositol kinases, which transfers a phosphate from ATP to the 4-position of the inositol part of the molecule to produce phosphatidylinositol 4-phosphate. Another inositide kinase can further phosphorylate phosphatidylinositol 4-monophosphate in the 5-position of the inositol to yield phosphatidylinositol 4,5-bisphosphate. The polyphosphoinositides, i.e. phosphatidylinositol 4-monophosphate and phosphatidylinositol 4,5-bisphosphate, can be dephosphorylated by specific phosphomonoesterases. These enzymes can remove the 5-phosphate of the inositol group of phosphatidylinositol 4,5-bisphosphate to produce phosphatidylinositol 4-monophosphate. This could be further dephosphorylated by another phosphomonoesterase to yield phosphatidylinositol.

Phosphatidylinositol, phosphatidylinositol 4-monophosphate and phosphatidylinositol 4,5-bisphosphate are hydrolyzed by phosphodiesterases or phospholipase C[1,5]. Most agonists produce a rapid and transient decrease of cell-associated phosphatidylinositol 4,5-bisphosphate[5,8] which occurs in parallel with the formation of 1,2-diacylglycerol[9] and inositol 1,4,5-trisphosphate[1]. Inositol 1,4-bisphosphate and inositol 1-monophosphate are also produced by the action of phospholipase C which hydrolyzes phosphatidylinositol 1,4-bisphosphate and phosphatidylinositol 1-monophosphate respectively. The polyphosphoinostides are preferentially hydrolyzed in stimulated cells leading to the mobilization of Ca^{2+} that might then trigger a calcium-dependent hydrolysis of phosphatidylinositol[10].

Metabolism of Inositol Phosphates

Inositol 1,4,5-trisphosphate is the second messenger molecule that is able to effect the release of Ca^{2+} from the endoplasmic reticulum to the cytosolic compartment in a wide variety of cells[11]. Therefore, the regulation of the metabolism of inositol 1,4,5-trisphosphate is relevant to sustain or stop the intracellular mobilization of Ca^{2+}. Inositol 1,4,5-trisphosphate is metabolized by dephosphorylation or phosphorylation to produce, in each case, inactive compounds[1,5,10]. Dephosphorylation involves the activity of inositol 1,4,5-trisphosphate 5-phosphatase that liberates the phosphate from the 5-position to yield inositol 1,4-bisphosphate[12,13,14]. The enzyme seems to be regulated by protein kinase C since it is phosphorylated by brain protein kinase C[14], resulting in a fourfold increase in activity.

This agrees with information that shows that phorbol ester and 1,2-diacylglycerol stimulate the activity of the 5-phosphatase in human platelets[12].

Inositol 1,4,5-trisphosphate can be phosphorylated by a calmodulin-dependent 3-kinase to form inositol 1,3,4,5-tetrakisphosphate[15,16]. This tetrakisphosphate can be dephosphorylated by the 5-phosphatase to produce inositol 1,3,4-trisphosphate[15]. In many instances, during the stimulation of cell by agonists, the formation of inositol 1,4,5-trisphosphate and inositol 1,3,4,5 tetrakisphosphate is so transient that these products are hardly detectable. Therefore, the formation of the stable product inositol 1,3,4-trisphosphate represents a good indication that the liberated inositol 1,4,5-trisphosphate has been phosphorylated by the 3-kinase to inositol

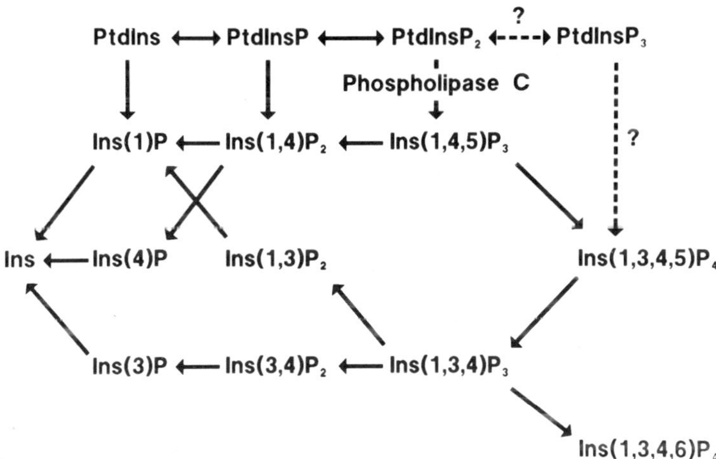

Figure 1. Metabolism of inositol phospholipids and inositol phosphates

Phosphatidylinositol (PtdIns) can be sequentially phosphorylated by specific kinases to phosphatidylinositol 4-monophosphate (PtdInsP) and phosphatidylinositol 4,5-bisphosphate ($PtdInsP_2$) and, perhaps, phosphatidylinositol 3,4,5-trisphosphate ($PtdInsP_3$). The polyphosphoinositides can also be dephosphorylated by specific phosphomonoesterases. Phospholipase C can hydrolyze the inositol phospholipids to the corresponding inositol phosphates (Ins P). The inositol phosphates can be phosphorylated and dephosphorylated by specific enzymes as shown in this figure.

1,3,4,5-tetrakisphosphate and that this compound has been dephosphorylated to inositol 1,3,4-trisphosphate. However, in few instances it has been reported that a small percentage of the inositol 1,3,4-trisphosphate or inositol 1,3,4,5-tetrakisphosphate are derived from specific related parent lipids by the action of phospholipase C[17,18]. It has also been reported that inositol 1,3,4-trisphosphate can be phosphorylated by a 6-kinase to inositol 1,3,4,6-tetrakisphosphate[19].

Further metabolism of inositol 1,3,4-trisphosphate and inositol 1,4-bisphosphate can be seen in Fig. 1. The various inositol phosphates can be properly separated on HPLC. The dephosphorylation of the three inositol monophosphates (see Fig. 1) is inhibited by Li^+. Whether these inositol monophosphates are dephosphorylated by the same enzyme or different enzymes is not known.

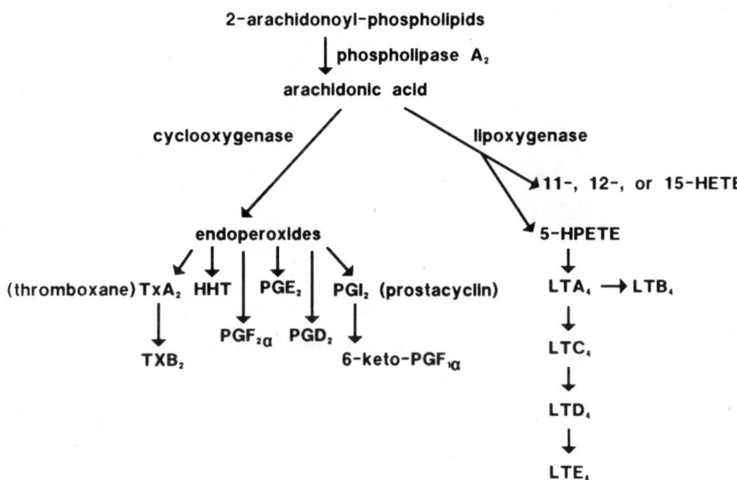

Figure 2. Biochemical reactions involved in the deacylation of arachidonoyl-containing phospholipids and the formation of prostaglandins (PG), prostacyclin, thromboxanes (TX), and leukotrienes (LT) from arachidonic acid.

Hydrolysis of esterified arachidonic acid from cellular phospholipids is the first rate-limiting step in the eicosanoid pathway. Cyclooxygenase activity produces endoperoxides, thromboxanes, prostaglandins and hydroxy acids (HHT). Lipoxygenase activity produces hydroxy acids (HETE) and leukotrienes (LT).

Liberation of Arachidonic Acid by Phospholipase A_2

The oxygenated derivatives of arachidonic acid which are biologically active are defined as eicosanoids. Among the eicosanoids are prostaglandins, including prostacyclin, thromboxanes, leukotrienes and various hydroxy acids (See Fig. 2).

The eicosanoid precursor, arachidonic acid, is esterified in the 2-position of several phospholipids and it must be hydrolyzed before the eicosanoids can be synthesized (Fig. 2). The liberated arachidonic acid can be enzymatically oxygenated by a membrane-bound cyclooxygenase and/or a cytosolic lipoxygenase with the formation of unstable intermediate products (Fig. 2). These intermediate products include the endoperoxides for prostaglandin production and epoxides (LTA_4) and hydroperoxides for leukotriene and hydroxy acid formation (See Fig. 2). The enzymes each cell contains determines the type of arachidonate oxygenation.

The eicosanoids' precursors are not found as free substances in most cells and liberation of arachidonic acid from the _sn_-2-position of phospholipids by phospholipase A_2 must precede metabolic oxygenation. The generation of the free eicosanoids from phospholipids is thus a rate-limiting process and occurs as a consequence of the stimulation of specific cell-surface receptors[6]. Phosphatidylcholine, phosphatidylethanolamine, phosphatidylinositol, phosphatidic acid, plasmenylethanolamine, and 1-_O_-alkyl-2-arachidonoyl-sn-glycero-3-phosphocholine are all known to release arachidonic acid in different cells. Phospholipase A_2 has been detected in almost all cells in which its presence has been investigated. This activity requires an alkaline pH (7.8-9.5) and is stimulated by Ca^{2+} ions.

Regulation of Phospholipases

It is not yet well understood how receptor binding is able to activate phospholipases C and A_2. It has been shown that GTP-binding proteins are involved in the activation of phospholipases C and A_2[6,20]. These findings are based on the ability of GTP analogues to stimulate phospholipases C and A_2 in permeabilized cells and membrane preparations or by pertussis toxin to inhibit their activities[4,20]. Since pertussis toxin ADP-ribosylates and inactivates G_i (G-protein that inhibits adenylate cyclase) a role for G_i has been suggested in those cases where pertussis toxin inhibits agonist-induced stimulation of phospholipases. However, in those cells where pertussis toxin is ineffective in inhibiting phospholipases, another G-protein is believed to be involved[20]. The identity of the specific G-protein(s) that activate phospholipases has not yet been

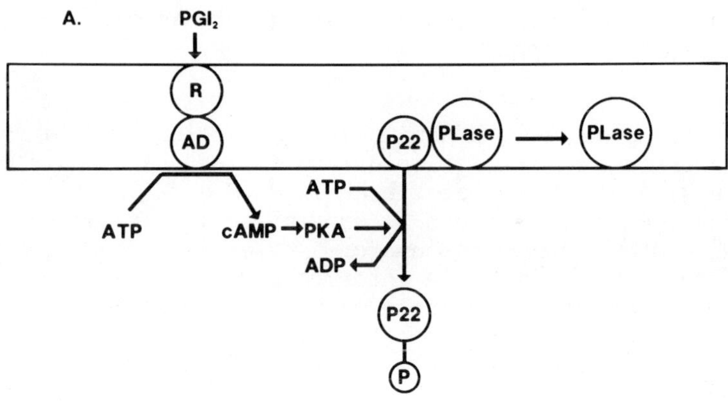

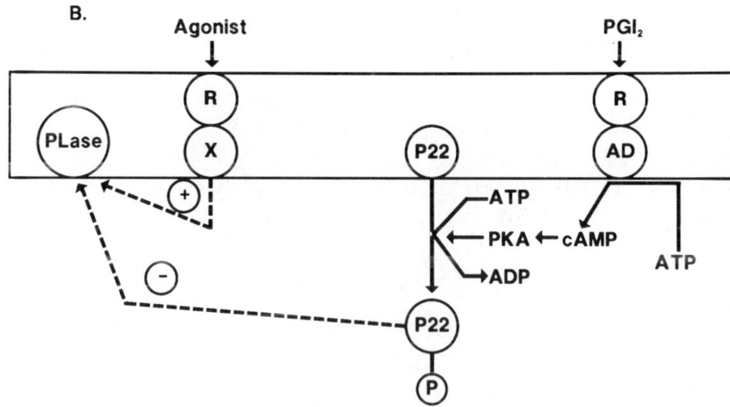

Figure 3. A *ras*-related protein (p22) might influence the activity of phospholipases

Cyclic AMP or agents that increase cyclic AMP levels such as prostacyclin (PGI_2) cause the A-kinase (PKA) phosphorylation of a *ras*-related protein (p22) which can then be translocated from the membrane to the cytosol. This might leave membrane-phospholipase in an inhibited state (A). Alternatively, the translocated and phosphorylated p22 protein might inhibit membrane-bound phospholipases. For details see text.

determined. Some of our recent information suggests that a G-protein that is affected by phosphorylation is related to regulation of phospholipases[21]. The increase of cyclic AMP in platelets causes the inhibition of phospholipases C and A_2[22]. We have recently found that cyclic AMP-dependent protein kinase phosphorylates a G-protein that is immunologically recognized by p21 *ras* antibodies[21]. This 22 kDa (p22) *ras*-related protein is present in the membrane and it is translocated to the cytosol after phosphorylation. Therefore, it is possible that phosphorylation and translocation of the 22 kDa (p22) *ras*-related protein might regulate phospholipases. In platelets, cyclic AMP levels can be increased by prostacyclin (PGI_2) or prostacyclin analogs such as iloprost. The interaction of prostacyclin with its platelet membrane receptor causes the activation of adenylate cyclase and the increase of cyclic AMP levels[5,22]. This increase of cyclic AMP correlates with the inhibition of phospholipases and the phosphorylation of the 22 kDa (p22) *ras*-related protein. The ways that the 22 kDa (p22) *ras*-related protein might be regulating phospholipases is depicted in Fig. 3.

The unphosphorylated 22 kDa (p22) *ras*-related protein might normally have a stimulatory effect on the phospholipases but its phosphorylation and translocation leaves phospholipases in an inhibited state (Fig. 3A). Alternatively, the phosphorylated 22 kDa (p22) *ras*-related protein might have an inhibitory effect on the membrane-bound phospholipases as shown in Fig. 3B. More work is needed to determine the exact influence of this *ras*-related protein on phospholipases and how they interplay with G_i in this regulation.

References

1. M.J. Berridge, Inositol trisphosphate and diacylglycerol: two interacting secondary messengers. Annu. Rev. Biochem., 56:159-193 (1987).
2. Y. Nishizuka, The role of protein kinase C in cell surface signal transduction and tumour promotion. Nature, 308:693-698 (1984).
3. S. Cockcroft and B.D. Gomperts, Role of guanine nucleotide binding protein in the activation of polyphosphoinositide phosphodiesterase. Nature, 314:534-536 (1985).
4. I. Litosch and J.N. Fain, Regulation of phosphoinositide breakdown by guanine nucleotides. Life Sci. 39:187-194 (1986).
5. E.G. Lapetina, Inositide-dependent and independent mechanisms in platelet activation. In: Phosphoinositides and Receptor Mechanisms, edited by J.W. Putney, Jr., p. 271. Alan R. Liss, New York (1986).
6. E.G. Lapetina, Regulation of arachidonic acid production: Role of phospholipases C and A_2, Trends in Pharmacol. Sci. 3:115-118, (1982).

7. M.F. Crouch and E.G. Lapetina, No direct correlation between Ca^{2+} mobilization and dissociation of G_i during phospholipase A_2 activation. Biochem. Biophys. Res. Commun. 153:21-30 (1988).
8. M.M. Billah and E.G. Lapetina, Rapid decrease of phosphatidylinositol 4,5-bisphosphate in thrombin-stimulated platelets. J. Biol. Chem., 257:12705-12708 (1982).
9. S. Rittenhouse-Simmons, Production of diglyceride from phosphatidylinositol in activated human platelets. J. Clin. Invest., 63:580-587 (1979).
10. P.W. Majerus, D.B. Wilson, T.M. Connolly, T.E. Bross and E.J. Neufeld, Phosphoinositide turnover provides a link in stimulus-response coupling. TIBS. 10:168-171 (1985).
11. H. Streb, R.F. Irvine, M.J. Berridge and I. Schulz, Release of Ca^{2+} from a nonmitochondrial intracellular store in pancreatic acinar cells by inositol-1,4,5-trisphosphate. Nature, 306:67-69 (1983).
12. L. Molina y Vedia and E.G. Lapetina, Phorbol 12,13-dibutyrate and 1-oleyl, 2-acetyl-diacylglycerol stimulate inositol trisphosphate dephosphorylation in human platelets. J. Biol. Chem. 261:10493-10495 (1986).
13. L. Molina y Vedia and E.G. Lapetina, Subcellular localization of the enzymes that dephosphorylate *myo*-inositol phosphates in human platelets. Biochem. J. 255:795-800 (1988).
14. T.M. Connolly, T.E. Bross and P.W. Majerus, Isolation of a phosphomonoesterase from human platelets that specifically hydrolyses the 5-phosphate of inositol 1,4,5-trisphosphate. J. Biol. Chem., 260:7868-7874 (1985).
15. R.F. Irvine, A.J. Letcher, J.P. Heslop and M.J. Berridge, The inositol tris/tetrakisphosphate pathway: demonstration of Ins (1,4,5) P_3 3-kinase activity in animal tissues. Nature, 320:631-634 (1986).
16. T.J. Giden, M. Comte, J.A. Cox and C.B. Wollheim, Calcium-calmodulin stimulates inositol 1,4,5-trisphosphate kinase activity from insulin-secreting RINm 5F cells. J. Biol. Chem., 262: 9437-9440 (1987).
17. A.E. Traynor-Kaplan, A.L. Harris, B.L. Thompson, P. Taylor and L.A. Sklar, An inositol tetrakisphosphate-containing phospholipid in activated neutrophils. Nature 334:353-356 (1988).
18. M. Whitman, C.P. Downes, M. Keeler, T. Keller and L. Cantley, Type I phosphatidylinositol kinase makes a novel inositol phospholipid, phosphatidylinositol-3-phosphate. Nature 332:644-646 (1988).
19. T. Balla, G. Guillemette, A.J. Baukal and K.J. Catt, Metabolism of inositol 1,3,4-trisphosphate to a new tetrakisphosphate isomer in angiotensin-stimulated adrenal glomerulosa cells. J. Biol. Chem. 262: 9952-9955 (1987).

20. M.F. Crouch and E.G. Lapetina, A role for G_i in control of thrombin receptor-phospholipase C coupling in human platelets. J. Biol Chem., 263:3363-3371 (1988).
21. E.G. Lapetina, J.C. Lacal, B.R. Reep and L. Molina y Vedia, A *ras*-related protein is phosphorylated and translocated by agonists that increase cyclic AMP levels in human platelets, Proc. Natl. Acad. Sci. U.S.A. 86:3131-3134 (1989).
22. S.P. Watson, R.T. McConnell and E.G. Lapetina, The rapid formation of inositol phosphates in human platelets by thrombin is inhibited by prostacyclin. J. Biol. Chem., 259:13199-13203 (1984).

THE ARACHIDONIC ACID SIGNAL SYSTEM IN THE THYROID: REGULATION BY THYROTROPIN AND INSULIN/IGF-I

Kazuo Tahara, Motoyasu Saji, Salvatore M. Aloj, and Leonard D. Kohn

Section on Cell Regulation
Laboratory of Biochemistry and Metabolism
National Institute of Diabetes, Digestive and Kidney Diseases
National Institutes of Health
Bethesda, MD 20892

INTRODUCTION

Previous reports (1-11) have defined the importance of the Ca/phosphoinositide/arachidonic acid signal system to both the function and growth of FRTL-5 rat thyroid cells and to the action of both thyrotropin (TSH) and alpha-1 adrenergic agents in these cells. Thus evidence has been presented that norepinephrine and TSH could increase degradation of phosphatidylinositol 4,5-bisphosphate (PIP_2) (1) with the concomitant formation of diacylglycerol and IP_3 (2). This action was accompanied by increases in cytosolic Ca^{++} (3), arachidonic acid release from the cells (4, 5) and the action of arachidonic acid metabolites in processes important to thyroid hormone formation and growth (4-11).

The importance of this signal system to FRTL-5 thyroid cell growth was emphasized in studies of the action of monoclonal antibodies to the TSH receptor (12-17). Thus it was noted that monoclonal antibodies to the TSH receptor could be divided into groups according to their ability to inhibit TSH binding and stimulate adenylate cyclase activity of thyroid cells (Table 1). Those antibodies which inhibited TSH binding but did not

TABLE 1

Representative Monoclonal Antibodies to the TSH Receptor

Clone Number	Receptor Source	"Activity"
13D11	Bovine	Inhibitor
11E8	Bovine	Inhibitor
59C9	Human	Inhibitor
60F5	Human	Inhibitor
129H8[a]	Human	Inhibitor
122G3[a]	Human	Inhibitor
22A6	Bovine	Stimulator
307H6[a]	Human	Stimulator
206H3[a]	Human	Stimulator
52A8	Humam	Mixed
208F7[a]	Human	Mixed

a) Heterohybridomas. Properties are derived from data in references 12-17.

TABLE 2

Effect of Monoclonal antibodies to the TSH receptor on the growth of FRTL-5 thyroid cells as measured by radiolabeled thymidine uptake into DNA (18, 19)

Monoclonal Antibody	$[^3H]$thymidine uptake into DNA (cpm/microgram DNA) Alone	+TSH $1x10^{-10}$ M	+Indomethacin
None	1600	6700	1400
Normal IgG	1450	5900	1510
TSH $1x10^{-10}$ M	6800	--	3500
$1x10^{-9}$ M	31000	--	14800
Stimulating Antibodies			
22A6	6800	11200	6900
307H6	8700	13200	9200
Mixed Antibodies			
52A8	18500	25100	7400
208F7	17200	23800	6500
Inhibiting Antibodies			
122G3	1350	2300	1460
59C9	1410	1900	1390
129H8	5600	14200	1480

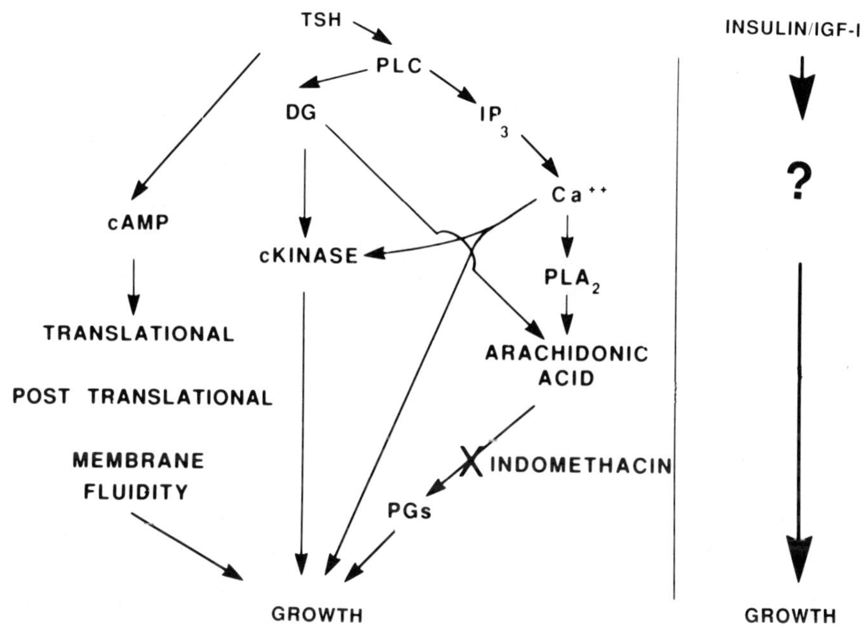

Figure 1. TSH uses multiple transmembrane signalling systems to promote growth,

stimulate adenylate cyclase activity were termed inhibiting antibodies; their properties were consistent with the thyrotropin binding inhibiting antibodies (TBIAbs) evident in the sera of patients with Graves' disease. A second group exhibited only weak inhibition of TSH binding but were able to stimulate adenylate cyclase activity; these antibodies were termed stimulators and were equivalent to the thyroid stimulating antibodies (TSAbs) in the sera of patients with Graves' disease. A last group had properties of both and were termed mixed antibodies. When these antibodies were tested for their ability to increase tritiated thymidine incorporation into DNA, a measurement which had been related to cell growth in separate studies of Graves' autoantibodies (18, 19), it was found, surprisingly, that all TSAbs could increase tritiated thymidine incorporation into DNA, some TBIAbs could also do this, and mixed antibodies were better than both (Table 2). Although these data clearly linked the cAMP signal to growth in these cells, they also indicated that another signal might be important and that this signal was also generated through the TSH receptor. The ability of indomethacin to completely inhibit the TBIAb activity, not affect the TSAb activity, and partially inhibit both TSH and mixed antibody activity, with respect to tritiated thymidine incorporation into DNA (Table 2), suggested that the second signal involved an arachidonic acid metabolite of the cyclooxygenase pathway.

These observations were consistent with the previous observations that TSH could increase phosphoinositide degradation, IP_3 formation, cytosolic free calcium levels, and arachidonic acid metabolite signalled thymidine incorporation into DNA, iodide efflux and iodination of thyroglobulin (1-11). They were consistent with the possibility that TSH activation of the Ca/phosphoinositide/arachidonic acid signal system and the formation of cyclooxygenase metabolites of arachidonic acid, as well as the cAMP, C-kinase and Ca^{++} signals, were important in the growth of thyroid cells (Fig. 1). Rat FRTL-5 thyroid cells (ATCC #CRL 8305) are a line of continuously growing cells whose growth and function requires TSH (18, 20, 21). It is, however, clear that the simultaneous action of other hormones, in particular insulin and IGF-I, is required for TSH regulation of FRTL-5 thyroid cell growth (22). The relationship of the insulin/ IGF-I action on growth to these multiple signal systems is, therefore, also of major interest.

The present report summarizes studies concerned with

the action of TSH, insulin, and IGF-I on the different steps involved in the formation of arachidonic acid and in the formation of the multiplicity of cyclooxygenase metabolites which are presumed related to the growth of FRTL-5 thyroid cells (Fig. 2). In this report we show that TSH stimulates the synthesis of arachidonic acid as well as its release from FRTL-5 cells. This TSH action does not require insulin or IGF-I. We show, also, that the major metabolic route taken by the arachidonic acid formed and released as a result of the TSH action involves the indomethacin-sensitive cyclooxygenase rather than the lipoxygenase or epoxygenase path. In contrast to the ability of TSH to increase arachidonic acid formation and release, we show that insulin/IGF-I plays an important role in the cyclooxygenase path. Thus insulin or IGF-I are required for TSH-induced expression of the cyclooxygenase activity; the hormonally enhanced cyclooxygenase activity, at least in part, reflects enhanced gene expression. Finally, we show that TSH and insulin/IGF-I also regulate the different isomerases or synthetases involved in the formation of the multiplicity of prostaglandins derived from the PGH_2 formed by the cyclooxygenase (Fig. 2).

The present data explicitly link the ability of TSH to alter arachidonic acid metabolism to the complex array of events needed for the growth of FRTL-5 thyroid cells.

TSH AFFECT ON ARACHIDONIC ACID FORMATION AND RELEASE IN FRTL-5 THYROID CELLS

TSH is important in the synthesis of fatty acids by FRTL-5 cells. This can be demonstrated when cells, deprived of TSH, insulin, and serum for several days, are rechallenged with TSH (Fig. 3), then, at different times after TSH challenge, given [^{14}C]acetate during the last two hours of culture. When lipids are extracted from the cell and radioactivity incorporated into free fatty acids is measured after thin layer chromatography (Fig. 4 Top), it is evident that TSH causes at least a 4-fold increase in incorporation of radioactivity into fatty acids. The increase in labeling is a function of the time of TSH treatment: the maximal effect of TSH is evident 24 hours following its readdition to the cells. Several further observations were made related to this phenomenon.

First, a major portion of the radioactivity in the fatty acid spot on thin layer chromatograms was in arachidonic acid, as evidenced by HPLC analysis of the

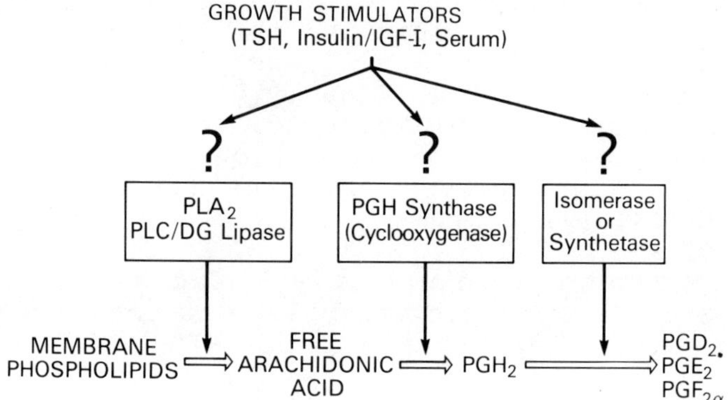

Figure 2. Prostaglandins are produced through three steps. The first step is the release of free arachidonic acid, the second is the production of PGH_2 by PGH synthase (cyclooxygenase) and the third is the conversion of PGH_2 to various prostaglandins by specific isomerases, synthetases, or other mechanisms.

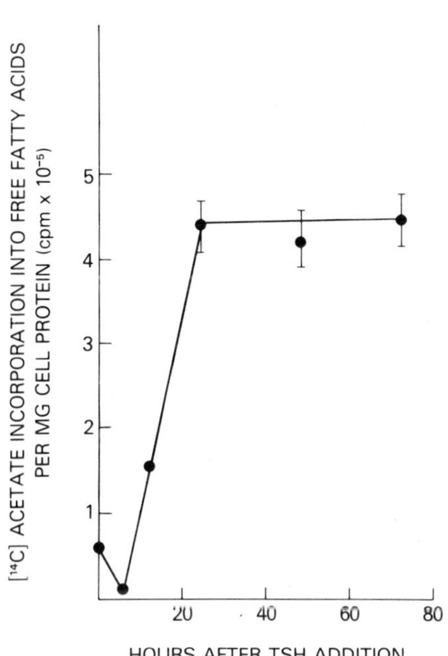

Figure 3. Radioactivity incorporated into free fatty acids extracted from FRTL-5 rat thyroid cells as a function of time after TSH ($1x10^{-10}$ M) addition when cells were maintained in medium without insulin and exposed to [^{14}C]acetate 2 hours prior to the end of the experiment. Cells were maintained 4 days in 5H (no TSH) medium and an additional three days in 4H medium (no TSH, no insulin) before they were rechallenged with TSH. During the last three days before TSH rechallenge, the serum content of the medium was also reduced to 0.2%. Lipids were extracted (26) and subjected to thin layer chromatography (27) along with an authentic standard to identify the free fatty acid spot. Radioactivity was quantitated with a Berthold scanning detector. Points represent the mean of three individual experiments with three different batches of cells plus or minus SE.

material extracted from thin layer plates (Fig. 4, bottom). Second, a significant portion of the radioactivity was being released into the medium in the presence of TSH (Fig 4, TOP).

To further confirm the last observation we measured the effect of TSH on the release of arachidonic acid from FRTL-5 thyroid cells prelabeled with [^{3}H]arachidonic acid as described in an earlier study of the action of alpha-1 adrenergic agents (4, 6), i. e. cells incubated overnight with [^{3}H]arachidonic acid wherein the radiolabeled arachidonic acid was >98% incorporated into cellular lipid (Fig. 5). In this experiment FRTL-5 thyroid cells were incubated for 4 days in 5H medium with 5% serum, then an additional 3 days in medium without insulin as well as TSH (4H medium) and only 0.2% serum. TSH, $1x10^{-10}$ M, caused statistically significant release 5 minutes after its addition to the cells prelabeled overnight with the [^{3}H] arachidonic acid (Fig. 5A). Higher concentrations of TSH increased the amount of radiolabeled arachidonic acid released when measured 5 minutes after the addition of the agonist (Fig. 5B) and shifted the time point at which statistically significant increases ($p < 0.05$) could be measured to 1 minute (data not shown).

As was the case for the action of alpha-1 adrenergic agents, pertussis toxin treatment of the prelabeled cells for four hours before adding the agonist (6), inhibited the ability of TSH to stimulate arachidonic acid release (Table 3). The same treatment only minimally affected the ability of TSH to elevate cAMP levels in the cells (Table 3).

Certain conclusions could be drawn from these data relatively easily. The data indicated that TSH was able to stimulate the synthesis of arachidonic acid and its release from FRTL-5 thyroid cells. A pertussis toxin-sensitive G protein and a non cAMP transducing signal appeared to be important for release since pertussis toxin blocked the release but not the increase in cAMP levels induced by TSH (Table 3). The effect of TSH on arachidonic acid release is, therefore, similar to that described for alpha-1 adrenergic agents in these cells.

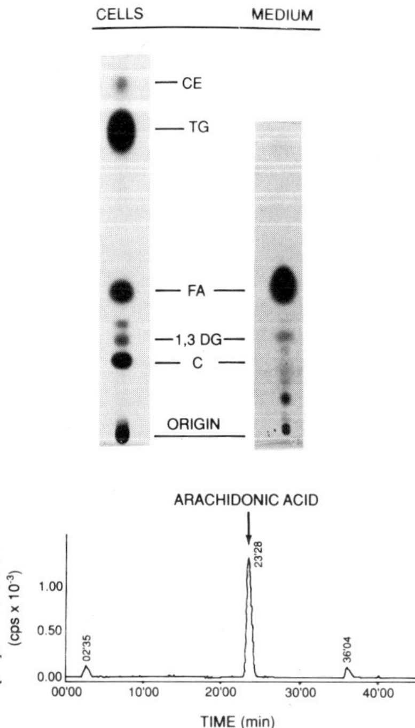

Figure 4. (TOP) Autoradiograph of thin layer chromatogram of lipids labeled with [^{14}C]acetate and extracted from cells and medium 24 hours after rechallenge with TSH as described in Figure 3. The FRTL-5 cells were maintained for 4 days in 5H medium (no TSH) with 5% calf serum and an additional 3 days in 4H medium (no TSH, no insulin) with 0.2% calf serum before the readdition of 1×10^{-10} M TSH. Lipids were extracted and chromatographed as described in Fig. 3 and references 26 and 27. Identification of radioactive lipids as cholesterol (C), 1,3-diacylglycerol (1,3 DG), fatty acid (FA), triglyceride (TG) or cholesterol ester (CE) was by cochromatography with unlabeled standards. (BOTTOM) HPLC analysis of the radioactivity in the fatty acid (FA) spot after thin layer chromatographic separation of the lipids extracted from the medium 24 hours after TSH challenge. The FA spot identified in the autoradiograph in the top of this figure was scraped, reextracted with chloroform-methanol, and subjected to reverse-phase HPLC analysis using an octadecyl silica column. Isocratic elution was carried out using a solvent system of acetonitrile/water/acetic acid (72:28:0.01, v/v/v).

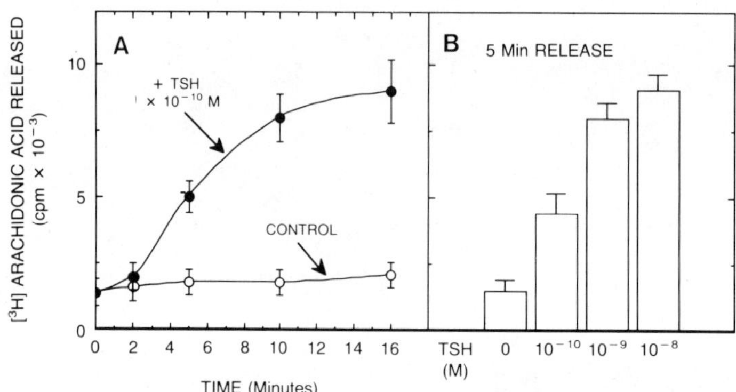

Figure 5. Radiolabeled arachidonic acid released into the medium from FRTL-5 rat thyroid cells after TSH challenge measured both as a function of time (A) and TSH concentration (B). Cells were maintained 4 days in 5H (no TSH) medium with 5% calf serum and an additional 3 days in 4H medium (no TSH, no insulin) with 0.2% serum before overnight incubation with [^{3}H]arachidonic acid as described (6). Release was measured as detailed (6) after challenge with 1x10^{-10} M TSH at the times noted in (A) or 5 minutes after challenge with the noted concentration of TSH in (B). All experimental points were in quadruplicate; values are the mean of these values plus or minus SE from a representative experiment. In this experiment each well contained 24±3 micrograms DNA per well. Similar data were obtained on three separate occasions involving different batches of cells.

TABLE 3

Effect of pertussis toxin preincubation on TSH-stimulated release of $[^3H]$arachidonic acid from FRTL-5 rat thyroid cells and on TSH-stimulated increases in cAMP levels.

TSH	PERTUSSIS TOXIN	ARACHIDONIC ACID RELEASED (cpm x 10^{-3})	cAMP LEVEL (pmol/ugDNA)
-	-	1250 + 210	0.2 + 0.1
-	+	1110 + 194	0.6 + 0.2
+	-	8608 + 419	17.4 + 1.3
+	+	1425 + 314	15.8 + 0.9

FRTL-5 thyroid cells in 12 well plates were maintained in 5H medium with 5% calf serum for 4 days and 4H medium with 0.2% serum for 3 additional days before preincubation with $[^3H]$arachidonic acid overnight as described (6). When present, pertussis toxin (10 nM) was added to cells 4 hours before they were washed and exposed to 1 x 10^{-10} M TSH for 15 minutes as described (7). Control incubations with no TSH contained only the HBSS-albumin buffer mixture. After the supernatant solution was removed for analysis of $[^3H]$arachidonic acid released, 1 ml of ice cold ethanol was added, and the plates left overnight at -20°C. The ethanol was removed, evaporated, and the residue used to measure cAMP levels (18). The pellet residue in the plates was incubated with diphenylamine reagent (18) to measure DNA values. DNA content of each well in this experiment was 20.4 + 2.2 micrograms. All assays were in quadruplicate and were performed on 4 separate occassions with 3 different batches of cells. The values are the mean of one experiment + SE; similar results were obtained in each experiment.

METABOLISM OF ARACHIDONIC ACID IN FRTL-5 THYROID CELLS BY PGH SYNTHASE (CYCLOOXYGENASE)

The assay of cyclooxygenase metabolites

One of two HPLC systems were used to evaluate metabolites of arachidonic acid. The first system (Fig. 6A) involves a step wise gradient system which identifies all major metabolites and takes nearly 90 minutes. The second, more simplified system, taking less than 60 minutes was used to evaluate the cyclooxygenase metabolites only (Fig. 6B). The first system was used in initial studies in whole cells and homogenates; the second for most subsequent studies.

The cyclooxygenase path is the major route in intact cells

Metabolites formed from arachidonic acid in intact FRTL-5 cells incubated in 6H medium containing TSH, insulin, and 5% serum were determined in cells prelabeled with [^{3}H]arachidonic acid for 2 hours, washed repeatedly with Hanks balanced salt solution, then stimulated with A23187 (10 microM, 5 min, 37 C) to release the metabolites. The choice of a 2 hour rather than overnight incubation reflected a desire to minimize autooxidation of [^{3}H]arachidonic acid; the use of A23187 as a releasing agent for arachidonic acid metabolites in FRTL-5 cells has already been demonstrated (6). In the presence of TSH, A23187 did cause a 15-fold increase in the release of radioactivity; however, only three metabolites of arachidonic acid were evident by HPLC analysis (Fig. 7A). The metabolites had the retention times of standard PGF_{2alpha}, PGE_2, and PGD_2 and were not present in cells pretreated with indomethacin (Fig. 7B). In separate prelabeling experiments, analysis of samples with the step gradient system in Figure 6A confirmed that PGE_2 was a major peak and also showed that there were no obvious peaks of HHT, 15-HETE, or 11-HETE which could be detected, in contrast to results in the homogenate system of FRTL-5 cells (see below). The release of arachidonic acid itself was unaffected by indomethacin.

The radioactivity detected in the metabolite peak was only approximately 1% that in the peak of released arachidonic acid despite the fact that 50% of the added radiolabeled arachidonic acid had been incorporated into the cell during the 2 hour preincubation. This result may be explained by the data in Figures 3 and 4; TSH-treated FRTL-5 cells synthesize and accumulate arachidonic acid making the endogenous pool of arachidonic acid large

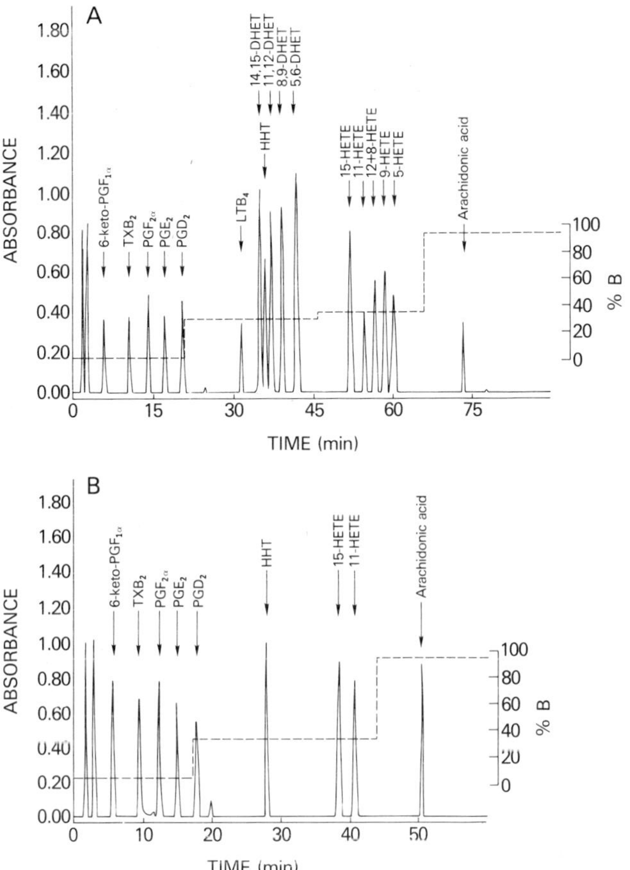

Figure 6. Reverse-phase HPLC analysis of all major metabolites of arachidonic acid using octadecyl silica columns. In both cases the solvent system is a mixture of acetonitrile and water containing 0.1% acetic acid. Mixtures of arachidonic acid metabolites are eluted from the column by changing the % acetonitrile in stepwise fashion. Using the system in (A) all five primary prostaglandins, leukotriene B_4, HHT, all stable epoxygenase metabolites, and five different isomers of HETEs can be separated. System (B) uses a modified step gradient for the rapid analysis of cyclooxygenase products to quantitate cyclooxygenase activity. The two solvents used to create the gradients in both panels were acetonitrile/water/acetic acid (30/70/0.1) and acetonitrile (100); in both cases the flow rate is 1 ml/min. In (A) the stepwise mixture, expressed as the % of the second solvent (%B), is as follows: 0 min., 3%; 22 min., 30%; 47 min., 35%; 67 min., 95%. In (B) the stepwise mixture was as follows: 0 min., 4%; 17 min., 37%; 44 min., 95%.

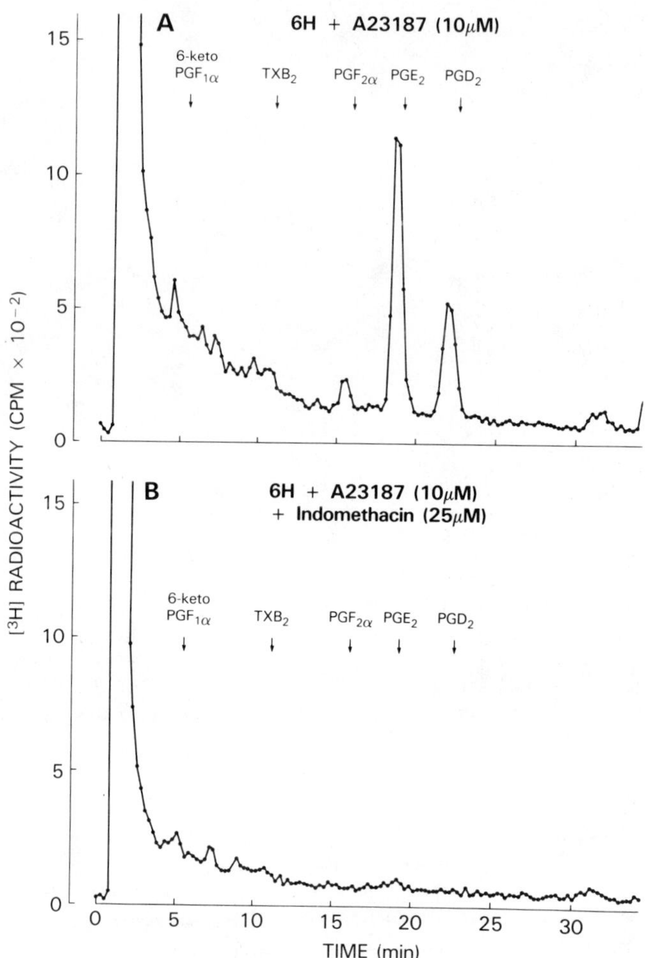

Figure 7. HPLC profile of arachidonic acid metabolites released from cells maintained in the presence of the 6H complement of hormones (including TSH and insulin) plus 5% calf serum and prelabeled with [3H]arachidonic acid for 2 hours. After the 2 hour labeling period in the presence or absence of 25 microM indomethacin, cells were washed 4-times with HBSS and stimulated for 5 minutes with A23187 as described (6) in order to effect maximal release of the metabolites. Metabolites released into the media were evaluated using reverse-phase HPLC with isocratic elution, a flow rate of 1.7 ml/min., and a solvent mixture of acetonitrile/water/acetic acid (28:72:0.1, v/v/v). Fractions were collected every 15 seconds and radioactivity measured in a scintillation spectrometer.

relative to the added radiolabel. The results did indicate (a) that arachidonic acid metabolism was an active process in intact FRTL-5 thyroid cells treated with TSH and (b) that the cyclooxygenase pathway was a major metabolic path. They also indicated, however, (c) that studies to evaluate the hormonal regulation of cyclooxygenase activity in intact cells would be clouded by the low level of radiolabeled metabolites formed in prelabeling experiments.

The cyclooxygenase path also is the major metabolic route for arachidonic acid in homogenates

To further evaluate the cyclooxygenase path and the metabolism of arachidonic acid we tried a homogenate system rather than the whole cell. The successful use of cell homogenates to measure cyclooxygenase activity has recently been reported in studies of epidermal growth factor actions in amnion cells (23). The homogenate from FRTL-5 thyroid cells maintained in the standard 6H medium containing TSH, insulin, and 5% serum, was incubated in 50 mM sodium phosphate, pH 7.4, with 0.2 microM [^{3}H]arachidonic acid. Ten to 20% of the radiolabel was converted to metabolites, six of which were consistently and clearly detected by HPLC (Fig. 8A). The retention times of these 6 metabolites were identical to those of standard PGF_{2alpha}, PGE_2, PGD_2, HHT, 15-HETE, and 11-HETE; separate studies have already established the validity of these identifications by gas chromatography/ mass spectra analysis (6). The specific cyclooxygenase inhibitor, indomethacin, inhibited the production of all 6 metabolites to less than 10% of control (Fig. 8C). ETYA, an inhibitor of both the cyclooxygenase and lipoxygenase, inhibited the production of all the metabolites to the same extent as indomethacin (Fig. 8B). The lipoxygenase inhibitor, NDGA, had no effect (Fig. 8D) at a concentration known to inhibit iodide efflux and thyroglobulin iodination by the cells (5). These data indicated that all 6 metabolites are produced by the cyclooxygenase pathway illustrated in Figure 9. The presence of the PGE_2 and other isomerases in the homogenate, as well as the cyclooxygenase, can be presumed (Fig. 8 and 9). Although the proportion of individual metabolites may vary according to the activity of these isomerases or the nonenzymatic conversion of PGH_2, and may even vary with homogenate concentration, the sum of all the metabolites produced could accurately be estimated by HPLC (Fig. 6A or 6B) and was used to estimate cyclooxygenase activity using the calculations below (Equations I and II):

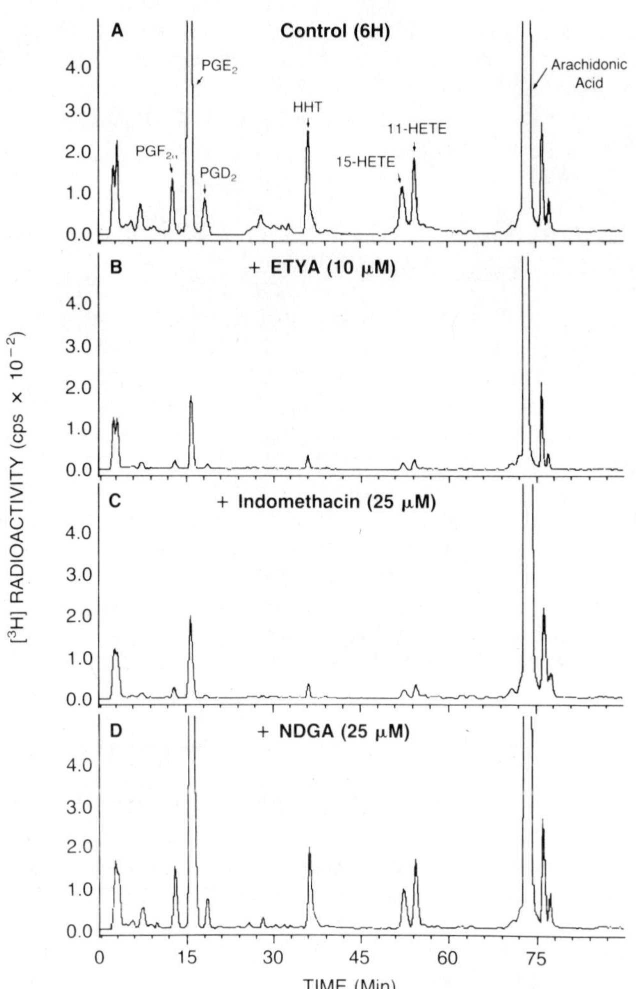

Figure 8. HPLC profiles of arachidonic acid metabolites produced by a total homogenate of FRTL-5 rat thyroid cells maintained in the 6H hormone mixture (including TSH and insulin) plus 5% calf serum. The total homogenate, 10 mg protein, was incubated with [^{3}H]arachidonic acid for 5 min. in the presence or absence of inhibitors: (A) no inhibitor; (B) 10 microM ETYA; (C) 25 microM indomethacin; (D) 25 microM NDGA. Organic solvent extracts of the reaction mixtures were analyzed by the reverse-phase HPLC system in Figure 6A.

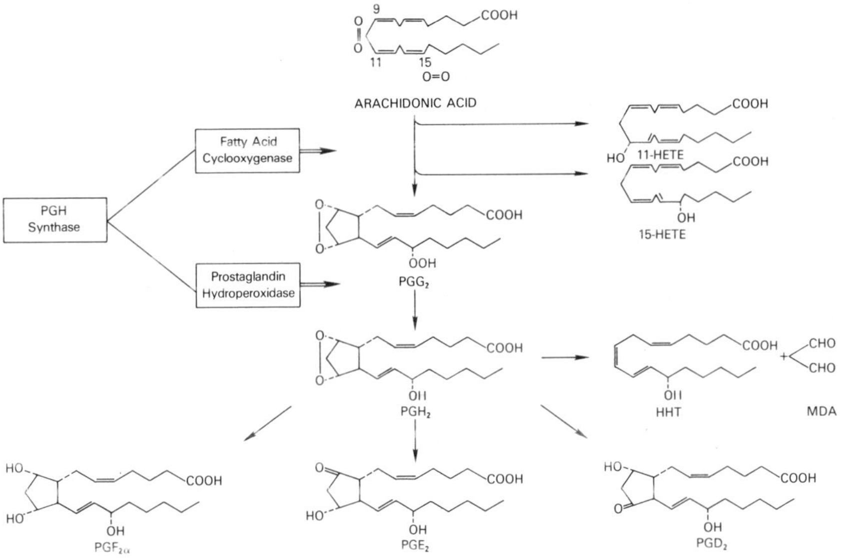

Figure 9. The 6 metabolites evident in Figure 8 can be accounted for as products of the cyclooxygenase pathway as detailed. The presence of appropriate isomerases or synthetases is presumed. PGF_{2alpha} and HHT can form from PGH_2 by a nonenzymatic route.

(I) Total metabolites per tube (nmol/tube) =

$$\frac{\text{radioactivity of the 6 metabolites (cps)x100 (nmol/tube)}}{\text{total radioactivity (cps)}}$$

(II) Cyclooxygenase activity (nmol/min/mg protein) =

$$\frac{\text{total amount of metabolites per tube (nmol/tube)}}{\text{(incubation time in minutes) x (mg protein per tube)}}$$

Optimal conditions to measure cyclooxygenase activity in FRTL-5 cell homogenates

Using the above procedure to estimate activity, the properties of the cyclooxygenase in the homogenate from FRTL-5 thyroid cells chronically maintained in complete medium (including TSH, insulin, and 5% serum) were defined before the individual effects of TSH, insulin, or IGF-I in the serum were tested. All assays were carried out at 30° C. Activity was dependent on the concentration of homogenate protein added to the assay (Fig. 10A) and was abolished if the homogenate was boiled (Fig. 10A). The pattern of metabolites did shift as the protein concentration was shifted to lower values (data not shown) suggesting differences in isomerase activity as a function of protein concentration. Nevertheless, all further characterization results (Figure 10 and Table 4) were the same at low (1 mg/ml) and high (5 mg/ml) protein concentrations, indicating this procedure could reasonably measure total cyclooxygenase activity. Activity was linear with time over the first 5 minutes of incubation (Fig. 10B); was optimal at pH 8 (Fig. 10C); and was optimal in 50 mM sodium phosphate, changing only slightly (20% decrease) with alterations in the ionic strength of the buffer from 25 to 200 mM. Activity was dependent on the concentration of substrate added to the incubation; a Vmax, 0.46 nmol/min/mg protein, and Km, approximately 10 microM, in the total homogenate from these cells could be determined.

In other systems, the cyclooxygenase activity of homogenates has been dependent on tryptophan and hematin. Maximal activity of the FRTL-5 homogenate from these 6H cells was very much dependent on tryptophan but was minimally affected by hematin (Table 4). Nevertheless, hematin, as well as tryptophan, was included in all assays measuring hormonal effects on cyclooxygenase activity unless otherwise noted.

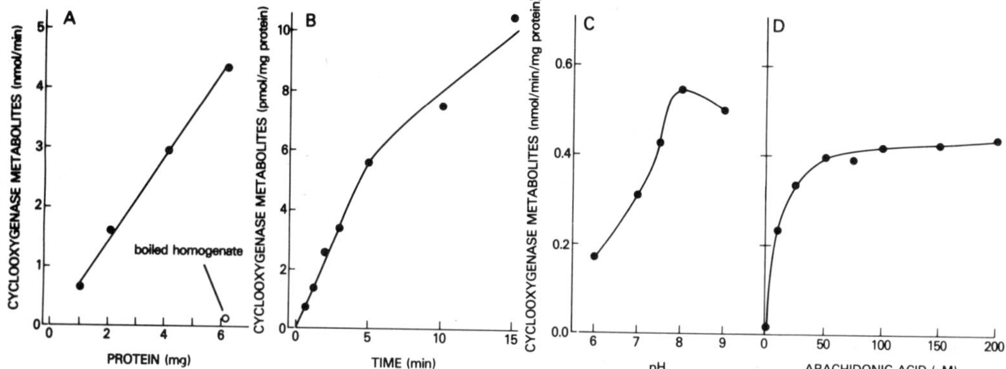

Figure 10. Optimal conditions to measure the cyclooxygenase activity of FRTL-5 homogenates determined by examining the reactivity of the homogenate with [^{3}H]arachidonic acid as a function of (A) protein concentration, (B) time, (C) pH, and (D) substrate concentration. The homogenate in this case is from FRTL-5 cells maintained in the 6 hormone mixture plus 5% calf serum. In (A), (C), and (D) optimal conditions were used with the exception that tryptophan was only 4 mM. In (B) only 1 microM arachidonic acid, rather than 100 microM, was present. From these data, the routine assay to evaluate hormone effects was determined to be best measured with reaction mixtures containing 1 to 5 mg protein/ml, for 5 min. at a pH of 8.0, and including 100 micromolar arachidonic acid. Also included is 20 mM tryptophan and 1 micromolar hematin as determined from the data in Table 4.

TABLE 4

Effect of tryptophan and hematin on cyclooxygenase activity of homogenates from FRTL-5 rat thyroid cells.

TRYPTOPHAN CONCENTRATION (mM)	ACTIVITY (nmol/min/ mg protein)	HEMATIN CONCENTRATION (microM)	ACTIVITY (nmol/min/ mg protein)
0	0.1	0	0.1
2.0	0.4	0.1	0.1
4.0	0.6	0.5	0.1
8.0	0.8	2.0	0.1
10.0	0.9		
20.0	0.9		
40.0	1.0		

Assays were performed using homogenates from cells exposed to 6H medium plus 5% calf serum for 7 days under otherwise optimal conditions.

Effect of TSH, Insulin/IGF-I and serum on cyclooxygenase activity

FRTL-5 thyroid cells were depleted of insulin, TSH, and serum by incubation in 4H medium with 0.2% serum for 7 days then rechallenged with complete medium containing TSH, insulin and 5% serum. Cyclooxygenase activity was measured as a function of time of hormone addition under the optimal assay conditions defined above: 50 mM sodium phosphate, pH 8, 100 microM [^{3}H]arachidonic acid, 1 microM hematin, and 20 mM tryptophan and 3 mg/ml homogenate protein (Fig.11). It is evident that there is a time dependent increase in cyclooxygenase activity whether measured per cell (per microgram DNA) or as a function of cell protein. The activity is maximal at 36 hours.

The effect of individual hormones on cyclooxygenase activity was investigated using homogenates from "hormonally depleted" cells maintained in 4H medium (no insulin, no TSH) and 0.2% serum for 7 days. As noted in Figure 12, neither TSH nor insulin alone could increase cyclooxygenase activity. In contrast, the presence of TSH plus insulin was able to increase cyclooxygenase activity (Fig. 12) and the addition of calf serum plus insulin further enhanced the action of TSH (Fig. 12). This result is similar to studies of the effect of TSH and insulin on glycosaminoglycan synthesis by FRTL-5 thyroid cells rather than on thyroglobulin biosynthesis and gene expression (22). Thus insulin has no independent effect in the present case and in the GAG situation but is active in thyroglobulin biosynthesis. This pattern is also similar to the action of these agents on growth in that TSH requires insulin for activity and the action of TSH plus insulin is further enhanced by calf-serum (22).

The inclusion of insulin or 5% calf serum in the medium during the 7 day depletion period results in a lesser loss of cyclooxygenase activity (Fig. 13) and preserves the TSH responsiveness (Fig. 13).

Hormonal effects on cyclooxygenase gene expression

The data above indicated that cyclooxygenase activity was regulated by insulin/IGF-I as well as TSH and that TSH effects on cyclooxygenase activity require insulin/IGF-I. This conclusion was validated by studies showing that the ability of insulin/IGF-I and TSH to

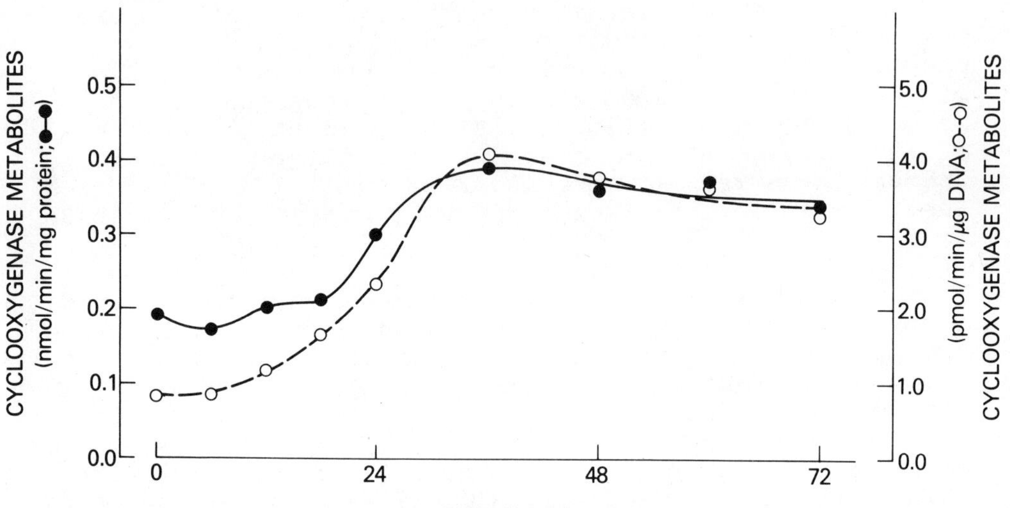

Figure 11. Effect of the 6 hormone mixture (including insulin plus TSH) with 5% calf serum on cyclooxygenase activity as a function of time of treatment and expressed per mg homogenate protein or per microgram cell DNA. FRTL-5 thyroid cells grown to confluency in the 6H mixture plus 5% calf serum were deprived of insulin, TSH, and serum for 7 days, then rechallenged with the complete 6H hormone mixture plus 5% serum. At the times indicated homogenates of the cells were made and assayed for cyclooxygenase metabolites using optimal assay conditions (Fig. 10) and reverse-phase HPLC analysis (Fig. 6B).

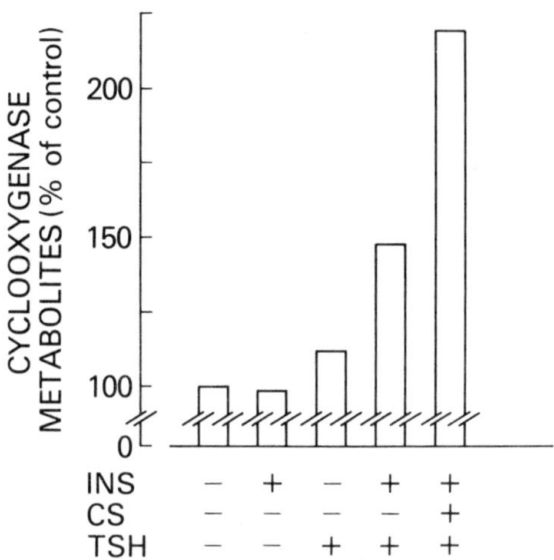

Figure 12. Effect of TSH and insulin on cyclooxygenase activity using the same protocol as defined in Figure 11. Cells were depleted of insulin, TSH, and serum for a 7 day period, then exposed to TSH and insulin, alone or in combination, at the concentrations normally present in the medium, $1x10^{-10}$ M and 10 micrograms per ml, respectively. The insulin plus TSH combination was also supplemented with 5% serum in one set of cells. Homogenates were made 36 hours after hormone treatment and included in the standard assay mixture; arachidonic acid metabolites formed by the cyclooxygenase were measured by reverse-phase HPLC as described in Figure 6B.

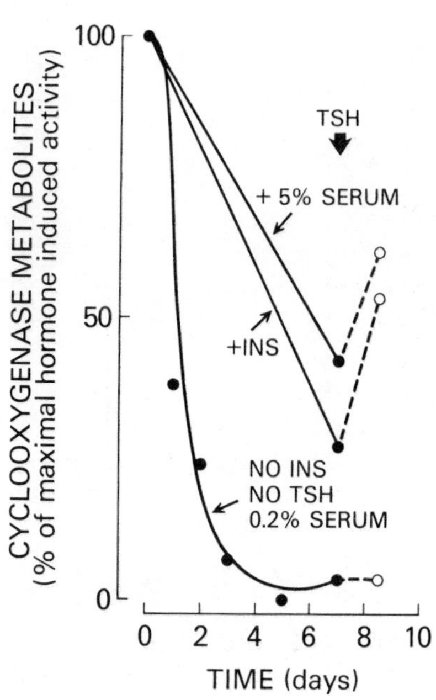

Figure 13. Effect of withdrawing insulin and TSH from the medium and depleting the medium of serum (to 0.2% from 5%) on cyclooxygenase activity of FRTL-5 cell homogenates by comparison to the effect of keeping either the insulin or the 5% calf serum in the medium during the 7 day withdrawal period. The ability of $1x10^{-10}$ M TSH to increase cyclooxygenase activity on each of the groups of cells maintained in different depletion conditions is also measured. Homogenate preparation, cyclooxygenase assay, and HPLC analysis was otherwise identical to Figure 12.

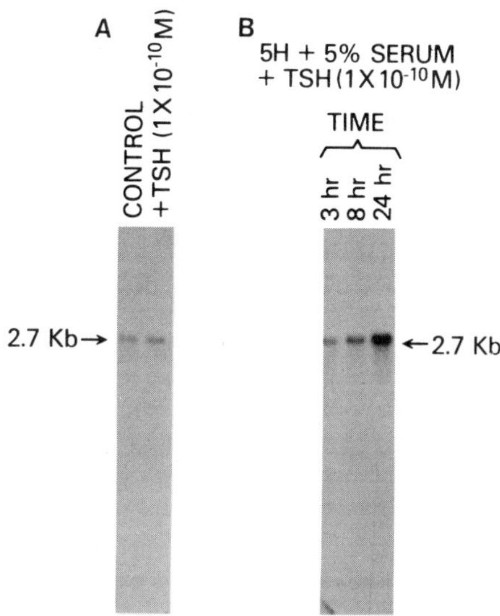

Figure 14. Ability of $1x10^{-10}$ M TSH to increase the level of cyclooxygenase mRNA in the absence (A) or presence (B) of insulin as measured by Northern blot analysis. In (A) cells were maintained for 7 days with no insulin, no TSH and in 0.2% serum before TSH was added for a 24 hour period. In (B) cells were maintained in medium with no TSH but with insulin and 5% serum for 7 days before TSH was added for the times noted. RNA was extracted by a standard procedure (28) and poly A+RNA prepared (29). Northern blot analysis (30) was performed using Nytran membranes(Schleicher and Schuell), stringent conditions recommended by the manufacturer (Schleicher and Schuell) and using a 860 bp insert from the FRTL-5 cell cyclooxygenase cDNA which was labeled by random priming (31). The size of the cyclooxygenase mRNA is 2.7 kb. Each lane contains 5 micrograms of polyA+ RNA; blots were stripped and rehybridized with a beta-actin probe to confirm that each lane contained identical amounts of the poly A+ RNA.

increase cyclooxygenase activity reflected, at least in part, their action on gene expression.

The nucleotide sequence of sheep cyclooxygenase mRNA has been reported (24). Using an oligonucleotide defined by the aspirin binding site of the enzyme, a rat FRTL-5 thyroid lambda gt11 expression library was screened and an 0.86 kb cDNA insert containing the aspirin binding site coding sequence was obtained. The sequence exhibited 80% homology (amino acid) with the comparable sheep sequence. Using this insert as a probe, the effect of physiologic concentration of TSH ($1x10^{-10}$ M) on cyclooxygenase transcript expression were determined in cells maintained in "hormonally depleted" medium (4H, 0.2% serum) for 5 days (Fig. 14A). TSH did not increase transcript expression under these conditions, consistent with the data above.

The effect of TSH was, however, evident when cells, maintained in the presence of insulin (5H, 5% serum), were exposed to TSH (Figure 14B). The effect of TSH on cyclooxygenase gene expression in cells maintained in insulin containing medium is not only evident, it is shown to have a time dependency consistent with its affect on cyclooxygenase activity.

THE ACTION OF INSULIN AND TSH ON THE CONVERSION OF PGH_2 TO PGD_2, PGE_2, AND PGF_{2alpha}

Figure 15 presents the HPLC radiochromatograms matching the data in Figure 12. When cells are maintained for 7 days in 4H medium (no insulin, no TSH) and only 0.2% serum, the homogenate produces PGF_{2alpha} but little PGE_2 or PGD_2. Despite the absence of a statistically significant increase in total cyclooxygenase products, it is evident that TSH alone, and to a lesser extent insulin or IGF-I alone, can change the ratio of production of PGF_{2alpha}, PGE_2, and PGD_2. The addition of TSH, insulin or IGF-I (Fig. 15B) alone increases the production of PGD_2. The combination of insulin plus TSH (Fig. 15D) increases PGE_2 as well as PGD_2; the further addition of 5% serum to the cells treated with insulin plus TSH (Fig. 15E) exaggerates the production of PGE_2 relative to PGD_2.

These results suggest that there is a constitutive level of cyclooxygenase activity after the 7 day hormone depletion period but that the primary product of the PGH_2 formed by the PGH_2 synthase, PGF_{2alpha} and HHT, may result from nonenzymatic conversion of PGH_2. In the presence of

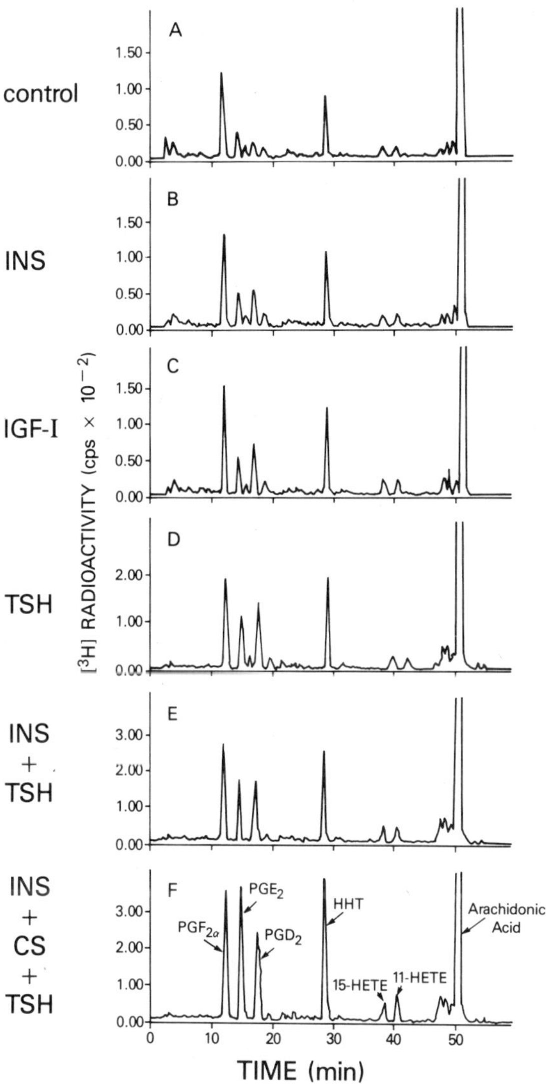

Figure 15. HPLC analysis of the cyclooxygenase metabolites produced by the treatment of cells with insulin (10 micrograms/ml), IGF-I (100 ng/ml) or TSH ($1x10^{-10}$ M) alone or in combination as in Figure 12. HPLC analysis used the procedure in Figure 6B. Total recovery of metabolites is >90% under these conditions; assays used optimal conditions (Fig. 10 and Table 4).

TSH, insulin or IGF-I alone, despite the absence of an increase in PGH_2 synthase activity, the PGD_2 isomerase/synthetase is presumably induced, decreasing the amount of PGF_{2alpha} while increasing the amount of PGD_2. The mixture of insulin plus TSH, or insulin plus TSH plus serum, may increase the PGE_2 isomerase as well as the PGH_2 synthase activities. These results suggest the hormones (a) regulate the activity of the isomerases as well as the PGH_2 synthase (cyclooxygenase) activities and (b) regulate the PGD_2 and PGE_2 isomerases differently. Definitive examination of this point will require studies of the action of homogenates on PGH_2 and the characterization of PGE_2 and PGD_2 isomerases or synthetases; these studies are in progress.

SUMMARY

The present study and the previous report (6) show that the cyclooxygenase path is a primary route of metabolism of arachidonic acid in FRTL-5 rat thyroid cells. The production of PGD_2 and PGE_2 is an active process in intact cells treated with complete medium including TSH, insulin and 5% calf serum. In contrast, PGF_{2alpha} and HHT are probably nonenzymatic degradation products of an unstable intermediate, PGH_2, since the two compounds are produced and occupy a significant proportion of the cyclooxygenase metabolites only in the homogenate system; this is true in other cells (25).

Although the production of prostaglandins involves three steps, i. e. the release of free arachidonic acid, the production of PGH_2 by PGH synthase (cyclooxygenase) and the conversion of PGH_2 to various prostaglandins by specific isomerases or synthetases (Fig. 2), the first step, the release of free arachidonic acid, has been, until recently, believed to be the sole step important for the regulation of prostaglandin synthesis. This presumption rested on the following observations. Only the free form of arachidonic acid is converted to prostaglandins and the intracellular free arachidonic acid pool is very small compared to the esterified form in phospholipids. The size of the free arachidonic acid pool is regulated by the balance between release from phospholipids by phospholipases and reacylation into phospholipids. When resting cells are stimulated, the release of arachidonic acid and the production of prostaglandins increase concomitantly.

The present study shows, however, that all three steps of prostaglandin synthesis are under regulatory control in FRTL-5 rat thyroid cells and that the control is a complex process involving TSH, insulin/IGF-I, and serum. The first step is primarily under the control of TSH. TSH increases the synthesis of arachidonic acid and also, like norepinephrine (5, 6) induces the release of arachidonic acid from the cell by a mechanism involving a pertussis toxin-sensitive G protein. Regulation of the second step can be estimated by measuring cyclooxygenase activity. The present report shows that TSH increases cyclooxygenase activity, presumably by increasing gene expression, but that the TSH effect on cyclooxygenase activity requires insulin/IGF-I or serum. This result is similar to studies showing the effect of TSH and insulin/IGF-I on glycosaminoglycan synthesis, thyroglobulin synthesis, and growth in FRTL-5 thyroid cells (22).

Finally, the present report suggests that the TSH and insulin also regulate PGD_2 and PGE_2 isomerase activities, that they regulate them differently when alone or in combination, and that PGD_2 isomerase activity, unlike cyclooxygenase or PGE_2 isomerase activity, can be regulated by either hormone alone rather than requiring the presence of both hormones.

The sum of these studies suggest that TSH and insulin, or IGF-I presumably, regulate the synthesis of prostaglandins in thyroid cells. The actions of prostaglandins on thyroid or other cells makes this a potent autocrine or paracrine regulatory system which may have profound regulatory effects on thyroid hormone formation, cell growth, thyroid blood flow, and even lymphocyte interactions in the thyroid.

REFERENCES

1. N. J. Philp and E. F. Grollman, Thyrotropin and norepinephrine stimulate the metabolism of phosphoinositides in FRTL-5 thyroid cells, FEBS Letters, 202: 193 (1986).
2. E. A. Bone, D. W. Alling and E. F. Grollman, Norepinephrine and thyroid-stimulating hormone induce inositol phosphate accumulation in FRTL-5 cells, Endocrinology, 119: 2193 (1986).
3. S. J. Weiss, N. J. Philp and E. F. Grollman, Effect of thyrotropin on iodide efflux in FRTL-5 cells is mediated by Ca^{2+}, Endocrinology, 114: 1108 (1984).
4. D. Corda, C. Marcocci, L. D. Kohn, J. Axelrod, and A. Luini, Association of the changes in cytosolic

Ca^{2+} and iodide efflux induced by thyrotropin and by the stimulation of alpha 1 adrenergic receptors in cultured rat thyroid cells, J. Biol. Chem., 260: 9230 (1985).

5. C. Marcocci, A. Luini, P. Santisteban and E. F. Grollman, Norepinephrine and thyrotropin stimulation of iodide efflux in FRTL-5 thyroid cells involves metabolites of arachidonic acid and is associated with the iodination of thyroglobulin, Endocrinology 120: 1127 (1987).
6. R. M. Burch, A. Luini, D. E. Mais, D. Corda, J. Y. Vanderhoek, L. D. Kohn and J. Axelrod, Alpha-1 adrenergic stimulation of arachidonic acid release and metabolism in a rat thyroid cell line, J. Biol. Chem., 261: 11236 (1986).
7. D. Corda and L. D. Kohn, Role of pertussis toxin sensitive G proteins in the alpha-1 adrenergic receptor mediated activation of membrane phospholipases and iodide fluxes in FRTL-5 thyroid cells, Biochem. Biophys. Res. Commun., 141: 1000 (1986).
8. D. Corda and L. D. Kohn, Phorbol myristate acetate inhibits alpha-1 adrenergically but not thyrotropin regulated functions in FRTL-5 rat thyroid cells, Endocrinology, 120: 1152 (1986).
9. P. Santisteban, M. DeLuca, D. Corda, E.F. Grollman and L. D. Kohn, Regulation of thyroglobulin iodination and thyroid hormone formation in FRTL-5 thyroid cells, in: "Fronteirs in Thyroidology, v. 2," G. Medeiros-Neto and E. Gaitan, Plenum Press, New York (1986).
10. L. D. Kohn, E. A. Bone, J. Y. Chan, D. Corda, O. Isozaki, A. Luini, C.Marcocci, P. Santisteban and E. F. Grollman, Interactions of peptinergic hormone and biogenic amine signals in the regulation of thyroid function and growth, in: "Tansduction of Neuronal Signals," P. J. Magistretti, J. H. Morrison and T.D. Reisine, eds., Foundation for the study of the Nervous system, Geneva (1986).
11. J. Axelrod, Transducing mechanism in pituitary, thyroid and visual system, in: "Tansduction of Neuronal Signals," P. J. Magistretti, J. H. Morrison and T.D. Reisine, eds., Foundation for the study of the Nervous system, Geneva (1986).
12. E. Yavin, Z. Yavin, M. D. Schneider and L. D. Kohn, Monoclonal antibodies to the thyrotropin receptor: implications for receptor structure and the action of autoantibodies in Graves' disease, Proc. Natl. Acad. Sci. USA, 78: 3180 (1981).
13. W. A. Valente, P. Vitti, E. Yavin, C. M. Rotella, E. F. Grollman, R. Toccafondi and L. D. Kohn,

Monoclonal antibodies derived from the lymphocytes of patients with Graves' disease, Proc. Natl. Acad. Sci. USA, 79: 6680 (1982).

14. L. D. Kohn, E. Yavin, Z. Yavin, P. Laccetti, P. Vitti, E. F. Grollman and W. A. Valente, Autoimmune thyroid disease studied with monoclonal antibodies to the TSH receptor, in: "Monoclonal Antibodies: Probes for the Study of Autoimmunity and Immunodeficiency," B. F. Haynes and G. S. Eisenbarth, eds., Academic Press, New York (1983).
15. L. D. Kohn, D. Tombaccini, M. De Luca, M. Bifulco, E. F. Grollman and W. A. Valente, Monoclonal antibodies and the thyrotropin receptor, in: "Monoclonal Antibodies to Receptors: Probes for Receptor Structure and Function," M. F. Greaves, ed., Receptors and Recognition, Series B, 17: 201 (1984).
16. L. D. Kohn, F. V. Alvarez, C. Marcocci, A. D. Kohn, A. Chen, W. E. Hoffman, D. Tombaccini, W. A. Valente, M. De Luca, P. Santisteban and E. F. Grollman, Monoclonal antibody studies defining the origin and properties of Graves' autoantibodies, Ann. N. Y. Acad. Sci., 475: 157 (1986).
17. J. Y. Chan, M. De Luca, P. Santisteban, O. Isozaki, S. Shifrin, S. M. Aloj, E. F. Grollman and L. D. Kohn, Nature of thyroid autoantigens: the TSH receptor, in: Thyroid Autoimmunity," A. Pinchera, S. H. Ingbar and J. M. McKenzie, eds., Plenum Press, New York (1987).
18. L. D. Kohn, W. A. Valente, E. F. Grollman, S. M. Aloj and P. Vitti, Clinical determination and/or quantification of thyrotropin and a variety of thyroid stimulatory or inhibitory factors performed in vitro with an improved thyroid cell line FRTL-5, U. S. Patent 4,609,622, Sep. 2 (1986).
19. W. A. Valente, P. Vitti, C. M. Rotella, M. M. Vaughan, S. M. Aloj, E. F. Grollman, F. S. Ambesi-Impiombato and L. D. Kohn, Antibodies that promote thyroid growth: a distinct population of thyroid stimulating autoantibodies, N. Engl. J. Med., 309: 1028 (1983).
20. F. S. Ambesi-Impiombato, L. A. M. Parks and H. G. Coon, Culture of Hormone dependent epithelial cells from rat thyroids, Proc. Natl. Acad. Sci. USA, 77: 3455 (1980).
21. F. S. Ambesi-Impiombato, Living, fast growing thyroid cell strain, FRTL-5, U. S. Patent 4,608,341, August 26 (1986).
22. L. D. Kohn, M. Saji, T. Akamizu, S. Ikuyama, O. Isozaki, A. D. Kohn, P. Santisteban, J. Y. Chan, S. Bellur, C. M. Rotella, F. V. Alvarez and S. M. Aloj,

Receptors of the thyroid: the thyrotropin receptor is only the first violinist of a symphony orchestra, in: "The Thyroid: Regulation of its Normal Growth and Function," R. Ekholm, L. D. Kohn and S. Wollman, eds., Plenum Press, New York (1989).

23. M. L. Casey, K. Korte and P. C. MacDonald, Epidermal growth factor stimulation of prostaglandin E_2 biosynthesis in amnion cells: induction of prostaglandin H_2 synthase, J. Biol. Chem., 263: 7846 (1988).

24. J. P. Merlie, D. Fagan, J. Mudd and P. Needleman, Isolation and characterization of the complimentary DNA for sheep seminal vesicle prostaglandin endoperoxide synthase (cyclooxygenase), J. Biol. Chem., 263: 3550 (1988).

25. D. H. Nugteren and E. Hazelhof, Isolation and properties of intermediates in prostaglandin biosynthesis, Biochimica et Biophysica Acta, 326: 448 (1973).

26. J. G. Heider and R. L. Boyett, The picomole determination of free and total cholesterol in cells in culture, J. Lipid Res., 19: 514 (1978).

27. M. A. Kaluzny, L. A. Duncan, M. V. Merrit and D. E. Epps, Rapid separation of lipid classes in high yield and purity using bonded phase columns, J. Lipid Res., 26: 135 (1985).

28. J. M. Chirgwin, A. E. Przybyla, R. J. MacDonald and W. J. Utter, Isolation of biologically active ribonucleic acid from sources enriched in ribonuclease, Biochemistry 18: 5294 (1979).

29. H. Aviv and P. Leder, Purification of biologically active globin messenger RNA by chromatography on oligo thymidilic acid-cellulose, Proc. Natl. Acad. Sci. USA, 69: 1408 (1972).

30. P. S. Thomas, Hybridization of denatured RNA and small DNA fragments transferred to nitrocellulose, Proc. Natl. Acad. Sci. USA, 77: 5201 (1980).

31. A. P. Feinberg and B. Vogelstein, A technique for radiolabeling DNA restriction endonuclease fragments to high specific activity, Anal. Biochem., 137: 266 (1984).

INTEGRATED REGULATION OF GROWTH AND OF FUNCTION

Margaret C. Eggo and Gerard N. Burrow

M013K
Department of Medicine
University California, San Diego
La Jolla, CA 92093-0613

INTRODUCTION

In vivo studies have shown that thyrotropin regulates thyroid growth and function. How TSH is able to exert these dramatic effects is not clear. The last decade has seen such refinements in cell culture systems that this question can finally be addressed. The major advance in cell culture technology has been the removal of serum from the culture medium of primary cultures of thyroid cells released from tissues. Serum can be replaced by a cocktail of hormones and other factors which have been determined empirically to be essential for the maintenance of most cells in culture.[1] This chemically-defined medium permits researchers to add hormones both individually and in combination to examine direct, cooperative, and indirect interactions between them. Another unanticipated benefit from serum-free culture of thyroid cells has been that thyroid cell conditioned medium has been found to contain several proteins of potential biological importance.[2-5] This finding has opened up a new area examining potential endocrine functions other than thyroid hormone production for the thyroid. Alternatively, these newly discovered products could be for autocrine or paracrine use. In this brief review we shall discuss the direct ways in which TSH is thought to regulate thyroid growth and function and how TSH interacts with other hormones and growth factors to influence these parameters. We shall examine the intracellular pathways thought to be activated by TSH, growth factors and by agents known to be capable of discretely activating second messengers of some partially defined intracellular pathways. We shall use as a model system data we have obtained with the sheep thyroid cell culture system. This culture system differs from FRTL5, dog and human thyroid cells in culture because cells reorganize to form 3D follicles[6] and synthesize and secrete physiologic quantities of thyroid hormones.[7]

TSH IN THYROID GROWTH AND FUNCTION

Chronic stimulation by endogenous TSH causes marked but usually limited hyperplasia. In vivo studies in rats using antithyroid drugs to cause hypothyroidism and hence relieve the negative feedback of T_3 and T_4 on the pituitary show that mesenchymal cells, endothelial cells as well as follicular cells in the thyroid undergo growth.[8] The growth response in adult man is limited leading to suggestions that the thyroid cell population turns over slowly. Thyroid cells may become insensitive to the growth stimulatory effects of TSH[9] which may in part explain the difficulty experienced in demonstrating a substantial growth response in culture of primary thyroid explants. However the consensus appears to be that for many thyroid cell culture systems, TSH is mitogenic when (and probably only when) insulin or IGF-I is included in the culture media. By itself TSH is not mitogenic for FRTL5 cells[10] or for sheep thyroid cells[11] and human thyroid cells in culture.

TSH is known to activate adenylate cyclase with the production of cyclic AMP. In fact the levels of cyclic AMP in cells acutely stimulated with TSH are barely detectable in sensitive assays for cyclic AMP unless the phosphodiesterase inhibitor, methyl isobutyl xanthine is included. This may reflect the transient nature of the signal as well as its compartmentalisation. Protein substrates for this kinase have been identified but their functions are unknown. However the TSH receptor, whose structure remains elusive, could potentially be coupled to second messengers other than cyclic AMP e.g inositol phospholipid hydrolysis. For FRTL5 cells there is evidence that supraphysiologic concentrations of TSH can stimulate the production of one of the products of inositol phospholipid breakdown.[12,13] TSH is not as potent in this regard as norepinephrine. Bone et al[12] showed that inositol trisphosphate (IP_3) production was increased modestly in FRTL5 cells following challenge of TSH-treated cells with supraphysiologic concentrations of TSH. Subsequently Field et al[13] showed that these cells in supraphysiologic concentrations of TSH did show an increase in IP_3 production and suggest that there are two classes of TSH receptor. They postulate that when the TSH receptor coupled to inositol phospholipid hydrolysis is activated, it is able to cause the phenomenon of desensitization of the cyclic AMP-coupled receptor.[13] Although we observed that preincubation with TPA reduced the cumulative concentration of cyclic AMP in TSH-treated sheep thyroid cells, the decrease was modest (50%) and the inhibitory effects of protein kinase C activation were not reversed by addition of cyclic AMP analogs.[14] Until the turnover of TSH receptors is known the significance of the effects observed with extremely high TSH concentrations is speculative. For dog thyroid slices there is some controversy over whether TSH does in fact stimulate this production and again supraphysiologic TSH concentrations were required.[15,16] TSH has not been shown to increase intracellular calcium levels in dog cells and in sheep thyroid cells we did not find that TSH at any concentration was able to increase inositol trisphosphate production in the time periods where this is usually detected.

The effects of TSH on thyroid function are largely reproduced by cyclic AMP or agents such as forskolin. Again, as for growth, TSH is effective in functional assays only if insulin or IGF-I is included.[10,17,18] TSH could be acting by enhancing the binding of IGF-I as has been shown in granulosa cells cultured in the presence of follicle stimulating hormone.[19] However, in the thyroid, studies examining this relationship have been controversial. Saji found that TSH had no effect on IGF-I binding to porcine thyroid cells[20] whereas Tramontano et al[21] found decreased binding to FRTL5 cells cultured in high concentrations of TSH. Polychronakos et al[22] showed an increased number of type II IGF receptors during goitrogen-induced hyperplasia in rats. The mechanism of action of the somatomedins and insulin and the possible way that second messengers of these pathways could interact with the cyclic AMP-dependent protein kinase is discussed in the next section.

THE INSULIN-LIKE GROWTH FACTORS AND INSULIN IN THYROID GROWTH AND FUNCTION

The effect of insulin in vivo on thyroid gland histology was investigated by Catz[23] more than thirty years ago. Rats injected with insulin showed thyroid follicular cell hypertrophy. In common with TSH,[24] insulin is known to stimulate sugar, ion and amino acid transport.[25] In addition there are several enzymes whose activity is regulated by insulin and insulin action has been shown to include redistribution of membrane proteins e.g the glucose transporter and the receptors for IGF-II and transferrin.[25] In vitro studies have shown synergism between the effects of TSH and insulin or IGF-I on FRTL5 cell growth.[10,26] Whether insulin or IGF-I are able stimulate growth independent from TSH and vice versa in these cells is unclear. In FRTL5 cells preincubation in TSH produced an exaggerated response to subsequent addition of IGF-I suggesting that TSH is a competence factor and IGF-I a progression factor through the cell cycle.[21] The synergism between the pathways activated by insulin or IGF-I and TSH on growth is remarkable and has also been shown for human,[27] dog[28] and sheep[18] thyroid cells in culture. In these primary cultures both insulin and IGF-I were growth factors independent of TSH. Similarly in another differentiated strain of rat cells[29] insulin itself is mitogenic.

Santisteban et al[10] showed that in FRTL5 cells insulin and IGF-I were able to induce thyroglobulin mRNA accumulation and thyroglobulin protein synthesis. TSH by itself at physiological concentrations was unable to stimulate thyroglobulin mRNA production or thyroglobulin synthesis but in the presence of insulin or IGF-I these parameters were stimulated five fold. Similarly Aouani et al[30] found that hormones other than TSH were capable of regulating thyroglobulin synthesis. Using iodide organification as a measure of differentiated thyroid function Sho and Kondo[17] found that in pig follicles insulin was not stimulatory but markedly stimulated TSH-mediated iodide organification. From these data TSH can be summarized as being necessary but not sufficient for optimal expression of thyroid differentiated function and growth. Similarly insulin and IGF-I can share the same definition. Clearly there is integrated regulation of growth and function.

<u>Second messengers for insulin and IGF-I action</u>

a) Tyrosine kinase

Whether insulin and IGF-I are acting through the same intracellular pathways to synergise with the TSH-stimulated pathway is not known. However the receptors for insulin and IGF-I share considerable sequence homology. The highest degree of homology (84%) is in the tyrosine kinase domains of these receptors.[31] This domain is located on the beta subunit of the receptor which also contains a membrane spanning domain. Several tyrosine residues on the receptor are autophosphorylated. Tyrosine kinase activity was thought to be essential for the observed effects of insulin but recent data using monoclonal antibodies have resurrected a controversy.[32] A search for substrates for this kinase has not yielded conclusive information. Various proteins of differing molecular weights on SDS polyacrylamide gels have been shown to be phosphorylated on tyrosine but no common, universal protein has been identified.[31] Possibly these phosphorylated intermediates are rare proteins whose phosphorylated state is only transient.

b) Diacylglycerol and inositol phospholipid hydrolysis

Diacylglycerol is the endogenous activator of protein kinase C and is one of the products of inositol phospholipid hydrolysis. Insulin (and presumably IGF-I) does not appear to stimulate rapid inositol phospholipid hydrolysis in most systems studied.[33] However in FRTL5 cells diacylglycerol production was increased on long-term (6d) treatment with insulin or IGF-I.[34] TSH also was able to stimulate an increase in diacylglycerol production in this long-term assay and synergism between insulin- or IGF-I- and TSH-stimulated production was seen. This synergism between TSH and insulin is unusual because in smooth muscle, increased cyclic AMP is associated with inhibition of phosphoinositide hydrolysis.[35] In pig thyroid cells in culture, Munari-Silem et al[36] showed translocation of only 10-15% of cytosolic protein kinase C following treatment with physiologic concentrations of TSH whereas active phorbol esters under the same conditions induced a 90% change. In other systems down-regulation of protein kinase C by preincubation with phorbol esters does not inhibit insulin action on phosphorylation of proteins.[33] Similarly the effects of phorbol ester on sheep thyroid cell growth are additive to those of insulin and TSH itself is not mitogenic.[37] Evidence that any or all of insulin, IGF-I or TSH are stimulating inositol phospholipid hydrolysis at physiologic TSH concentrations, is lacking.

c) Diacylglycerol from other sources

However diacylglycerol can also be produced from phosphatidylcholine catabolism[38] and from glycolipids involved in anchoring proteins to membranes.[39] One of these alternate pathways may be the source of diacylglycerol produced in FRTL5 cells by insulin, IGF-I or TSH action e.g insulin and the somatomedins are known to increase phosphatidylcholine synthesis. Beguinot et al[40] observed an increased relative proportion of phosphatidylcholine in FRTL5 cells growth-arrested in medium without TSH for 8 days. The rate-limiting enzyme in phosphatidylcholine synthesis is CTP:phosphocholine cytidyltransferase. The enzyme is activated following translocation from the cytosol to the endoplasmic reticulum. There is evidence that this enzyme is a substrate for the cAMP-dependent kinase and that phosphorylation on serine residues mediates its translocation from the endoplasmic reticulum to the cytosol and hence its inactivation.[38] Possibly the synergism observed between TSH and insulin and IGF-I is due to incresaed synthesis of phosphatidylcholine mediated by insulin and IGF-I coupled with increased catabolism mediated by TSH.

If diacylglycerol were produced from phosphatidylcholine cycles, no increase in inositol trisphosphate would be expected. Whether protein kinase C activation by diacylglycerol produced from phosphatidylcholine can occur without the concomitant rise in intracellular calcium mediated by inositol trisphosphate is not known although phorbol esters are able to activate protein kinase C under these conditions. The composition of the diacylglycerol generated from phosphatidylcholine may have a different composition than that from phosphoinositide hydrolysis. Similarly diacylglycerol produced by phospholipase C or D action on glycosyl-phosphatidylinositols may differ from that produced by the other two pathways. Low and Saltiel[39] postulate that since the fatty acid acid composition of diacylglycerol may influence its ability to activate protein kinase C and since several isoforms of this enzyme exist, complex regulation of protein kinase C can occur. A final comment on protein kinase C regulation (perhaps confirming this speculation) is the recent paper showing inhibition of protein kinase C by naturally occurring gangliosides.[41] Since there are reports that the TSH receptor has a ganglioside component, there could be regulation at the TSH receptor level of protein kinase C activity.[42] This would provide a pleasing explanation for the antagonistic effects of active phorbol esters on TSH-mediated iodine uptake and organification observed by ourselves and several other groups.

PROSTAGLANDINS

Another product of both inositol phospholipid hydrolysis and phosphatidylcholine catabolism is arachidonic acid. This product is the substrate in the cyclooxygenase pathway which ultimately produces prostaglandins, endoperoxides and thromboxane A2. This latter compound in platelets reinforces the breakdown of phosphatidylcholine and inositol phospholipids by binding to surface receptors and activating phospholipase C.[43] Prostacyclin and prostaglandin E_1 bind to receptors coupled to adenylyl cyclase activation. Cyclic AMP acts to decrease intracellular calcium by stimulating reuptake into an intracellular pool and, as mentioned before, it inhibits inositol phospholipid hydrolysis. Clearly the autocrine effects of the prostaglandins could regulate thyroid growth and function. Their production by primary cultures of pig thyroid cells has been documented[44] but knowledge of the eicosanoids produced by FRTL5 cells and other thyroid cells culture systems is not well disseminated. Noradrenaline induces release of arachidonic acid from FRTL5 cells and prostaglandin E_2 stimulates radiolabeled thymidine incorporation in these cells.[45]

EPIDERMAL GROWTH FACTOR

Epidermal growth factor (EGF), like insulin and IGF-I is coupled to a receptor with intrinsic tyrosine kinase activity. Its effects on thyroid cells in culture however bear more similarities to the effects of phorbol esters than insulin and the IGF's.[11,14] Whether EGF activates protein kinase C in the thyroid is uncertain although a recent report using pig cells in culture showed an increase in inositol trisphosphate production within minutes of its addition.[46] Diacylglycerol production and protein kinase C translocation were not measured. In our studies with the active tumor promoters and EGF we consistently showed that tumor promoters were more efficacious in inhibiting parameters of thyroid differentiated functions than EGF and we also showed additivity between the two compounds on their effects on iodide metabolism.[14] EGF pretreatment had no significant effect on the subsequent increase in cyclic AMP production induced by acute TSH treatment. However cumulative levels of cyclic AMP were reduced by 50% in cells cultured in both EGF and TSH. The inhibition of iodide metabolism was not prevented by addition of exogenous cyclic AMP analogues suggesting that this was an indirect effect of EGF action. We found no evidence that TSH was able to alter EGF receptor number[37] as reported by another group.[47]

OTHER FACTORS MEDIATING THYROID GROWTH AND FUNCTION

a) Autocrine factors

We first reported the secretion of both types of insulin-like growth factors from primary cultures of sheep thyroid cells.[2,3] These observations have been confirmed in human thyroid tissue[48] and, for IGF-II, in FRTL5 cells.[49] As discussed above, IGF-I has profound synergistic effects on TSH-mediated thyroid growth and function. While we found that IGF-II was able to stimulate thyroid cell growth in combination with TSH, we have not as yet observed any effects on thyroid iodide metabolism. In view of the multifunctional nature of the IGF-II receptor,[50] its autocrine roles may prove interesting. We have also shown that IGF binding proteins are secreted and that their production and distribution are regulated by hormones and growth factors.[5] The IGF binding proteins are proving to be heterogeneous and it may be that the various species have different functions. One type may be stimulatory and other inhibitory to binding and bioactivity of the IGF's. One question (of many) remaining is whether the thyroid follicular cells are producing the IGF's and their binding proteins or whether a cell of mesenchymal origin is responsible. While academically worthy the situation of thyroid follicular cells in vivo is that they are influenced profoundly by IGF-I both as a mediator of growth and function and that IGF-I, whether of autocrine or paracrine origin, is available to them. The IGF binding proteins may regulate the binding or presentation of the IGF's to the cells. Since TSH may regulate IGF production and appears to inhibit IGF binding protein production there are several levels of control of growth and function possible.

In an analogous manner thyroid cells in all probability secrete transforming growth factor beta. FRTL5 cells have recently been shown to secrete this factor in common with many epithelial cells.[51] This factor has been shown in pig thyroid cells to inhibit growth and to be a modest inhibitor of thyroid function.[52] Its effects in FRTL5 cells were to inhibit growth but stimulate iodine trapping. As for the IGF's there is a secondary level of control built in to this system in that transforming growth factor beta is usually secreted in a latent form that requires proteolytic action for activation. Sheep thyroid cells secrete plasminogen activators[4] which are putative activators of latent transforming growth factor beta.[53] Plasminogen activator production is regulated by EGF, active phorbol esters as well as TSH. Regulation of transforming growth factor production and the means to activate it could regulate both thyroid growth and function.

Organification of iodide also exerts autocrine regulation of both thyroid function and growth. Excess iodide results in inhibition of growth in FRTL5 and sheep cells[54] and in inhibition of thyroid hormone synthesis and secretion.[7] The mechanism of action of iodide inhibition is not known although organification of iodide is required. This has lead to speculation concerning an iodinated intermediate which is currently under research in many laboratories. Whether excess iodide could regulate production of the other autocrine factors discussed previously also awaits investigation.

b) Other factors found in serum

Although insulin and TSH produce marked effects on growth and function, the initial concoction reported by Ambesi-Impiombato et al[55] produces an even greater growth stimulus. This is probably due to the inclusion of transferrin which has profound effect on most cells in culture. In addition we have shown that serum increases the growth response of FRTL5 cells to hormones.[56] Other factors in serum include platelet-derived growth factor and interleukin-I. This latter factor has been reported to increase growth in FRTL5 cells.[57] In human thyroid primary cultures this same factor may be toxic.

c) Adrenergic regulation of thyroid cells

There are many papers defining the role of adrenergic receptors in FRTL5 growth and function which are described in an excellent review by Bidey et al.[57] However data from these cells are not compatible with those from primary cultures and these authors conclude that in the cloning of these cells an alteration in the coupling of adrenergic receptor to the adenylate cyclase system may have occurred.

Acknowledgments

We thank Dr LK Bachrach for helpful discussions. The financial support of the Medical Research Council of Canada (MA5949) is gratefully acknowledged.

References

1. D. Barnes and G. Sato, Methods for the growth of cultured cells in serum-free medium, Anal Biochem. 102:255 (1980).

2. W.W. Mak, B. Bhaumick, R.M. Bala, J.E. Kudlow, M.C. Eggo, and G.N. Burrow, Possible role of insulin-like growth factors in the regulation of thyroid growth, ICSU Short Reports, Advances in gene technology: Molecular biology of the endocrine system 4:50 (1985).
3. L.K. Bachrach, M.C. Eggo, W.W. Mak, and G.N. Burrow, Insulin-like growth factors in sheep thyroid cells: action, receptors and production, BBRC 154:861 (1988).
4. L.K. Bachrach, M.C. Eggo, W.W. Mak, and G.N. Burrow, Insulin-like growth factors in sheep thyroid cells: action, receptors and production, BBRC 154:861 (1988).
5. W.W. Mak, M.C. Eggo, G.N. Burrow, Thyrotropin regulation of plasminogen activator activity in primary culture of ovine thyroid cells, BBRC 123:633 (1984).
6. W.W. Mak, J.E. Errick, R.C. Chan, M.C. Eggo, and G.N. Burrow, Thyrotropin-induced formation of functional follicles in primary cultures of ovine thyroid cells, Exp. Cell Res. 164:311 (1986).
7. G.P. Becks, M.C. Eggo, and G.N. Burrow, Iodide regulation of differentiated thyroid function by iodide, Endocrinology 120:2560 (1986).
8. S. Wollman and T.R. Breitman, Changes in DNA weight of thyroid glands during hyperplasia and involution, Endocrinology 86:322 (1970).
9. F. Lamy, P. Roger, L. Contor, S. Reuse, E. Raspe, J. Vasn Sande, and J.E. Dumont, Control of thyroid cell proliferation: the example of the dog thyroid, Colloque Inserm Hormones and Cell Regulation, 11th European Symposium 153:169 (1987).
10. P. Santisteban, L.D. Kohn, and R. DiLauro, Thyroglobulin gene expression is regulated by insulin and insulin-like growth factor I, as well as thyrotropin, in FRTL5 cells, J.Biol.Chem. 262:4048 (1987).
11. M.C. Eggo, L.K. Bachrach, G. Fayet, J.Errick, J.E. Kudlow, M.F. Cohen, and G.N. Burrow, The effects of growth factors and serum on DNA synthesis and differentiation in thyroid cells in culture, Mol. Cell. Endocrinol. 38:141 (1984).
12. E.A. Bone, D.W. Alling, and E.F. Grollman, Norepinephrine and TSH induce inositol phosphate accumulation in FRTL5 cells, Endocrinology 11:2193 (1986).
13. J.B. Field, P.A. Ealey, N.J. Marshall, and S. Cockcroft, TSH stimulates increases in inositol phosphates as well as cyclic AMP in the FRTL5 rat thyroid cell lne, Biochem. J. 247: 519 (1987).
14. L.K. Bachrach, M.C. Eggo, W.W. Mak, and G.N. Burrow, Phorbol esters stimulate growth and inhibit differentiation in cultured thyroid cells, Endocrinology 116:1603 (1985).
15. I. Graff, E. Laurent, C. Erneux, and J. E. Dumont, Carbachol and sodium fluoride but not TSH, stimulate the generation of inositol phosphates in the dog thyroid. FEBS Lett. 210:204 (1987).

16. M. Taguchi, and J.B.Field, Effects of TSH, carbachol, norepinephrine, and adenosine 3'5'-monophosphate on polphosphatidylinositol phosphate hydrolysis in dog thyroid slices, Endocrinology 123:2019 (1988).
17. K. Sho and Y. Kondo, Insulin modulates thyrotropin-induced follicle reconstruction and iodine metabolism in hog thyroid cells in chemically defined medium, BBRC 118:385 (1985).
18. M.C. Eggo, L.K. Bachrach, and G.N. Burrow, Control of thyroid growth and function by insulin, insulin-like growth factors and TSH, Program of the 63rd meeting of the American Thyroid Association, Montreal #120 (1988).
19. E. Adashi, C.E. Resnick, M.E. Svoboda, and J.J. Van Wyk, FSH enhances somatomedin C binding to cultured rat granulosa cells, J. Biol. Chem. 261:3923 (1986).
20. H. Saji, T. Tsushima, O. Isozaki, H. Murakami, Y. Ohba, K. Sato, M. Arai, K. Shizume, Interaction of IGF-I with porcine thyroid cells cultured as a monolayer, Endocrinology 121: 749 (1987).
21. D. Tramontano, A.C. Moses, R. Piccone, and S.H. Ingbar, Characterization and regulation of the receptor for IGF-I in the FRTL5 rat thyroid follicular cell line, Endocrinology 120:785 (1987).
22. C. Polychronakos, H.J. Guyda, B. Patel, and B.I. Posner, Increase in the number of type II receptors during propylthiouracil-induced hyperplasia in the rat thyroid Endocrinology 119:1204 (1986).
23. B. Catz, Effect of insulin on thyroid gland microhistometric studies. Proc.Soc.Exp.Biol. Med. 95:62 (1957).
24. S. Filetti, G. Damante, D. Foti, Thyrotropin stimulates glucose transport in cultured rat thyroid cells, Endocrinology 120:2576 (1986).
25. O. Rosen, After insulin binds, Science 237:1452 (1987)
26. D. Tramontano, G.W. Cushing, A.C. Moses, and S.H. Ingbar, IGF-I stimulates the growth of rat thyroid cells in culture and synergises the stimulation of DNA synthesis induced by TSH and Graves' IgG, Endocrinology 119:940 (1986).
27. P. Roger and J.E. Dumont, Thyrotropin is a potent growth factor for normal human thyroid cells in primary culture, Biochem. Biophys. Res. Commun. 149:707 (1987).
28. P. Roger, P. Servais, and J.E. Dumont, Stimulation by thyrotropin and cAMP of the proliferation of quiescent canine thyroid cells cultured in a defined medium containing insulin, FEBS Lett. 157:323 (1983).
29. M.L. Brandi, C.M. Rotella, C. Mavilia, F. Franceschelli, A. Tanini, and R. Toccafondi, Insulin stimulates cell growth of a new strain of differentiated rat thyroid cells, Mol. Cell. Endocrinol. 54:91 (1987).
30. A. Aouani, S. Hovsepian, and G. Fayet, cAMP-dependent and independent regulation of thyroglobulin synthesis by two clones of the OVNIS thyroid cell line Mol. Cell. Endocrinol. 52:151 (1987).

31. J. Espina, What is the role of insulin receptor tyrosine kinase? TIBS 13: 367 (1988).
32. D.M. Hawley, A. Maddux, R.G. Patel, K-Y Wong, P.W. Mamula, G.L. Firestone, A. Brunetti, E. Verspohl, and I. Golfine, Insulin receptor monoclonal antibody that mimic insulin action without activating tyrosine kinase, J. Biol. Chem. 264:2438 (1989).
33. P.J. Blackshear, Insulin-stimulated protein biosynthesis as a paradigm of protein kinase C-independent growth factor action, Clinical Res. 37:15 (1988).
34. L. Brenner-Gati, K.A. Berg, M.C. Gershengorn, Thyroid stimulating hormone and IGF-I synergise to elevate 1,2 diacylglycerol in rat thyroid cells, J. Clin. Invest. 82:1144 (1988).
35. J.M. Madison, and J.K. Brown, Differential inhibitory effects of forskolin, isoproterenol and dibutyryl cAMP on phosphoinositide hydrolysis in canine tracheal smooth muscle, J. Clin. Invest. 82:1462 (1988).
36. Y. Munari-Silem, C. Audebet, and B. Rouset, Protein kinase C in pig thyroid cells:activation, translocation and endogenous substrate phosphorylating activity in response to phorbol esters. Mol. Cell. Endocrinol. 54:81 (1987).
37. M.C. Eggo, L.K. Bachrach, and G.N. Burrow, Role of non-TSH factors in thyroid cell growth, Acta Endocrinol. (Copenh) 281:231 (1987).
38. S.L. Pelech, and D.E. Vance, Signal transduction via phosphatidylcholine cycles, TIBS 14:28 (1989).
39. M.G. Saltiel, an A.R. Saltiel, Structural and functional roles of glycosylphosphatidyl inositol in membranes, Science 239:268 (1988).
40. F. Beguinot, L. Beguinot, D. Tramontabo, C. Duilio, S. Formisano, M. Bifulio, F.S. Ambesi-Impiombato, and S.M. Aloj, Thyrotropin regulation of membrane fluidity in the FRTL5 thyroid cell line, J. Biol. Chem. 262:1575 (1987).
41. D. Kreutter, J. Kim, J.R. Goldenring, H. Rasmussen, C. Ukomadu, R. DeLorenzo, and R.K. Yu, Regulation of protein kinase C activity by gangliosides, J. Biol. Chem. 262:1633 (1987).
42. P. Lacetti, E.F. Grollman, S.M. Aloj, and L.D. Kohn, Ganglioside-dependent return of TSH receptor function in a rat thyroid tumor with TSH receptor defect, BBRC 110:772 (1983).
43. F.A. Kuehl, J.H. Humes, V.J. Cirillo, and E.A. Ham, Cyclic AMP and prostaglandins in hormone action. Adv. Cyclic Nucl. Res. 1:493 (1972).
44. N. Takasu, L. Takashashi, T. Yamada, and S. Sato, Modulation of prostaglandin E_2, F_{2a} and I_2 content and synthesis in cultured porcine thyroid cells and intact rat thyroid glands, Biochim. Biophys. Acta 797:51 (1984).

45. R.M. Burch, A. Luini, D.E. Mais, D. Corda, J.Y. Vanderhoek, L.D. Kohn, and J. Alexrod, Alpha 1 adrenergic stimulation of prostaglandin release and metabolism in a rat thyroid cell line. Modulation of cell replication by prostaglandin E_2, J. Biol. Chem. 261:11236 (1986).
46. N. Takasu, M. Takasu, T. Yamada, and Y. Shimizu, EGF produces inositol phosphates and increases cytoplasmic-free calcium in cultured porcine thyroid cells, BBRC, 151:530 (1988).
47. K. Westermark, F.A. Karlsson, L.E. Ericson, and B. Westermark, EGF-a regulator of thyroid growth and function in: "Progress in Endocrine research and therapy, 2: Thyroglobulin the prothyroid hormone," M.C. Eggo and G.N Burrow, eds., Raven Press, New York, pp 225, (1985).
48. F. Minuto, A. Barreca, P. Del Monte, G. Cariola, G.C. Torre, and G. Giordano, Immunoreactive IGF-I and IGF binding protein content in human thyroid tissue. J.Clin. Endocrinol. Metab. 68:621 (1989).
49. R.M.B. Maciel, A.C. Moses, G. Villone, D. Tramontano, and S.H. Ingbar, Demonstration of the production and physiological role of IGF-II in rat thyroid follicular cells in culture, J. Clin. Invest. 82:1546 (1986).
50. D.O. Morgan, J.C. Edman, D.N. Standring, V.A. Fries, M.C. Smith, R.A. Roth, W.J. Rutter, Insulin-like growth factor II receptor as a multifunctional binding protein, Nature 329:301 1987).
51. J.C. Morris, G. Ranganathan, I.D. Hay, R.E. Nelson, and N-S Jiang, The effects of transforming growth factor beta on growth and differentiation of the continuous rat thyroid cells line, FRTL5, Endocrinology, 123:1385 (1988).
52. T. Tsushima, M. Arai, M. Saji, Y. Ohba, H. Murakami, E. Ohmura, K. Sato, and K. Shizume, Effects of transforming growth factor beta on DNA synthesis and iodine metabolism in porcine thyroid cells in culture, Endocrinology 123:1187 (1987).
53. J. Keski-Oja, M. Laiko, and I. Loki, The activation of latent transforming growth factor beta by the plasminogen activator urokinase. Program of joint meeting of ASBMB and American Society for Cell Biology, San Francisco #265 (1989).
54. G.P. Becks, M.C. Eggo, and G. N. Burrow, Organic iodide inhibits DNA synthesis and growth in FRTL5 cells, Endocrinology 123:545 (1988).
55. F.S. Ambesi-Impiombato, L.A.M. Parks, and H.G. Coon, Culture of hormone-dependent functional epithelial cells from rat thyroids, Proc. Natl. Acad. Sci. 77:3455 (1980).
56. M.C. Eggo, W.W. Mak, L.K. Bachrach, J.E. Errick, and G.N. Burrow, Cultured thyroids-is immortality the answer? in: "Progress in Endocrine research and therapy, 2: Thyroglobulin the prothyroid hormone," M.C. Eggo and G.N Burrow, eds., Raven Press, New York, pp 201, (1985).

57. S.P Bidey, A. Lambert, and W.R. Robertson, Thyroid cell growth, differentiation and function in the FRTL5 cell line: a survey, J. Endocrinol. 119:365 (1988).

REGULATION OF GROWTH AND DIFFERENTIATION IN FOLLICLE CELLS

Margaret C. Eggo, M.A. Christine Pratt*, Gregory P. Becks#, and Gerard N. Burrow

Department of Medicine
Univ. California, San Diego, La Jolla, CA 92093
*University of Ottawa, Ontario, Canada
#University of Western Ontario, Ontario, Canada

INTRODUCTION

Hypertrophy and hyperplasia follow chronic TSH stimulation in vivo. An early study by Matovinovic and Vickery[1] showed that the total number of cells in guinea pig thyroid glands was increased 2.5 times following 14 daily injections of TSH. Another study showed that the volume of the nucleus was increased threefold in guinea pigs within 2h of an injection of TSH although mitotic activity was not increased until the third day.[2,3] Data from rats suggest that in adults there is a very slow turnover of the thyroid cell population. Growth of endothelial and mesenchymal cells was observed to accompany that of thyroid follicular cells when rats were given goitrogens.[4] In man there are few in vivo studies examining direct effects of TSH on follicular cell growth. In patients expressing autoantibodies capable of stimulating the TSH receptor, hyperplasia rather than growth may account for the modest increase in size of the gland observed in some patients. The ability to culture cells in a hormone-free and serum-free environment has allowed a more minute examination of the growth process. In FRTL5 cells, a rat thyroid cell line maintaining some aspects of thyroid differentiated function, TSH was found to stimulate growth only when insulin or IGF-I was included in the incubation medium.[5] In dog and human thyroid cells insulin is required with TSH in order for optimum expression of thyroid growth.[6,7] In this paper we shall examine the synergism between insulin and IGF's in stimulating sheep thyroid cell growth and function. The sheep thyroid cell culture system differs significantly from FRTL5, dog and human thyroid cell culture systems in that cells synthesize and secrete physiologic quantities of thyroid hormones de novo.[8] In addition we have shown that these cultures condition the medium with relevant concentrations of both types of insulin-like growth factors,[9,10,11] as well as the insulin-like growth factor binding proteins. The production of these proteins is regulated by hormones and in particular growth factors.[10,11,12]

Increased thyroid function following TSH action is much better documented both in vivo and in vitro. In vitro many of the effects of TSH on increased metabolism and thyroid hormone synthesis and secretion can be reproduced by increases in intracellular cyclic AMP concentrations[13] suggesting that this is the principal manner by which TSH exerts its effects. However, as for studies on regulation on thyroid cell growth there is considerable evidence that insulin or IGF-I are also required for the stimulatory effects of TSH on differentiation to be manifest.[5,14] We shall examine this interdependence in the primary cultures of sheep thyroid cells.

Other autocrine (or paracrine) factors secreted by thyroid cells include plasminogen activator activity.[15] We have shown that both tissue-type plasminogen activator and urokinase-like plasminogen activator are secreted by thyroid cells and that their production is regulated by TSH and insulin. Plasminogen activators are also secreted by tumor cells and are reported to be associated with invasive growth. We have examined the regulation of their secretion by factors we have shown to be regulators of thyroid growth. Transforming growth factor beta has been reported to inhibit plasminogen activator production.[16] A further relationship between these two proteins has recently been proposed i.e that plasminogen activators could activate the latent form of transforming growth factor beta secreted by most cells in culture.[17] Plasmin itself can activate latent transforming growth factor beta. However regulation of its proteolytic activation is not well understood. The effects of transforming growth factor beta on sheep thyroid cell growth and function are described in this paper and its potential regulatory roles discussed.

Another enzyme frequently associated with cell growth and differentiation is ornithine decarboxylase which is the rate limiting enzyme in polyamine biosynthesis.[18] Inhibition of ornithine decarboxylase activity has been shown to inhibit growth and differentiation in vitro.[19] We have examined the induction of enzyme activity by growth factors in FRTL5 cells.

METHODS

Cell Culture

Sheep thyroids were collected from the abattoir and

transported back to the laboratory on ice in Hank's balanced salt solution (HBSS). Thyroids were trimmed free of connective tissue and chopped finely with scalpel blades. The chopped tissue was washed several times by decantation from 50 mL of ice-cold HBSS to remove fat and light tissue fragments. The chopped tissue was digested for 3h in HBSS containing 0.2% collagenase type 1 (Sigma). The tissue fragments were stirred slowly with a magnetic stirring bar throughout digestion. Following completion of incubation when most tissue fragments were digested, the mixture was filtered through stainless steel filters of 595 and 250 um respectively. The tissue was washed through the filters with ice-cold HBSS and centrifuged at 800xg for 10 minutes. The pellet containing the thyroid follicles was washed several times with HBSS and centrifuged at 400xg for 2 min to pellet the follicles. The follicular pellet was pink-brown in color and was easily distinguishable from layers of membrane debris (white) and red blood cells which layer on top of the follicular pellet following low speed centrifugation. If present, these contaminating layers were removed by suction. Follicles were plated at a density of 5×10^{-4} cells per cm^2 in the medium described by Ambesi-Impiombato et al[20] containing 0.5% bovine calf serum. Serum was removed at the first medium change following plating. TSH when included was used at a concentration of 100-300 uU per mL.

Plasminogen activator assays were prepared as described previously.[15] Protein content in cell layers was measured by dissolving the cell layer in 0.1 M NaOH and reading the A_{280nm} and A_{235nm} and applying the formula described by Whitaker and Granum.[21] RNA was isolated by the method of Chirgwin[22] and Northern blots on nitrocellose were probed with a cDNA to urokinase-like plasminogen activator kindly supplied by Dr F Blasi, Director, International Institute of Genetics and Biophysics, CNR, Naples, Italy.

C-myc proteins were detected on Western blots using an affinity purified polyclonal antiserum to human myc supplied by Oncor. cDNA to porcine thyroperoxidase was kindly supplied by Drs Magnusson and Rapoport, University of San Francisco. cDNA to goat thyroglobulin was kindly supplied by Dr JJM DeViljder, University of Amsterdam, The Netherlands.

RESULTS

Effects of TSH on thyroid hormone synthesis in sheep thyroid cells in culture

Primary cultures of sheep thyroid cells were incubated in 5H medium (5H=insulin (10ug/mL), transferrin (5ug/mL), cortisol (10^{-8}M), somatostatin (10ng/mL), G-H-L 10ng/mL) without serum. Increasing concentrations of TSH were added (6H medium) to triplicate wells and thyroid hormones were measured by radioimmunoassay as described previously.[8] The results shown in table 1 are from 0.5 mL medium from cells grown on a 2cm^2 culture well.

Table 1

Thyroid hormone synthesis in sheep thyroid cells-effect of TSH

TSH (mU per mL)	T3 (ng per mL)	T4 (ng per mL)
0.0	0.2	1.3+0.1
0.1	0.3+0.1	1.3+0.1
0.2	7.7+1.4	43.1+10.6
0.5	8.6+0.6	49.2+5.2
1.0	8.7+1.3	46.6+1.6

The data clearly show the TSH-dependence of thyroid hormone synthesis in cells cultured in 5H medium. There was a 30-40 fold increase in both T3 and T4 synthesis in cells cultured in TSH. Optimum TSH concentrations for thyroid hormone synthesis were between 0.1-1.0 mU per mL. Higher concentrations of TSH (10mU per mL) were inhibitory. This inhibitory effect has also been observed for iodine uptake and organification and for radiolabeled thymidine uptake.

Effect of insulin, IGF-I and IGF-II on radiolabeled thymidine incorporation into cultures of sheep thyroid cells

The effects of insulin, IGF-I and IGF-II on methyl ^{3}H-thymidine incorporation into DNA in secondary cultures of thyroid cells are shown in figure 1. Cells were incubated in TSH and insulin or IGF's at the concentrations indicated and incorporation of isotope over the next 60h measured. Methyl-^{3}H thymidine incorporation in acid-precipitable material is presented as fold increase over control. The addition of either IGF-I or IGF-II showed significant increases in labeled thymidine incorporation at 10 ng per mL. The response to insulin was biphasic, showing a plateau at low concentrations and a further increase at supraphysiologic concentrations. This may represent activation by insulin of the IGF-I receptor although we have not been able to show additivity in the effects of insulin andIGF-I on growth. Thyroid cells are sensitive to insulin at physiologic concentrations (<10ng per mL) both in growth and function assays implying activation of the insulin receptor. The dose response curves to the IGF's and insulin varied which may reflect the instability of these compounds, loss on glass and plastic, or regulation of receptor number or affinity.

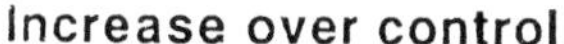

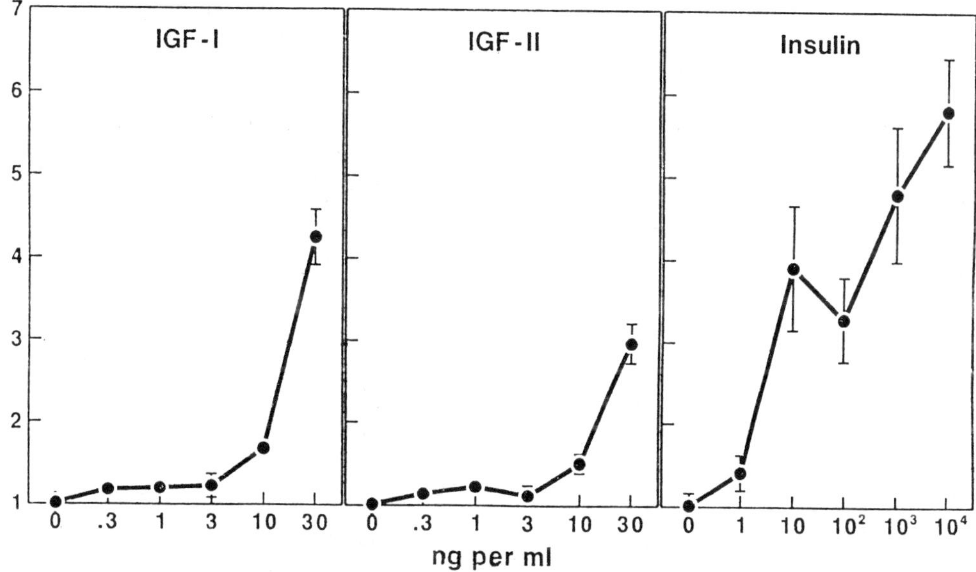

Figure 1. Effect of IGF-I, IGF-II and Insulin on ³H-Thymidine Incorporation in Sheep Thyroid Cells.

<u>Synergism between the effects of TSH with insulin and IGF-I</u>

The effects of TSH with and without insulin and IGF-I on protein content in sheep thyroid cell monolayers are shown in table 2. Estimates of protein content reflect increased cellular activity as well as growth.

Table 2

<u>Synergistic effects of TSH, IGF-I and Insulin on protein content in sheep thyroid cells</u>

	ng per ml	micrograms protein per $2cm^2$ well -TSH	+TSH
	0	108±7	134±2
IGF-I	10	107±4	148±2
	100	123±16	187±12
Insulin	10	127±11	191±4
	100	178±1	222±4

Mean ± S.E.M. n=3.

IGF-I at the concentrations tested in this assay was not stimulatory by itself in increasing protein content in sheep thyroid cell monolayers. However in the presence of TSH significant increases were seen. Insulin at 10 ng per mL did not significantly stimulate protein content of the monolayers but in the presence of TSH there was a marked increase over control values without insulin. At 100 ng per mL insulin by itself stimulated protein content and again the effect of insulin and TSH was greater than the effect of either agent alone.

Effects of TSH, Insulin and IGF-I on thyroglobulin mRNA expression

The effects of insulin, IGF-I and TSH on thyroglobulin, thyroperoxidase and actin mRNA are shown in figure 2. Cells were cultured in 6H medium. After reaching confluence the cultures were washed and incubated in medium containing no additives except the ones noted on the figure. Insulin and IGF-I were used at a concentration of 100 ng per mL, TSH was used at a concentration of 300uU per mL. Equal quantities of RNA were dot blotted onto Zetaprobe nylon membranes (BioRad) and hybridized with ^{32}P-labeled cDNA to thyroglobulin. Following stripping the blot was hybridised to ^{32}P-labeled cDNA to thyroperoxidase and again, following stripping, to cDNA to actin.

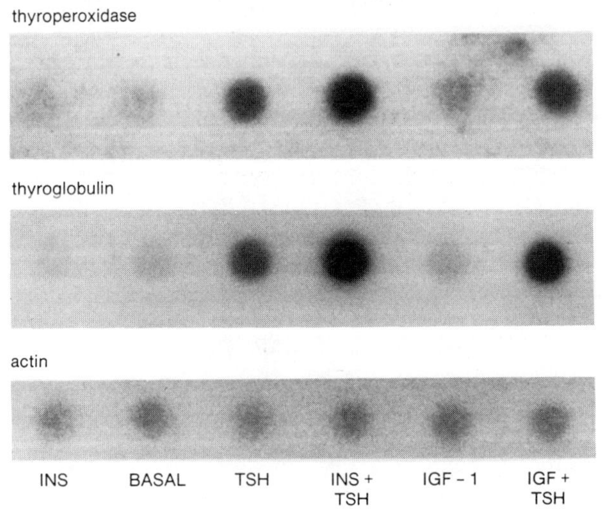

Figure 2. Effect of Insulin and TSH on Thyroperoxidase, Thyroglobulin and Actin mRNA Expression.

Neither insulin nor IGF-I-treated cells showed expression of thyroglobulin or thyroperoxidase mRNA. Cells treated with TSH showed a noticeable increase in expression of thyroglobulin and thyroperoxidase mRNA. However this increase was enhanced when IGF-I and in particular insulin were included in the incubation.

Effect of insulin and TSH on expression of c-myc protein in thyroid cells.

Induction of c-myc mRNA is frequently associated with DNA synthesis.[2,3] However transcriptional regulation does not necessarily translate into increases in protein. In these experiments we examined the expression of c-myc protein in sheep thyroid cells incubated with serum and TSH together and in combination as shown in figure 3.

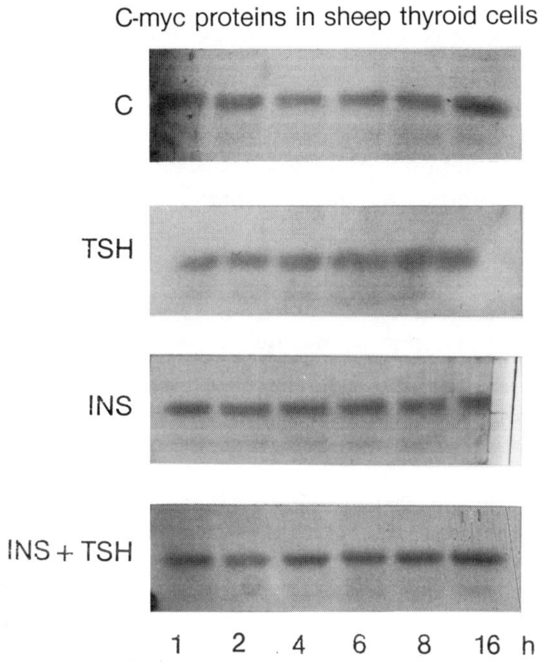

C-myc proteins in sheep thyroid cells

C

TSH

INS

INS + TSH

1 2 4 6 8 16 h

Figure 3.

The cell layers from cultures incubated with these hormones for the times indicated on the figure were dissolved in SDS-sample buffer. Samples were reduced with 100 mM dithiothreitol and were examined by SDS gel electrophoresis. Following electrophoresis the proteins on the gels were transferred electrophoretically to nitrocellulose and incubated with polyclonal antiserum to human c-myc protein. The bound antiserum was recognised by antibody to sheep gamma globulins conjugated to alkaline phosphatase. Color development using nitro blue tetrazolium at 0.3 mg per mL and 5-bromo-4-chloro-3-indoyl phosphate at 0.15 mg per mL as substrates was performed in 100 mM Tris buffer pH9.5 containing 5 mM $MgCl_2$ and 100mM NaCl. C-myc protein was identified as a single band of molecular weight 55,000. It was present in cells cultured in basal medium alone with no hormones or growth additives. Whether this is due to a pleiotrophic effect of the medium change or whether c-myc protein is continually produced throughout the cell cycle is not known. Alternatively expression may be high because of the endogenous production of thyroid-derived growth factors e.g IGF-I and IGF-II.[9-11] c-myc protein was not induced by TSH action alone. This finding is in agreement with our findings that by itself TSH is not a growth factor for these cells.[24] There was a noticeable increase in C-myc protein when cells were cultured in insulin, 6h folllowing its addition. In cells cultured in insulin and TSH C-myc protein was induced by 4h following treatment with growth factors and remained elevated through til 16h.

<u>Effects of TSH and serum on FRTL5 cell ornithine decarboxylase enzyme activity</u>

In a previous study we have shown that not only insulin but also serum can interact with TSH to induce growth in FRTL5 cells[24]. The enzyme ornithine decarboxylase (ODC) is markedly induced in several cells by trophic stimuli. Because the ability of FRTL5 cells to proliferate in response to growth stimuli far exceeds that of primary cultures of sheep thyroid cells we have examined induction of this enzyme in these cultures as shown in figure 4.

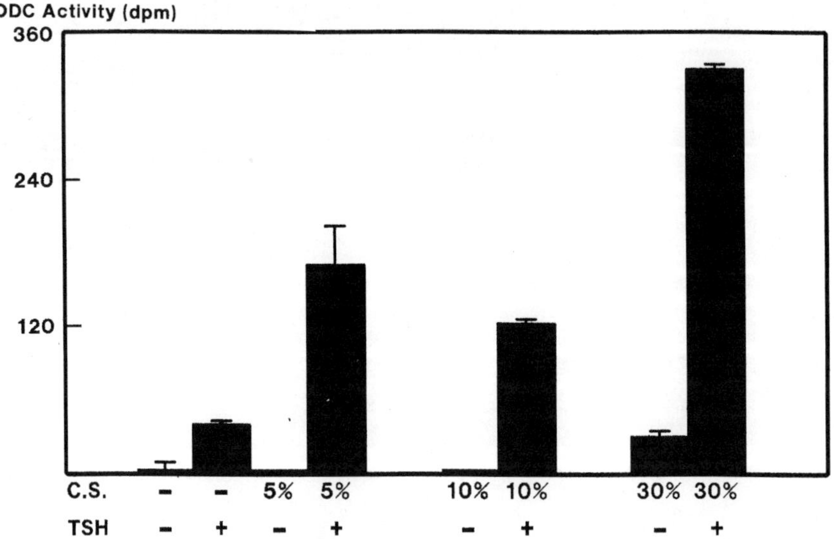

Figure 4. Synergism Between Serum and TSH on ODC Activity in FRTL5 Cells.

FRTL5 cells were grown in medium containing serum and all growth supplements (5H) with the exception of TSH for 5 days before the start of the experiment. 3h before the start of the incubation in growth factors, serum was removed from the culture medium. After 3h medium was changed and 0.5mM methyl isobutyl xanthine was added to inhibit phosphodiesterase activity. TSH and serum as noted in figure 4 were added and the incubation continued for 6h which we had previously determined to be optimal for expression of ODC activity. The incubation was terminated by removing the medium and washing the cells as described by Kudlow et al.[25] Extracts from cells centrifuged at 27,000 x g were prepared as described by Kudlow et al. Data presented in figure 4 show that TSH (1mU per mL) produced a significant but small increase in ODC activity. When 5% calf serum was included in the incubation, there was a marked increase in ODC activity. Increasing the serum concentration to 30% further increased activity in the presence of TSH while 30% serum by itself produced increases in the same order as TSH by itself. These data further show the synergism between the pathways stimulated by TSH and other trophic factors.

Effects of Growth factors on plasminogen activator activity

We have previously shown that cultures of sheep thyroid cells secrete large quantities of both types of plasminogen activators and that their secretion is regulated by TSH.[15] We examined plasminogen activator production when cells were cultured in the autocrine (or paracrine) factors IGF-I or IGF-II as well as insulin. Figure 5 shows that plasminogen activator was increased with IGF-I but not IGF-II at physiologic concentrations. Insulin was only effective at supraphysiologic concentrations suggesting that its effects in this regard were mediated through the type I IGF receptor.

Another growth factor for thyroid cells i.e the tumor promoting phorbol ester tetradecanoyl phorbol acetate (TPA) also increased plasminogen activator activity as shown in Table 3.

Table 3

Effect of TSH and TPA on Plasminogen Activator Activity

	Activity (Ploug units per mL)
Control	8.7
TSH (0.3mU/mL)	14.7
TPA (30nM)	15.9
TSH + TPA	32.0

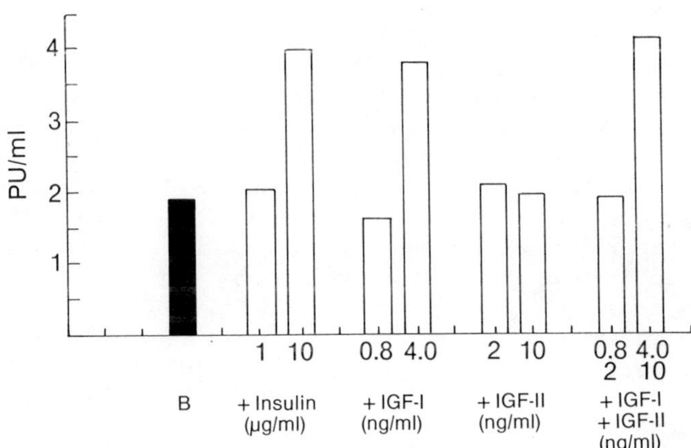

Figure 5. Effect of Insulin, IGF-I and IGF-II on Plasminogen Activator Production.

The additive effects of TPA and EGF on plasminogen activator production were also evident at the transcriptional level as shown in figure 6.

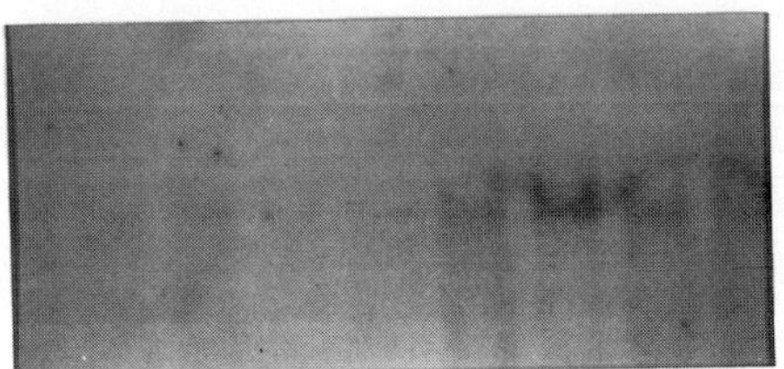

Figure 6. Plasminogen Activator mRNA in Sheep Thyroid Cells.

Cultures were incubated in the conditions as noted on the figure and RNA isolated by the method of Chirgwin et al.[22] Equal quantities of total RNA were fractionated on Northern gels and transferred to nitrocellulose. Blots were probed with ^{32}P-labeled cDNA to plasminogen activator (urokinase type) and exposed to Kodak X-Omat X-ray film. From the Northern blot TSH stimulates plasminogen activator mRNA activity both by itself and when added to 5H-treated cells. The combination producing the largest increase in plasminogen activator activity contained 6H and TPA. Interestingly insulin did not appear to induce plasminogen activator mRNA. EGF, which also stimulates growth in these cells, produced no marked increases in plasminogen activator mRNA and neither did iodide, used at a concentration optimal for thyroid hormone production.

<u>Effects of transforming growth factor beta on thyroid cell growth</u>

FRTL5 cells in culture in common with many epithelial cells have been shown to secrete transforming growth factor beta.[26] We examined the effects of this putative autocrine factor on sheep thyroid cell growth. In this experiment the effects of transforming growth factor beta (Collaborative Research Corporation) on DNA content in cells cultured in basal medium and medium supplemented with insulin or insulin and epidermal growth factor (EGF) were examined as shown in figure 7. Transforming growth factor beta was used at a concentration of 1 ng per mL and was added to secondary cultures of sheep thyroid cells. DNA content was assayed after 4 days incubation using a microdiphenylamine reaction. Transforming growth factor beta inhibited growth under all conditions examined.

Effects of TGF-β (1 ng per ml) on DNA Synthesis in Sheep Thyroid Cells.

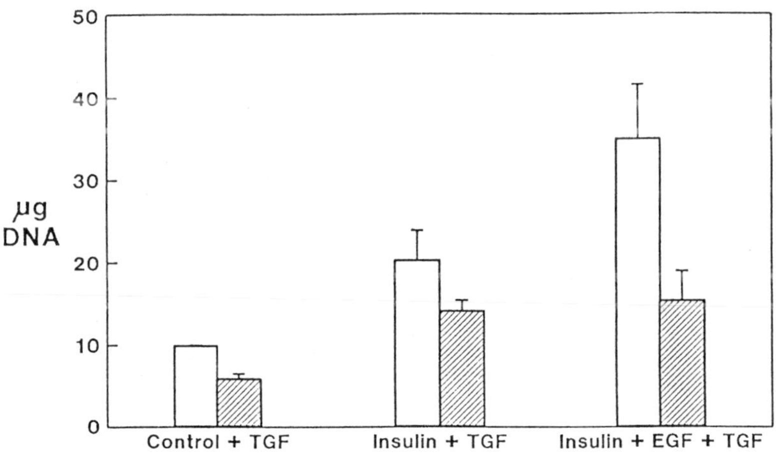

Secondary cultures of cells cultured in TSH incubated 4 days in factors as noted

Figure 7

In addition morphological changes were observed. In common with the data shown for pig thyroid cells in culture,[27] the effects of transforming growth factor beta on thyroid function showed a modest inhibition of iodide uptake and iodide organification. Whether this is due to an interaction with TSH-mediated processes leading to induction of thyroperoxidase and thyroglobulin synthesis or whether this is due to the toxicity of the protein, is unclear at this point. In FRTL5 cells, an increase in iodide uptake over control values which were extremely low, was observed.[26]

IGF binding protein production

We have previously shown that sheep thyroid cells in culture secrete both IGF-I and IGF-II. We have also found IGF binding protein activity in the condition medium. In figure 8 we show a dot blot of conditioned medium spotted onto nitrocelluose and incubated with radiolabeled IGF-I. The effects of 5H, 6H and 6H+EGF and 6H+TPA and TSH alone were examined.

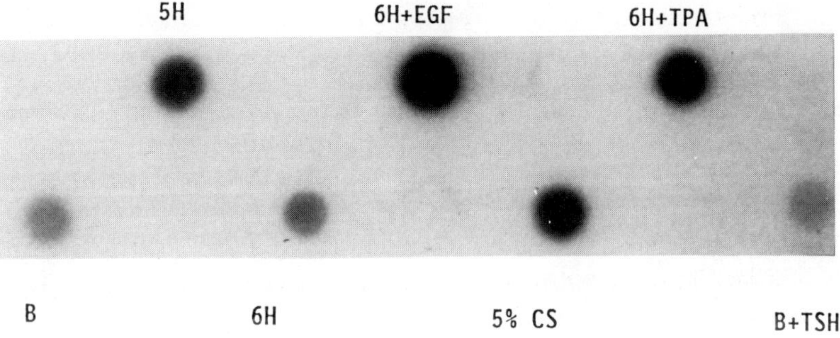

Figure 8. Regulation of IGF-Binding Protein Production by TSH, TPA and EGF.

5H-treated cells showed apparent increased binding protein activity. This increase was reduced by TSH. TPA and in particular EGF produced marked increases in IGF binding protein activity compared to 6H-treated cells alone. The role of the IGF binding proteins in regulating IGF bioactivity is still unclear, although both stimulatory and inhibitory functions have been proposed.[11]

CONCLUSIONS

In this study we have examined in vitro the regulation of thyroid hormone synthesis by TSH. We show that as in vivo thyroid hormone synthesis and secretion are dependent on TSH. However we also find that these primary cultures are secreting the insulin-like growth factors. After 3 days in culture the contents of a confluent well of thyroid cells can produce a concentration of IGF's sufficient for biological significance. We found that the effects of IGF-I frequently show synergism with those of TSH. This synergism was also seen with insulin when used at physiologic concentrations. We also show that the cells secrete the IGF binding proteins. Binding protein production appears to be hormonally regulated, inhibition of production being observed following TSH treatment. Even more intriguing is the marked stimulation of binding protein production by growth factors for the cells i.e EGF and TPA. We have previously shown that these factors induce the secretion of thyroglobulin and thyroid hormones from the cells.[28] Whether the binding proteins regulate the accessability of the hormone either positively or negatively to the receptors on thyroid cells is currently under examination in this laboratory.

We examined the regulation of other secreted products from thyroid cells. Synthesis of plasminogen activator (uPA) was found to be stimulated by EGF and TPA as well as by TSH. Plasminogen activators are serine proteases which have been implicated as possible activators of latent transforming growth beta.[17] In addition, because of their proteolytic activity, these enzymes could regulate other responsive elements of the thyroid cells. Transforming growth factor beta is in all liklihood secreted by sheep thyroid cells in culture. It has been found to be produced by FRTL5 cells[26] and human thyroid cells (data not shown) and other cells of epithelial origin.[29] We found that transforming growth factor beta at physiologic concentrations inhibited thyroid cell growth stimulated by other mitogens. Whether there is an interrelationship between regulation of transforming growth factor production (latent form), its activation to its active form and plasminogen activator production is currently under investigation in our laboratory. Similarly the relationship (if any) between plasminogen activator and IGF's and IGF binding proteins remains to be determined.

The data we have presented illustrate the potential complexity in regulation of thyroid cell growth and function. Not only is the thyroid receiving stimuli from other endocrine tissues e.g insulin and TSH but it is also proving to be a rich source of potentially biologically active compounds. There are receptors for some of these compounds on thyroid cells and we have shown that they regulate thyroid growth and differentiation in vitro. The intriguing interrelationships between these regulators in vitro will reveal important insights into anomalous clinical findings in the regulation of thyroid growth and function in vivo.

Acknowledgments

We thank Dr B Higgins, University of Toronto for the data shown in figure 4, Dr WW Mak, Seneca College, Toronto for the data shown in figure 5 and Mr D Tam, University of Toronto for the data shown in figure 6. We thank Dr Laura Bachrach for helpful discussions. The financial support of the Medical Research Council of Canada (MA 5949) is gratefully acknowledged.

References

1. J. Matinovic and A.L. Vickery, Relation of nucleic acids to the structure and function of the guinea pig thyroid gland, Endocrinology 64:149 (1959).
2. R. Ekholm and V. Pantic, Effect of thyrotropin on nucleic acid and protein contents of the thyroid, Nature 199:1203 (1963).
3. W. Tong, Actions of thyroid stimulating hormone, in: "Handbook of Physiology, section 7, Vol 3, The thyroid," M.A. Greer and D.H. Solomon, ed., Williams and Wilkins, Baltimore (1974).
4. S. Wollman and T.R. Breitman, Changes in DNA weight of thyroid glands during hyperplasia and involution, Endocrinology 86:322 (1970).
5. P. Santisteban, L.D. Kohn, and R. DiLauro, Thyroglobulin gene expression is regulated by insulin and insulin-like growth factor I, as well as thyrotropin, in FRTL5 cells, J.Biol.Chem. 262:4048 (1987).
6. P. Roger, P. Servais, and J.E. Dumont, Stimulation by thyrotropin and cAMP of the proliferation of quiescent canine thyroid cells cultured in a defined medium containing insulin, FEBS Lett 157:323 (1983).
7. P. Roger and J.E. Dumont, Thyrotropin is a potent growth factor for normal human thyroid cells in primary culture, Biochem. Biophys. Res. Commun. 149:707 (1987).
8. G.P. Becks, M.C. Eggo, and G.N. Burrow, Regulation of differentiated thyroid function by iodide, Endocrinology 120:2569 (1987).
9. W.W. Mak, B. Bhaumick, R.M. Bala, J.E. Kudlow, M.C. Eggo, and G.N. Burrow, Possible role of insulin-like growth factors in the regulation of thyroid growth, ICSU Short Reports, Advances in gene technology: Molecular biology of the endocrine system 4:50 (1985).
10. M.C. Eggo, L.K. Bachrach, and G.N. Burrow, Role of non-TSH factors in thyroid cell growth, Acta Endocrinol. (Copenh) 281:231 (1987).
11. L.K. Bachrach, M.C. Eggo, W.W. Mak, and G.N. Burrow, Insulin-

like growth factors in sheep thyroid cells: action, receptors and production, BBRC 154:861 (1988).
12. M.C. Eggo, L.K. Bachrach, and G.N. Burrow, Modulation at insulin-like growth factor binding proteins by growth hormone and growth factors in sheep thyroid cells. Program of 70th Annual Meeting of the Endocrine Society, New Orleans #525 (1988).
13. K. Sho and Y. Kondo, Insulin modulates thyrotropin-induced follicle reconstruction and iodine metabolism in hog thyroid cells in chemically defined medium, BBRC 118:385 (1985).
14. M.C. Eggo, L.K. Bachrach, and G.N. Burrow, Control of thyroid growth and function by insulin, insulin-like growth factors and TSH, Program of the 63rd meeting of the American Thyroid Association, Montreal #120 (1988).
15. W.W. Mak, M.C. Eggo, G.N.Burrow, Thyrotropin regulation of plasminogen activator activity in primary culture of ovine thyroid cells, BBRC 123:633 (1984).
16. O. Saksela, D. Moscatelli, and D.B. Rifkin, The opposing effects of basic fibroblasts growth factor and transforming growth factor beta on the regulation of plasminogen activator activity in capillary endothelial cells, J. Cell Biol. 105:957 (1987).
17. J. Keski-Oja, M. Laiko, and I. Loki, The activation of latent transforming growth factor beta by the plasminogen activator urokinase. Program of joint meeting of ASBMB and American Society for Cell Biology, San Francisco #265 (1989).
18. C. W. Tabor, and H. Tabor, The Polyamines, Ann Review Biochem. 53:749 (1984).
19. A.E. Pegg, Recent advances in the biochemistry of polyamines in eukaryotes, Biochem. J. 234:249 (1986).
20. F.S. Ambesi-Impiombato, L.A.M. Parks, and H.G. Coon, Culture of hormone-dependent functional epithelial cells from rat thyroids, Proc. Natl. Acad. Sci. 77:3455 (1980).
21. J.R. Whitaker, and P.E Granum, An absolute method for protein determination based on difference in absorbance at 235 and 280 nm, Anal. Biochem. 109:156 (1980).
22. J.M. Chirgwin, A.E. Przybyla, and R.J MacDonald, Isolation of biologically active RNA from sources rich with ribonucleases, Biochemistry 18:5294 (1979).
23. W.H. Dere, H. Hirayu, and B. Rapoport, TSH and cAMP enhance expression of the myc proto oncogene in cultured thyroid cells, Endocrinology 117:2249 (1985).
24. M.C. Eggo, L.K. Bachrach, G. Fayet, J.Errick, J.E. Kudlow, M.F. Cohen, and G.N. Burrow, The effects of growth factors and serum on DNA synthesis and differentiation in thyroid cells in culture, Mol. Cell. Endocrinol. 38141 (1984).
25. J.E.K. Kudlow, P.A. Rae, N.S. Gutman, B.P. Schimmer and G.N. Burrow, Regulation of ornithine decarboxylase activity by corticotropin and adrencortical tumor cell clones:

Roles of cAMP and cAMP-dependent protein kinase, _Proc. Natl. Acad. Sci._ 77:2676 (1980).

26. J.C. Morris, G. Ranganathan, I.D. Hay, R.E. Nelson, and N-S Jiang, The effects of transforming growth factor beta on growth and differentiation of the continuous rat thyroid cells line, FRTL5, _Endocrinology_ 123:1385 (1988).
27. T. Tsushima, M. Arai, M. Saji, Y. Ohba, H. Murakami, E. Ohmura, K. Sato, and K. Shizume, Effects of transforming growth factor beta on DNA synthesis and iodine metabolism in porcine thyroid cells in culture, _Endocrinology_ 123:1187 (1987).
28. M.C. Eggo, L.K. Bachrach, M.A.C. Pratt, H. Lippes, G. Becks, and G.N. Burrow, Regulation of the secetion of various proteins and thyroid hormones by sheep thyroid cells, Program of 62nd annual meeting of the American Thyroid Association, Washington, D.C. p33 (1987).
29. A. Rizzino, Transforming growth factor-beta, _Develop. Biol._ 130:411 (1988).

TRANSDUCING SYSTEMS IN THE CONTROL OF HUMAN THYROID CELL FUNCTION, PROLIFERATION AND DIFFERENTIATION

J.E. Dumont, A. Lefort, F. Libert, M. Parmentier, E. Raspé, S. Reuse, C. Maenhaut, P. Roger, B. Corvilain, E. Laurent, J. Mockel, F. Lamy, J. Van Sande, G. Vassart

Institute of Interdisciplinary Research (IRIBHN), Free University of Brussels, School of Medicine, Campus Erasme, 1070-Brussels, Belgium

INTRODUCTION

Our laboratory has been involved in the study of thyroid regulation at the cellular level for many years. The complex picture emerging from these studies leads to conclusions of general relevance. The regulation of the thyroid cell was once a classical example of the concept one hormone - one cell type - one intracellular secondary messenger with its pleiotypic effects. It should now rather be considered as a network of crosslinked regulatory steps where the extracellular and intracellular signal-molecules act on their receptors as bits of information in an electronic circuit, i.e., express on/off regulations with no definite general physiological meaning per se. Such networks differ from one cell type to another and for a given cell type from one species to another. In the case of the thyroid many apparent discrepancies in the literature are explained if this is taken into account. In this presentation, we wish to draw mainly on the results of our group to illustrate this point with regard to the regulation of function, proliferation and differentiation of the thyroid cell.

I. THE CASCADES INVOLVED IN THYROID CELL REGULATION

Although we are aware that it might not be a good model for the FRTL5 cell line, our main interest is the regulation of the human thyrocytes. However as dog tissue is still easier to obtain than human tissue (until when ?), our main experimental object is the dog thyrocyte. We therefore develop our methods and concepts on the dog thyroid, to adapt them to the human tissue thereafter. In fact apart from a few differences that I shall mention, the two tissues are similar. In the dog thyroid the main and best known circuit involves thyrotropin (TSH) stimulation of plasma membrane adenylate cyclase (1,2). Cyclic AMP produced by the cyclase is the intracellular signal molecule, which by activating cAMP-dependent protein kinases will enhance the main functions of the gland: the iodination of thyroglobulin and iodothyronine formation, i.e., the synthesis of thyroid hormones, and the uptake of thyroglobulin and its hydrolysis, i.e., the secretion of thyroid hormones and the synthesis of

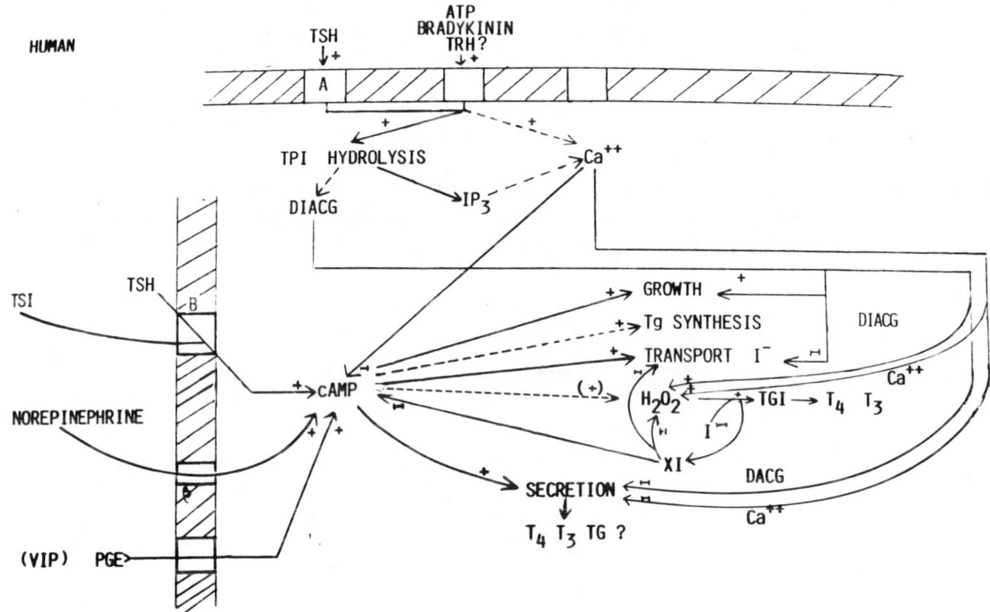

Fig. 1. Controls in the human thyrocyte.
Abbreviations : Ach : acetylcholine; DIACG : diacylglycerol; IP_3 : myo-inositol 1,4,5 phosphate; PG : prostaglandin; TG : thyroglobulin; TGI : iodinated thyroglobulin; TPI : phosphatidylinositol 5-biphosphate; TSI : thyroid stimulating immunoglobulins; XI : unknown iodinated inhibitor. Lines indicate controls : straight lines : proved controls; interrupted lines : postulated: controls; + : positive control = stimulation; ⊢ : negative control = inhibition.

thyroglobulin at the level of gene transcription. We have now shown that effects on iodination in fact reflect the control of H_2O_2 generation, i.e. the substrate supply of thyroperoxidase (3,4). The high generation of H_2O_2 in the stimulated thyroid raises the question of its toxicity. This might be involved in the pathogenesis of endemic cretinism, as selenium deficiency and consequently GSH peroxidase deficiency has been observed in Central Africa, i.e. in the geographical zone of endemic cretinism. In the dog thyroid the main fundamental effects of TSH are reproduced by cyclic AMP analogs and agents such as forskolin and cholera toxin which increase cyclic AMP accumulation in many tissues by activating adenylate cyclase and its GTP binding stimulating transducing protein Ns. They are thus mediated by cyclic AMP. By analogy with the β-receptor mediated action of norepinephrine they have been called B-effects.

Other extracellular signal molecules, prostaglandins of the E type and to a lesser extent norepinephrine through β receptors activate thyroid adenylate cyclase and mimic the TSH effects. The abnormal thyroid stimulating immunoglobulins (TSI), which appear in the serum of patients with Graves'disease, also activate adenylate cyclase, presumably by binding to the TSH receptors. In thyroid as in other systems, adenylate cyclase is negatively regulated by receptor activated inhibitory GTP binding transducing protein Ni. In the dog thyrocyte, norepinephrine through α2-receptors exerts this control. Negative feedback is also exerted on the TSH stimulatory pathway by the substrate of thyroid specialized metabolism : iodide (through a not yet defined oxidized derivative XI). Negative feedbacks by the thyroid hormones themselves and even thyroglobulin has been suggested, but their physiological relevance is still unknown.

The second major cell signalling system, the Ca^{++}-phosphatidylinositol cascade has also been demonstrated in the dog thyroid cells. Acetylcholine through a muscarinic receptor enhances free calcium intracellular concentration (as shown by Quin 2 fluorescence), $^{45}Ca^{++}$ translocation and the generation of Ins P1, Ins(1,4)P2 and Ins(1,4,5)P3 (5,6,7). The first phase of intracellular free Ca^{++} rise is independent of extracellular Ca^{++} and thus presumably originates from intracellular stores. The second phase is dependent of extracellular Ca^{++} which suggests that it is caused by an influx of this Ca^{++}. By analogy with other cell models, it is therefore inferred that acetylcholine activates, through its muscarinic receptor and a GTP binding transducing protein, a membrane phospholipase C. This enzyme hydrolyses phosphatidyl-inositol 4,5 phosphate (PtdIns(4,5)P2) and thus generates two intracellular signal molecules : myo-inositol 1,4,5 phosphate (Ins(1,4,5)P3) and diacylglycerol (DAG). IP3 would then cause the release by endoplasmic reticulum of stored Ca^{++} and be responsible for the first phase of Ca^{++} rise. DAG would activate thyroid protein kinase C. The role of the two branches of this cascade can be evaluated using as probes Ca^{++} ionophore A23187, and phorbol esters. The ionophore A23187 allows the influx of extracellular Ca^{++} and thus the activation of Ca^{++} dependent systems; phorbol esters are specific long acting analogs of DAG. In the dog thyroid, all the effects of acetylcholine appear to be mediated by Ca^{++}: they are reproduced by the ionophore A23187 in the presence of extracellular Ca^{++}, or by high concentrations of extracellular Ca^{++}; they are inhibited in Ca^{++} depleted cells or by Ca^{++}-channel blockers such as Co^{++} or Mn^{++}. These effects are: the activation of protein iodination and glucose oxidation, the enhancement of cyclic GMP accumulation, the prostaglandin synthesis and the inhibition of cyclic AMP accumulation and thyroid hormone secretion (8). The inhibition of cyclic AMP accumulation is caused by an activation by Ca^{++} of Ca^{++} calmodulin-dependent cyclic nucleotide phosphodiesterase. The inhibition of thyroid hormone secretion is caused both by this inhibition of cyclic AMP accumulation and by a direct effect on the secretory mechanism (9). The effects of the other intracellular signal generated by phospholipase C, diacylglycerol, can be inferred from the action of phorbol esters. These tumor promoters, as Ca^{++}, enhance protein iodination and inhibit thyroid hormone secretion. On the other hand, they appear to inhibit the first steps of the Ca^{++}-phosphatidylinositol cascade (IP_3 generation and Ca^{++} influx) and a consequence of the free intracellular Ca^{++} rise : the enhancement of cyclic GMP accumulation. DAG could therefore exert a negative feedback on the cascade (10). PGF_2 *, TRH and NaF reproduce some of the effects of acetylcholine in the dog thyrocyte. In dog thyroid cells, TSH enhances ^{32}P phosphate and ^{3}H inositol incorporation into phosphoinositides. It also stimulates $^{45}Ca^{++}$ efflux from prelabelled dog thyroid cells. These have been called A effects. This may suggest that TSH also activates the Ca^{++}-phosphatidylinostol cascade. However, TSH fails to enhance IP_3 generation in dog thyroid slices. The meaning of the TSH A effects on dog thyrocyte Ca^{++} and phosphatidylinositol metabolism remains therefore obscure.

Figure 1 is a scheme summarizing the regulation of the human thyrocyte as we know it now (11,12). Thyrotropin (TSH) through cyclic AMP activates all specialized functions of the tissue: the transport of iodide, its oxidation, thyroid hormone secretion and growth. Some of these stimulations are acute (within minutes) and require no prior protein synthesis (thyroid hormone synthesis and secretion) while others (iodide transport and growth) require just such a step. In the human thyrocytes, TSH and some neurotransmitters (ATP, bradykinin, etc) also activate the phosphatidylinositol 4-5 phosphate (PiP_2) cascade releasing $Ins(1,4,5)P_3$ and DAG in the cell (13). IP_3 elicits the release of calcium from endoplasmic reticulum and raises intracellular free calcium levels ($Ca^{++}i$). DAG and Ca^{++} act in parallel on function, inhibiting secretion and activating iodination and thyroid hormone synthesis. The dual action of thyrotropin may involve two different receptors as drawn on Fig. 1, or one receptor activating the GTP binding transducing proteins (G proteins) controlling the two cascades. The effect of TSH on the $PtdIns(4,5)P_2$ cascade is less sensitive to the hormone and slower than the action on cyclic AMP accumulation.

This general scheme applies to other species we have studied, except for a few important differences :

1) the action of TSH on the Pi cascade does not occur at physiological hormone levels in some species, among which dog
2) the neurotransmitters acting on the two cascades differ from one species to another. For example the Pi cascade is activated by acetylcholine in dog but not in human thyrocytes. β adrenergic cyclic AMP response also varies much between species (small in dog, higher in human)
3) iodination and thyroid hormone synthesis catalyzed by the same thyroperoxidase H_2O_2 generating system is controlled by H_2O_2 generation. This step is activated by cyclic AMP in dog thyrocytes, but only barely if at all by cyclic AMP in human thyrocytes. Ca^{++} and DAG activate H_2O_2 generation and iodination in both species.

As others, we are trying to clone the human TSH receptors and until now have failed. However using an approach based on homology with known receptors controlling G proteins we have managed to clone 7 such receptors : two were known : the $_2$ adrenergic receptor and the 5HT1 serotonine receptor; one is the dog correspondent of the α_1 adrenergic receptor cloned at the same time; the four others RDC_1, RDC_4, RDC_7 and RDC_8 are unknown. RDC_4 is clearly related to the known serotonin receptors; by Northern blot analysis, its expression has not been detected in any dog tissue ! RDC_1 has some homology to substance K receptor; it is expressed in heart, kidney and thyroid. RDC_7 and RDC_8 belong to a new family of receptors with little extracellular NH_2 terminal peptide and no glycosylation site; they are expressed in brain and for RDC_7 also in thyroid. We are now busy trying to identify and characterize these receptors. But as none of them is expressed exclusively in the thyroid we doubt that the TSH receptor is one of them (14).

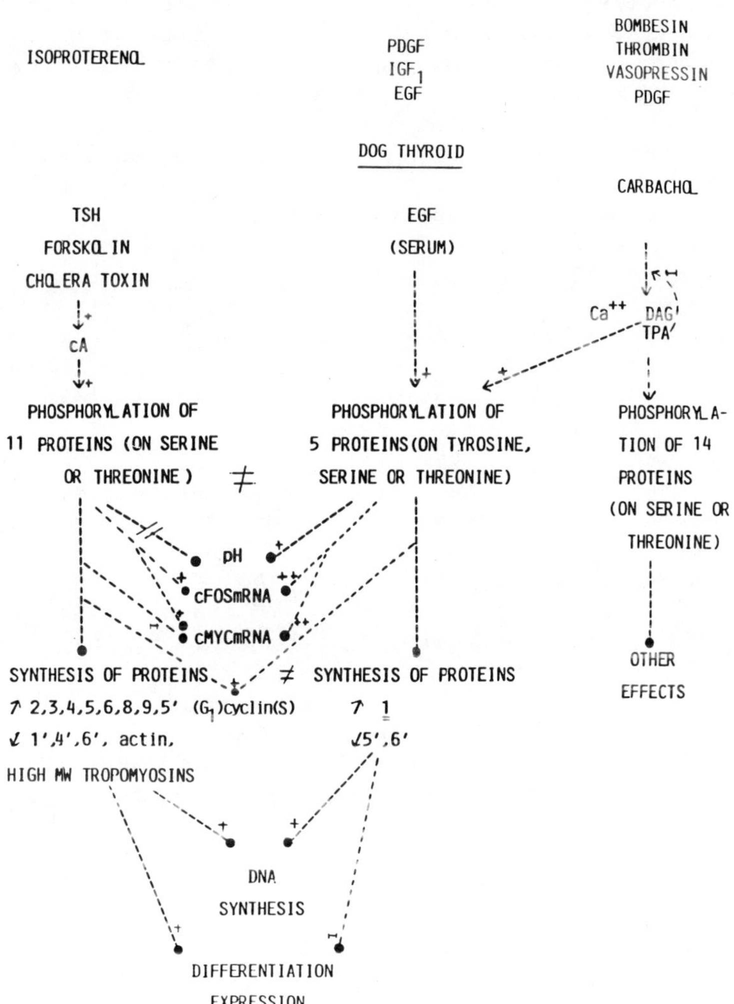

Fig. 2. Mitogenic pathways operating in model systems and in the thyroid.
Abbreviations : EGF : epidermal growth factor; IGF : insulin like growth factors; PDGF : platelet derived growth factor. --> causal relationships; ---0 sequential, possibly causal relationships; + positive i.e. stimulations; ↦ negative i.e. inhibitions
1, 2, 3 ...protein signals on 2D gel autoradiograms.

II. CONTROL OF THYROID CELL GROWTH

Many extracellular signal molecules, such as hormones, neurotransmitters, and growth factors acting as autocrine or paracrine stimulants, elicit the replication response by activating their membrane receptors and the intracellular biochemical cascade that they control. The study of conventional model systems of established fibroblastic cell lines has allowed a partial characterization of two such pathways (Fig. 2) : (i) Receptors for some growth factors (e.g. epidermal growth factor, EGF) possess an intrinsic protein tyrosine kinase activity as is the case for one class of transforming proteins encoded by oncogenes. The identity and function of many substrates for tyrosine kinase remain elusive and there is no direct proof that this activity is sufficient in normal cells to induce mitogenesis; (ii) other membrane receptors are coupled via a GTP-binding protein to a phospholipase C that cleaves phosphatidylinositol 4,5 bisphosphate into diacylglycerol and inositol 1,4,5 triphosphate (IP_3). The analogs of diacylglycerol, the phorbol esters tumor promoters, activate in some cell types, mitogenesis. Intracellular Ca^{++} also triggers cell proliferation in specific cells by little known mechanisms. Although recently shown to be clearly distinct in their initial part (receptor, transducer, first intracellular signal) both pathways rapidly converge on several events such as activation of Na+/H+ exchange and of several transporters, phosphorylation on tyrosine residues of 42K proteins and increase in c-fos and c-myc protooncogene mRNA. These early events are assumed to be necessary for growth stimulation, but causative relationship with late commitment to DNA replication remains unclear.

A third major regulatory cascade involved in the regulation of cell proliferation is the cyclic AMP system (15). Despite some early evidence to the contrary, in the seventies, there was an overwhelming acceptance of the concept that cAMP was a negative regulator of cell proliferation. This was based on the evidence, mostly obtained with established cell lines of fibroblastic or tumoral origins, that cAMP derivatives or cAMP elevating agents inhibited growth, and that cAMP levels in such cells in culture inversely correlated with proliferation. Although in some systems these observations are correct and confirmed by genetic analysis of resistant mutants, many other similar studies are questionable because they are based on the use of high concentrations of cAMP analogs with no suitable controls. Nevertheless, the concept of cAMP as a negative growth signal persists to this day and any evidence against it is often regarded as an exception to the rule. Perhaps because of these discrepancies, the role of cAMP in the control of growth is often ignored in general reviews on this subject (16).

In sharp contrast with this background, there is a series of cells in which cAMP enhances or initiates proliferation. Moreover, the demonstrated role of cAMP as an intracellular signal for replication in yeast Saccharomyces Cerevisiae is now giving respectability to such a control in upper eucaryotic cells.

Although there is no doubt that TSH in vivo stimulates the proliferation of thyroid cells, there was in the 1970s no evidence that this was a direct effect. Indeed, the ACTH trophic effect on the adrenal appears to be indirect. The first results obtained in cultures were quite contradictory. Indeed, even now, while in dog thyroid cells in primary culture, in rat thyroid follicles in suspension, in ovine cell lines (OVNI), and in rat cell line (FRTL) thyrotropin has been demonstrated to enhance or induce cell proliferation, to our knowledge, no such effect had been obtained in porcine, calf or ovine thyroid cells in primary culture. Whether this is due to inaccessibility of the TSH receptor(s), lack of an essential element in the culture medium, alteration of cell program in culture or true unresponsiveness to direct TSH action is not known. In dog thyroid cells in primary culture, TSH enhances proliferation in the presence of serum and induces it in its absence. This has been demonstrated using several methods. Thus in this species at least, TSH directly induces thyroid cell proliferation. In FRTL cell line, TSH is also required for proliferation, however the fact that such cells may die in the absence of TSH and serum might not allow to distinguish between a general trophic effect of the hormone or a definite proliferation signal. It should be noted that, in dog thyroid cells, TSH stimulates proliferation while maintaining the expression of differentiation. Differentiation expression, as evaluated by iodide transport, or thyroperoxidase and thyroglobulin mRNA content, or nuclear transcription, is induced by TSH, forskolin, cholera toxin and cyclic AMP analogs, in dog thyroid cells. Similar results, albeit partial, have been obtained in human and calf cells. These effects are obtained in all cells of a culture, as shown by in situ hybridization experiments. They are reversible; they can be obtained after the arrest of proliferation. Some of these effects, thyroglobulin but not thyroperoxidase gene expression, require the presence of insulin or IGF_1. Epidermal growth factor (EGF) also induces proliferation of dog thyroid cells. This effect is of the same order of magnitude as the effect of TSH. However, the action of EGF is accompanied by a general and reversible loss of differentiation expression as assessed above. The effects of EGF on differentiation can be dissociated from their proliferative action. Indeed, they are obtained in cells that do not proliferate in the absence of insulin. EGF also stimulates the growth of thyroid cells from other species in culture (eg. porcine, ovine, bovine and human but not of the FRTL cell line which lacks EGF receptors). In dog thyroid cells, insulin is necessary for growth in the presence of EGF and in half the cultures in the presence of TSH. A requirement for insulin has also been observed in rat cells in primary culture and for the FRTL5 rat thyroid cell line. Serum and fibroblast growth factor also induce growth in dog and calf thyroid cells. Finally, phorbols esters, the pharmacological probes of the protein kinase C system also enhance the proliferation and the dedifferentiation of dog thyroids cells. These effects are transient owing to desensitization of the system by protein kinase C inactivation (2).

Thyrotropin induces within minutes a striking morphological change in dog thyroid cells in culture : a rounding up following the disruption of the actin network. All the cells are affected. TSH also enhances the accumulation of cyclic AMP in these cells within less than five minutes. Cyclic AMP remains elevated for 48 hours in the continuous presence of TSH. The question arises of the role of cyclic AMP in all these TSH effects. In the dog thyroid cells, analogs of cyclic AMP as well as general cyclase activators (forskolin, cholera toxin) reproduce all the effects of TSH : acute morphological changes, proliferation, expression of differentiation. Moreover, combinations of cyclic AMP analogs which are synergistic on the two cyclic AMP dependent kinases isoenzymes are also synergistic on these effects. Cyclic AMP is therefore a general intracellular signal for function, proliferation and differentiation in the dog thyroid cells. For proliferation, similar results have been obtained with rat thyroid cells in culture and, despite a first contradictory report (17), in FRTL5 cells (18).

There are indications that TSH may stimulate the Ca^{++} phosphatidylinositol cascade in thyroid cells. In our dog thyroid cells, TSH, contrary to acetylcholine, does not enhance the generation of inositol phosphates. There is therefore little evidence that the A pathway of TSH action may be involved in the growth effect of TSH in this system.

The effects of EGF on dog thyroid cell (proliferation, inhibition of differentiation expression) are mimicked by phorbol esters tumor promoters. However, these compounds also inhibit EGF action : combined with EGF, they lower the proliferation level to the level induced by them. In several cell types, EGF, not only activates a tyrosine specific protein kinase, but also induces a rapid rise in cytoplasmic free Ca^{++} concentration. This rise in Ca^{++} concentration following EGF stimulation has been linked to an activation of the phosphatidylinositol Ca^{++} cascade although it has been suggested recently that it might result from an entry of extracellular Ca^{++} through the plasma membrane. It would therefore be conceivable that EGF action in the thyroid cell might result from an increase in Ca^{++} entry or from an activation of the phosphatidylinositol Ca^{++} cascade with generation of diacylglycerol, the action of which is mimicked by phorbol esters. Indeed EGF induces a rise in intracellular Ca^{++} in porcine thyroid cells, but it definitively fails to do so in dog cells. On the other hand, neither EGF nor phorbol esters enhance cyclic AMP accumulation in these cells. It is therefore likely that EGF acts through the phosphorylation of key proteins on tyrosyl residues. We have studied the phenomenology of EGF and TSH proliferative action on quiescent cells with the aim to identify common steps in this action. Three biochemical aspects of the proliferative response occurring at different times of the prereplicative phase have been studied. The pattern of protein phosphorylation induced within minutes by TSH is reproduced by cyclic AMP analogs (19). The phosphorylation of at least 11 proteins is increased or induced. NaOH treatment of the gels does not reveal any remaining phosphorylation on these proteins suggestive of tyrosine phosphorylation. In EGF stimulated cells, the phosphorylation of 5 proteins is stimulated, two of which become phosphorylated on tyrosines (42K). These two proteins are similar (isoelectric points, approximate molecular weight, composition in phosphorylated amino acids) to the two 42K proteins described in other systems and which have been implicated in the mitogenic response to diverse agents. Phorbol esters induce the phosphorylation of 19 proteins, including the tyrosine phosphorylated proteins mentioned above. There is no overlap in the patterns of protein phosphorylation induced by TSH and cyclic AMP enhancers on the one hand and by EGF and phorbol esters on the other hand.

The expression of c-myc and c-fos mRNA has been studied by Northern analysis of RNA extracts. As in other types of cells EGF and TPA enhance first c-fos, then c-myc mRNA concentrations. On the other hand, TSH or forskolin enhance strongly but shortly c-myc mRNA concentration and with the same kinetics as for EGF/TPA c-fos mRNA concentration. In fact cyclic AMP first enhances, then depresses c-myc mRNA accumulation. This second phenomenon is akin to what has been observed in fibroblasts in which cyclic AMP negatively regulates growth. In TSH and cyclic AMP action on the thyrocyte the first stimulation might be necessary to trigger the proliferation cascade while the later shut off might be necessary for the retention of the differentiated phenotype.

The pattern of proteins synthesized in response to the various proliferation stimuli has been studied (20). Again two patterns emerge. TSH and forskolin induce the synthesis of at least 8 proteins and decrease the synthesis of 5 proteins. Epidermal growth factor, phorbol ester and serum induce the synthesis of at least 1 protein and decrease the synthesis of 2 proteins. The only overlap between the two patterns concerns the decrease in the synthesis of a protein (18K) which is also reduced by EGF after proliferation has stopped. Only one protein has been shown to be synthesized in response to the three pathways : cyclin, but the kinetics of this synthesis are very different, with an early synthesis in the cyclic AMP cascade, (consistent with a role of signal) and a late, S phase synthesis in the other cascades. Thus, obviously two different phenomenologies are involved in the proliferation response to TSH through cyclic AMP on the one hand and epidermal growth factor and phorbol ester, presumably through protein tyrosine phosphorylation, on the other hand. Although this conclusion needs to be further substantiated, it certainly suggests that the proliferation of dog thyroid cells is controlled by at least two largely independent pathways.

While the TSH cyclic AMP pathway stimulates function and promotes both the expression of differentiation and proliferation, the converging EGF tyrosine protein kinase and phorbol esters - protein kinase C pathways induce proliferation but inhibit differentiation expression. A priori, it would therefore be tempting to relate hyperthyroidism caused by thyroid stimulating immunoglobulins or by an hyperfunctioning adenoma to an enhancement of the cAMP cascade and dedifferentiating tumors to the activation of the growth factor and phorbol esters cascades. In this regard it is interesting that TSI, at the concentration existing in pathological sera, in human thyrocytes only activates the cyclic AMP system and not, contrary to TSH, the phospholipase C pathway. Similarly, in preliminary experiments, TSH only stimulates the cyclic AMP system, but ,ot phospholipase C, in autonomous nodules !

Previous studies of human thyroid cells in culture (mostly from pathological tissues) failed to demonstrate a mitogenic effect of thyrotropin (TSH), leading to the proposal that the growth effect of TSH in vivo might be indirect. In order to reexamine the influence of TSH on DNA synthesis and cell proliferation, we established primary cultures of normal thyroid tissue from 9 subjects (21). When seeded in a 1%-serum-supplemented medium, thyroid follicles released by collagenase/dispase digestion developed as a cell monolayer that responded to TSH by rounding up and by cytoplasmic retraction. When seeded in serum-free medium, the cells remained associated in dense aggregates surrounded by few slowly spreading cells. In the latter condition, the cells responded to TSH and to other stimulators of cyclic AMP production such as cholera toxin and forskolin by displaying very high iodide trapping levels. Exposure to serum irreversibly abolished this differentiated function. TSH stimulated the proliferation (as shown by DNA content per culture dish) of 1% serum cultured cells (doubling times were reduced from 106h to 76h) and increased by 100% the ^{3}H-thymidine labelling indices. In serum-free cultured cells (dense aggregates or cell monolayers after seeding with serum), control levels of DNA synthesis were lower and up to 8-fold stimulation of DNA synthesis occurred in response to 100 μU/ml TSH (stimulation was consistently detected with 20 μU/ml), based on measurements of ^{3}H-thymidine incorporation into acid-precipitable material and counts of labelled nuclei on autoradiographs (up to 40% labelled nuclei within 24h). The mitogenic effect of TSH required a high insulin concentration (8.3×10^{-7}mol/L) or a low insulin-like growth factor-1 concentration. The mitogenic effects of TSH were mimicked by cholera toxin, forskolin and dibutyryl cAMP. Thus there is no doubt that TSH through cyclic AMP is mitogenic on human thyroid cells. Epidermal growth factor and phorbol myristate ester also stimulated thyroid cell proliferation and DNA synthesis, but they potently inhibited TSH-stimulated iodide transport.

Thus in human thyrocytes the regulation of growth and differentiation expression seems to operate through the same pathways as in the dog thyrocyte. However, our knowledge of the human cell is much less advanced. For instance, we know nothing of the patterns of protein phosphorylation or synthesis, or on protooncogene expression in this model. Moreover our experiments suggest that TSH action on proliferation may involve more than cyclic AMP, perhaps the Ca^{++}-phosphatidylinositol cascade. Before analyzing the alterations of the control systems which may be involved in the pathogenesis of goiter or thyroid tumors, a lot more work on the human thyrocytes is necessary (22).

III. CALCYPHOSIN

Another distinction between the two types of mitogenic pathways in dog thyroid cells is the synthesis of a 23K protein, which is enhanced by the cAMP pathway, and depressed by EGF, serum and TPA, even after cessation of growth. This protein thus appears as a possible marker of differentiation. Interestingly this protein is acutely phosphorylated in response to TSH or cyclic AMP enhancers, which suggests a role in functional activation (Fig. 3).

With antibodies raised against protein 23K we have screened a λgt11 dog thyroid cDNA expression library and obtained corresponding clones. The longuest cDNA insert has been cloned and sequenced . The sequence reveals a striking analogy with calmodulin with 4 EF hands; the first contains a putative cAMP

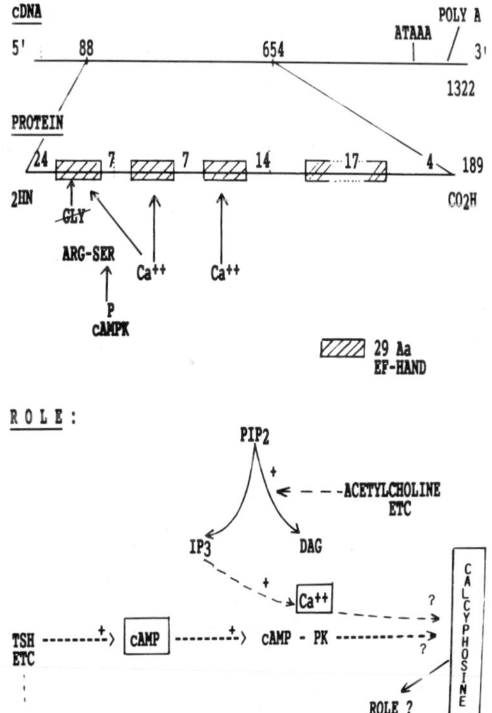

Fig. 3. cDNA, protein sequences and role of dog thyroid calcyphosin (2,4,7,.. number of aminoacids before, between, in and after the EF-hands).

dependent protein kinase phosphorylation site, the fourth one is interrupted by a non related aminoacid sequence. This suggested that the 23K protein might be a calcium binding protein. INdeed in Western blot this protein, identified by immunoblotting was shown to bind Ca^{++}. The 23K protein, a marker of differentiation of dog thyrocytes therefore binds calcium, and is phosphorylated in response to cyclic AMP; it has been named : calcyphosin. Calcyphosin has also been identified in the human thyroid and in other dog organs such as brain and salivary gland. It is the only protein known which is phosphorylated in response to cyclic AMP on the same peptide which binds Ca^{++}. Phosphorylase kinase presents similar properties but on different subunits. It is hypothesized that calcyphosin as a common target of the cyclic AMP and the Ca^{++} phosphatidylinositol cascade, might be involved in the control of a general cell biology process (such as ion transport or motility) or in the reciprocal control of these two cascades. Whatever its role, this protein presents a great interest as such !! (23).

Thus quite apart from the insights they give on the control of thyroid cell function, proliferation and differentiation and on the role of these controls in disease, our results have led, by serependity to interesting new general findings which may have a larger medical interest : the discovery of severe selenium deficiency in Central Africa (24), the cloning of 4 new receptors, the cloning of calcyphosin, a common protein target of the cyclic AMP and the Ca^{++} phosphatidylinositol cascades.

REFERENCES

1. Dumont, J.E., Takeuchi, A., Lamy, F., Gervy-Decoster, C., Cochaux, P., Roger, P., Van Sande, J., Lecocq, R., and Mockel, J. Thyroid control: an example of a complex cell regulation network. Adv. Cyclic Nucl. Res., 14:479 (1981).
2. Lamy, F., Roger, P., Contor, L., Reuse, S., Raspé, E., Van Sande, J., and Dumont, Control of thyroid cell proliferation: the example of the dog thyrocyte, Horm. Cell Regul.153(11):169 (1987)
3. Björkman, U, and Ekholm R. Accelerated exocytosis and H_2O_2 generation in isolated thyroid follicles enhance protein iodination, Endocrinology 122:488 (1988)
4. Corvilain, B., Van Sande, J. and Dumont, J.E. Inhibition by iodide of iodide binding to porteins: the "Wolff-Chaikoff-effect" is caused by inhibition of H_2O_2 generation. Biochem. Biophys. Res. Commun. 154:1287 (1988)

5. Sheela Rani C.S., Boyd A.E., and Field, J.B. Effects of acetylcholine, TSH and other stimulators on intracellular calcium concentration in dog thyroid cells. Biochem. Biophys. Res. Commun. 131:1041 (1985)
6. Raspé, E., Roger, P., and Dumont, J.E. Carbamylcholine, TRH, PGF_2 and fluoride enhance free intracellular Ca^{++} and Ca^{++} translocation in dog thyroid cells. Biochem. Biophys. Res. Commun. 141:569 (1986)
7. Graff, I., Mockel, J., Laurent, E., Erneux, C., and Dumont, J.E. Carbachol and sodium fluoride, but not TSH, stimulate the generation of inositol phosphates in the dog thyroid. FEBS Letters 210:204 (1987)
8. Decoster, C., Mockel, J., Van Sande, J., Unger, J., and Dumont, J.E. The role of calcium and guanosine 3':5'-monophosphate in the action of acetylcholine on thyroid metabolism. Eur. J. Biochem. 104:199 (1980)
9. Unger, J., Ketelbant, P., Erneux, C., Mockel, J., and Dumont, J.E. Mechanism of cholinergic inhibition of dog thyroid secretion in vitro. Endocrinology 114:1266 (1984)
10. Mockel, J., Van Sande, J., Decoster, C., and Dumont, J.E. Tumor promoters as probes of protein kinase C in dog thyroid cell : inhibition of the primary effects of carbamylcholine and reproduction of some distal effects. Metabolism 36:137 (1987).
11. Van Sande, J., Mockel, Boeynaems, J.M., Dor, P., Andry, G., and Dumont, J.E. Regulation of cyclic nucleotide and prostaglandin formation in normal human thyroid tissue and in autonomous nodules. J. Clin. Endocrinol. Metab. 50:776 (1980)
12. Van Sande, J., Lamy, F., Lecocq, R., Mirkine, N., Rocmans, P., Cochaux, P., Mockel, J. and Dumont J.E. Pathogenesis of autonomous thyroid nodules : in vitro study of iodine and adenosine 3',5'-monophosphate metabolism. J. Clin. Endocrinol. metab. 66:570 (1988)
13. Laurent, E., Mockel, J., Van Sande, J., Graff, I., and Dumont, J.E. Dual activation by thyrotropin of the phospholipase C and cyclic AMP cascades in human thyroid. Mol. Cell. Endocr. 52:273 (1987)
14. Libert, F., Parmentier, M;, Lefort, A., Dinsart, C., Van Sande, J., Maenhaut, C., Simons, M.J., Dumont, J.E., and Vassart, G. Selective amplification and cloning of four new members of the G protein-coupled receptor family. Science (in press) (1989)
15. Dumont, J.E., Jauniaux, J.C., Roger, P.P. The cyclic AMP-mediated stimulation of cell proliferation. Trends Biochem. Sci. 14:67 (1989)

16. Baserga, R. 1985 The Biology of Cell Reproduction, Harvard University Press.
17. Valente, W.A., Vitti, P., Kohn, L.D., Brandi, M.L., Rotella, C.M., Toccafondi, R., Tramontano, D., Aloj, S.M., Ambesi-Impiombato, F.S. The relationship of growth and adenylate cyclase activity in cultured thyroid cells. Separate bioeffects of thyrotropin. Endocrinology 112:71 (1983)
18. Dere, W.H., and Rapoport, B. Control of growth in cultured rat thyroid cells. Mol. Cell. Endocrinol. 44:195 (1986)
19. Contor, L., Lamy, F., Lecocq, R., Roger, P.P. and Dumont, J.E. Differential protein phosphorylation in induction of thyroid cell proliferation by thyrotropin, epidermal growth factor, or phorbol ester. Mol. Cell. Endocrinol 8:2494 (1988)
20. Lamy, F., Roger, P.P., Lecocq, R., and Dumont, J.E. Differential protein synthesis in the induction of thyroid cell proliferation by thyrotropin, epidermal growth factor or serum. Eur. J. Biochem. 155:265 (1986)
21. Roger, P.P., Taton, M., Van Sande, J., and Dumont J.E. Mitogenic effects of thyrotropin and cyclic AMP in differentiated human thyroid cells in vitro. J. Clin. Endocrinol. Metab. 66:1158 (1988)
22. Roger, P.P., Servais, P., and Dumont, J.E. Induction of DNA synthesis in dog thyrocytes in primary culture : synergistic effects of thyrotropin and cyclic AMP with epidermal growth factor and insulin. J. Cell. Physiol. 130:587 (1987)
23. Lefort, A., Lecocq, R., Libert, F., Lamy, F., Swillens, S., Vassart, G., and Dumont, J.E. Cloning and sequencing of a calcium-binding protein regulated by cyclic AMP in the thyroid. EMBO J. 8:111 (1989)
24. Goyens, P., Golstein, J., Nsombola, B., Vis, H., and Dumont, J.E. Selenium deficiency as a possible factor in the pathogenesis of myxoedematous endemic cretinism. Acta Endocrinol. 114:497 (1987)

THYROID SPECIFIC GENE EXPRESSION

Alison J. Sinclair, Renata Lonigro,
Donato Civitareale and Roberto Di Lauro

European Molecular Biology Laboratory
Heidelberg, FRG

INTRODUCTION

The biosynthesis of thyroid hormones requires the iodination and coupling of two tyrosine residues. During evolution specialized cells within the thyroid gland have developed to accomplish this task. The follicular cells of the thyroid gland are arranged in a characteristic tridimensional structure which consists of a sphere of follicular cells surrounding a lumen. Iodine is transported from the bloodstream into the follicular cells by a thyroid specific iodine channel, and subsequently reaches the lumen of the follicle. Two further thyroid specific functions are present in the follicle to assist hormone synthesis: a thyroid specific peroxidase (TPO) and thyroglobulin (Tg). The peroxidase has two functions: it catalyzes the incorporation of iodine onto some of the tyrosyl residues of the thyroglobulin molecule and it is required for the coupling of a subset of the iodinated residues to form the hormones. Upon interaction of Thyroid Stimulating Hormone (TSH) with its receptor the modified thyroglobulin is reabsorbed from the follicular lumen, then it is degraded within the follicular cells and free hormone is released in the bloodstream[1].

Several of the important functions in thyroid hormone formation indicated in this summary are thought to be specific for the thyroid gland, i. e. thyroglobulin, peroxidase, the iodide transport system and the receptor for TSH. Over the past few years we have been interested in how the cell type specific expression of these functions is determined in the thyroid, using as a model system the thyroid specific expression of the thyroglobulin gene. The choice of thyroglobulin has been dictated by several considerations: i) it is the most abundant mRNA expressed in thyroid; ii) the protein has been extensively characterized[2], iii) well characterized antibodies against thyroglobulin are available. The studies described here have been facillitated by the use of a cell line that closely resembles the thyroid tissue. The FRTL-5[3] cell line expresses in culture most of differentiated functions of the thyroid. It responds to TSH, produces and secretes thyroglobulin, expresses peroxidase and concentrates iodidine from the culture medium. The only differentiated thyroid phenotype that the FRTL-5 cells are unable to reproduce is the characteristic polarity and tridimensional organization of the follicular cells in vivo. It may be a consequence of this lack of intra- and intercellular organization that has made it very difficult to clearly demonstrate and analyse thyroid hormone synthesis in cultured FRTL-5 cells. It will certainly be challenging in the future to closely analyse the differences between the phenotypes of the FRTL-5 cell line and the thyroid gland to determine how the morphology of the cells and the gland influence the differentiated functions, but at present there are no reagents available to address this point.

THYROID SPECIFIC EXPRESSION OF THE THYROGLOBULIN GENE

Thyroid Specific Expression of Thyroglobulin is Regulated at the Level of Transcription

Several years ago we cloned cDNA copies of the rat thyroglobulin mRNA[4]. As an initial attempt at defining the nature of the mechanism that restricts the presence of thyroglobulin to the thyroid tissue we analysed the distibution of thyroglobulin mRNA in several tissues and cell lines. The cloned cDNA fragments were hybridized with RNA from many sources and the unequivocal answer was that thyroglobulin mRNA was only detected in the thyroid gland and the thyroid cell line FRTL-5[5]. This correlation between the pattern of expression of the protein and the mRNA indicates that the restriction of thyroglobulin expression to the thyroid gland is due to either transcriptional or post-transcriptional (differential stability or processing) regulation of the level of mRNA. Conclusive evidence in favor of transcriptional control came several years later, after the cloning of the rat thyroglobulin gene[6]. The availability of the FRTL-5 cell line and of gene transfer methods prompted us to ask whether the cloned Tg gene would behave as the endogenous one, i.e. whether its expression would lead to mRNA accumulation only in the FRTL-5 cell line.

It had been shown that for some genes intragenic signals are necessary for cell-type specific mRNA accumulation[7,8,9], while for other genes signals in the 5' flanking region are responsible[10]. The unusually large size of the thyroglobulin gene (> 200 kbp) forced us to ask whether fragments of the gene could confer thyroid specific mRNA accumulation onto a heterologous marker gene. We decided to test a segment of the 5' flanking region of the thyroglobulin gene which included 827 nucleotides before, and 36 nucleotides after, the transcriptional start site [6]. This segment of the thyroglobulin gene was fused to the bacterial gene for chloramphenicol acetyl transferase (CAT)[11], and introduced into FRTL-5 cells and into three control lines (FRT, FRA, and BRL), which are unable to express the endogenous thyroglobulin gene. The control cell lines were chosen in order to represent different ways to be "non-thyroid". The FRT cell line is derived from normal rat thyroid and is epithelial in morphology, but it does not express any thyroid differentiated function[12] and if it was derived from thyroid follicular cells it probably lost the differentiated phenotype during the establishment of the cell line. The FRA cell line is derived from a rat thyroid tumor[13] and it expresses low levels of thyroglobulin mRNA[5], but it does not express any other thyroid differentiated function. The BRL cell line is derived from rat liver[14] and so it has totally "non-thyroid" origins. As shown in Figure 1 the chimeric Tg-CAT gene was only expressed in FRTL-5 cells, with a degree of specificity of about 100[15]. This exciting result indicated that a fragment of the thyroglobulin gene of only 850 bp was able to function as a promoter, and that its expression was restricted to the FRTL-5 cell line. This suggests that at least part of the biochemical mechanisms responsible for the restriction of thyroglobulin mRNA to the thyroid tissue are transcriptional, but we are aware that some other transcriptional or post-transcriptional signals may contribute to the thyroid specific expression of the Tg gene. The task of examining the rest of the gene and the flanking sequences for transcription control signals is feasible, even if it is

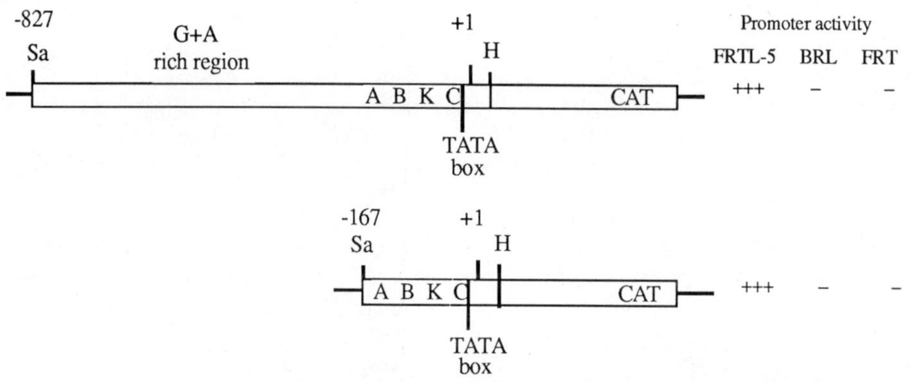

Fig. 1. Chimeric Tg-CAT constructs. The DNA sequence co-ordinates of the Tg 5' flanking sequence are marked relative to the transcription initiation start site at +1. Sequence features are marked (not to scale). The promoter activity is represented on the right: +++ 100 fold above background, - background level.

a formidable one, however the segment of DNA that we have described is responsible for promoting transcription in FRTL-5 at least 100 fold more than in other cells tested, and consequently the signals that we are going to describe in the next sections must be of great relevance in the extablishment or maintenance the expression of the differentiated phenotype in the FRTL-5 cells.

A Segment of 168 Nucleotides is Necessary and Sufficient to Promote Thyroid Specific Transcription

The transfection assay described before allowed us to establish that not all of the DNA sequence in our initial Tg gene fragment was necessary to promote transcription in the FRTL-5 cell line. Sequential deletion analysis indicated that the DNA sequence of a fragment extending from -167 to +1 was sufficient to promote FRTL-5 specific transcription[15] (Figure 1). This sequence contains a three fold repetition of a sequence motif (indicated as A, B and C regions in Figure 1 and Figure 2). Interestingly, only a two fold repetition can be found in the human[16] and calf[17] Tg promoters which correspond in position to the A and C region of the rat Tg promoter[18]. This repeated motif has a biological

I

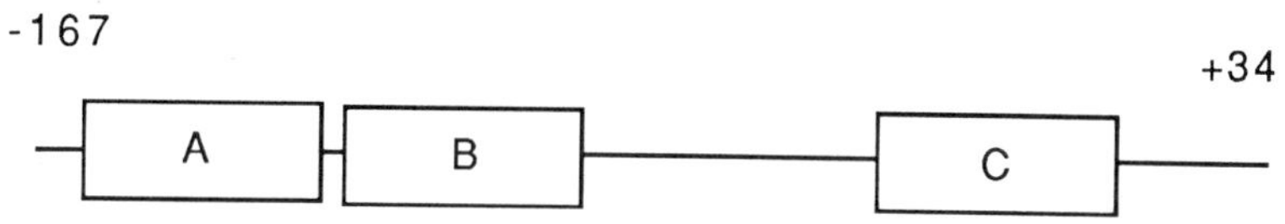

-167 +34

A B C

II

A a c t g a t t A c T C A A G T a t t c t t a g

B g g a g c a g A c T C A A G T a g a g g g a g

C a c t g c c c A g T C A A G T g t t c t t g a

Fig. 2. Repeated sequence motif in thyroglobulin promoter. I. The repeated motif is marked by a box. The three positions where it is found are marked A, B, and C. II. The sequences in the A, B, and C regions are aligned: conserved nucleotides are shown in upper case, and non-conserved nucleotides are shown in lower case.

significance, as will be discussed later. The region characterized by an asymmetrical distribution of purines and pyrimidines (Figure 1), which is observed in different positions in the promoter in all the three species[15, 16, 17] ,lies outside the minimal promoter and no function has been assigned to it.

At Least Three Regions Within the Minimal Promoter Necessary for FRTL-5 Specific Expression are Required for Efficient Transcription.

In order to assess which part(s) of the 167 base pairs are required for full transcription in our assay we undertook a systematic mutagenesis of this sequence by site directed mutagenesis[19]. We first constructed a pseudo-wild type promoter (pTACAT3) containing two single point mutations at -42 and -101 which generated an NheI and an Spe I restriction site respectively. This artificial promoter displays an activity very similar to the wild type one and allows an easy exchange of DNA fragments among the different mutants, in addition to the exchange of DNA fragments between the Tg promoter

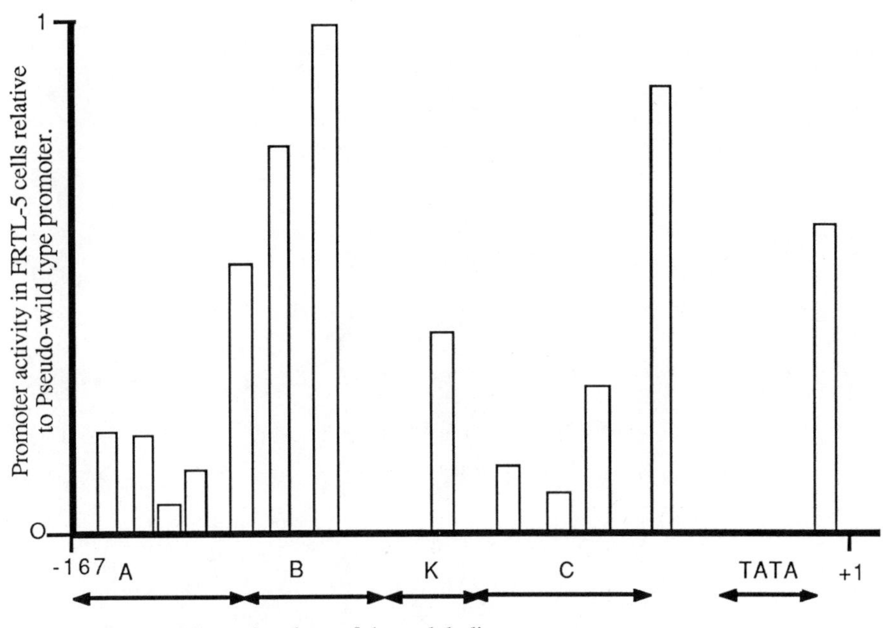

Fig. 3. Activity of Tg promoter mutants in FRTL-5 cells. The promoter activity of each mutant is expressed relative to the pseudo-wild type promoter (1). The position of each mutant is aligned on horizontal scale. The position of the sequence elements in the promoter is shown below.

and other promoters. Subsequently, we constructed a series of regularly spaced clustered point mutations which were individually assayed in FRTL-5 cells for transcriptional activity. The results of these assays are shown in Figure 3. It appears from these results that changing the DNA sequence in three regions of the promoter dramatically reduces the transcriptional ability in FRTL-5 cells. Two of the regions coincide with the A and C regions described before which contain an highly homologous DNA sequence motif. The B region, which shows a similar DNA sequence, does not seem to be required for efficient transcription. The third region important for promoter function (region K) maps between nucleotides -80/-102, and has no homology to the repeated sequence. None of the promoter mutants assayed displayed detectable activity in "non-thyroid" cells.

At Least Three FRTL-5 Nuclear Proteins Bind to the Thyroglobulin Promoter.

From the data described above we postulated that the DNA sequence elements of regions A, K and C of the thyroglobulin promoter must be involved in interactions with cellular factors. The specific expression of the promoter in FRTL-5 cells could be explained by the presence of negative controlling elements in non thyroid cells, or by the presence of activators exclusively in FRTL-5 cells, or a combination of the two. The evidence derived from the study of the mutant promoters suggested that the first model was unlikely because none of the mutations activated transcription in non thyroid cells, as one would have expected if one mutated a repressor binding site. More direct evidence in favour of the existence of FRTL-5 specific activator(s) came from extensive protein binding studies with nuclear extracts from FRTL-5, FRT and Rat1 (a fibroblastic cell line[20]) cell lines. As illustrated in Figure 4 we have characterised at least three proteins able to recognize the thyroglobulin promoter. Two of them are present as active DNA binding proteins only in nuclear extracts of FRTL-5 cells, and for this reason we call them Thyroid Transcription Factor 1 (TTF-1) and Thyroid Transcription Factor 2 (TTF-2). The third activity is present in nuclear extracts from all cell lines examined, hence the name Ubiquitous Factor A (UFA). TTF-1 binds in vitro to the three regions displaying sequence homology (regions A, B and C), TTF-2 binds in vitro to region K, while UFA binds in vitro to a sequence in the A region.

At the moment we are unable to distinguish the DNA sequences required for TTF-1 and UFA to bind to the A region, but we know that they are different because TTF-1 can also recognize the B and C regions while UFA cannot. Our model is that TTF-1 is able to recognize the common sequence in the three repeated regions while UFA must interact with some sequence unique to the A region, but possibly overlapping the repeated region. The interpretation of the relative role of TTF-1 and UFA in the A region is difficult. This region is clearly very important for promoter function, but whether UFA, TTF-1 or both are necessary for promoter function is not clear. Preliminary analysis of several mutations in the A region suggest that promoter activty is greatly reduced by

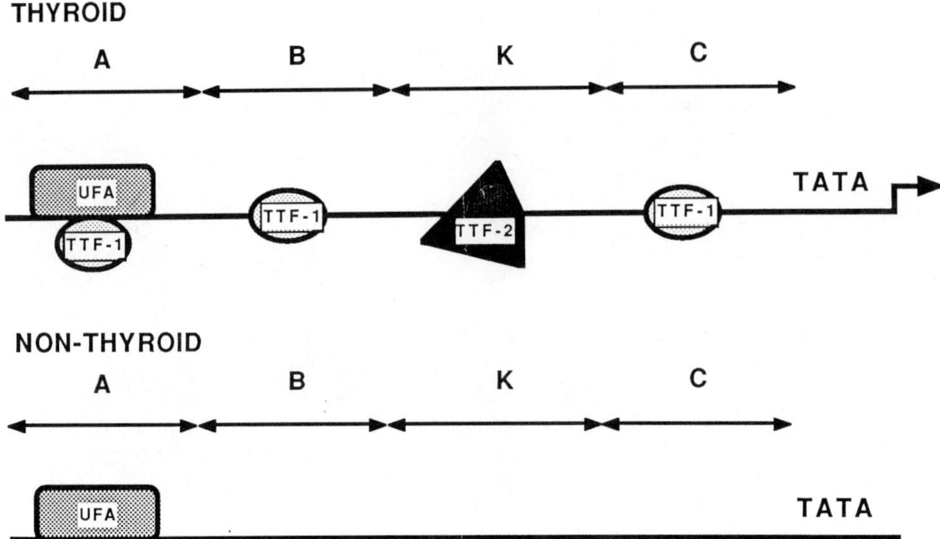

Fig. 4. Sequence specific interactions between nuclear proteins and the Tg promoter. The Tg promoter is represented from -167 to +1. The regions of this sequence that interact with nuclear proteins of thyroid and non-thyroid origins are shown (to scale).

mutations that reduce the binding of either protein, which indicates that both proteins may have a role (A. J. S. and R. D. L., unpublished). A mutant in the B region interfered with TTF-1 binding but had no effect on promoter function, suggesting that the binding of TTF-1 at the B site either does not occur in vivo, or is not required for promoter activity. Mutants in the C region, which decreased promoter activity by at least 10 fold, abolished TTF-1 binding, which shows that this interaction is essential for promoter activity. The mutant in the K region, which decreased promoter activity 2 fold also decreased the binding of TTF-2.

In conclusion, in order for the thyroglobulin promoter to function the binding of TTF-1 to the C and possibly to the A region is necessary. The binding of TTF-2 to the K region further increases this expression at least two fold. Figure 4 summarizes the interactions between these nuclear factors and the thyroglobulin minimal promoter and illustrates our model on the bio-

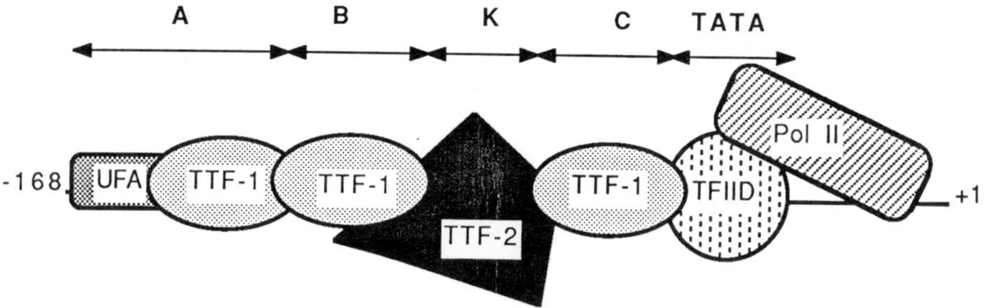

Fig. 5. Model of the transcriptionally active Tg promoter. One set of possible interactions between the transcription factors and the Tg promoter are shown.

chemical mechanisms that allow FRTL-5 specific expression of the thyroglobulin gene. In this model TTF-1 is the primary mediator of FRTL-5 specific expression: its exclusive presence, at least in an active form, in FRTL-5 cells allows expression of the thyroglobulin promoter. By the same mechanism, TTF-2 further increases the FRTL-5 specific expression by a factor of two. In non thyroid cells, the presence of UFA alone is not sufficient to mediate promoter activity and because of the absence of both TTF-1 and TTF-2 the promoter is essentially inactive. In Figure 5 the active configuration of the promoter is shown with the addition of the TATA binding protein TFIID, the transcription factor proposed to be responsible for the transfer of positive effects from the upstream regulatory elements to RNA polymerase II[21]. The model shows some potential interactions between the transcription factors that could mediate the binding of TFIID and RNA polymerase II, and so allow transcription.

The model just presented postulates then that FRTL-5 specific expression of the thyroglobulin gene is a positive regulatory phenomenon dependent on the FRTL-5 specific presence of two activators of transcription, TTF-1 and 2. Further support for this model comes from studies on the effect of transformation on thyroid specific gene expression. It has been shown that the expression of some oncogenes in FRTL-5 cells leads to the extinction of the thyroid differentiated phenotype, as measured by the disappearance of thyroglobulin mRNA, the loss of the iodine trapping mechanism and the loss

Rat thyroglobulin	(C region)	C T G c C C A G T C A a G
Human TPO	(-155/-136)	C T G a C C A G T C A g G

Fig. 6. Homology between the rat Tg and the human TPO promoters. The sequence in the rat Tg C region and the human TPO (-155/-136) are aligned. Conserved nucleotides are shown in upper case, non-conserved nucleotides are shown in lower case.

of the dependence on TSH for growth[22,23]. Binding studies carried out with nuclear extract from transformed FRTL-5 cells demonstrate that both TTF-1[24] and TTF-2 (Helen Francis-Lang and R. D. L., unpublished) activity disappear, which establishes another correlation between the presence of the thyroid specific transcription factors and active expression of the thyroglobulin gene.

OTHER THYROID SPECIFIC GENES

Of the other thyroid specific genes, some information has recently been obtained for the thyroid specific peroxidase (TPO). The mRNA for TPO has been found exclusively in thyroid tissue[25], which suggests that the mechanism that restricts the product of TPO to the thyroid is either transcriptional or post-transcriptional. This similarity with thyroglobulin suggested that there may be common mechanism(s) controlling the expression of the two genes, which led us to search for sequences similar to the TTF-1, and TTF-II binding sites within the 5'-flanking region of the human TPO gene[26]. Interestingly, about 150 nucleotides 5' from the transcription start site of the human TPO gene a strong homology is observed with the binding site for TTF-1 (Figure 6). The functional relevance of this homology will have to be demonstrated by mutational and binding studies on the TPO promoter.

The genes for the other thyroid specific functions (TSH receptor and iodine carrier) have not yet been cloned and so no information about the level of control of their expression is available.

MODULATION OF THYROGLOBULIN PROMOTER FUNCTION

Studies performed either in vivo or in cultured cells have shown that the basal level of thyroglobulin synthesis can be modulated by TSH[27, 28, 29, 30] and by IGF-1 and/or insulin[30]. The magnitude of the TSH effect is still controversial. It has been shown that transcription of the thyroglobulin gene decreases by a factor of two when TSH is removed from the culture media[30] of FRTL-5 cells. A similar effect on the level of thyroglobulin mRNA was observed in the rat thyroid gland in vivo after chronic administration of T3, which suggests that the moderate effect of TSH on thyroglobulin synthesis observed in the FRTL-5 cells mimicks the physiological role of the hormone in vivo[27]. Results obtained in other laboratories with hypophisectomized rats[28] showed a much larger depression of thyroglobulin mRNA synthesis, which could be due to the more profound alteration of the hormonal homeostasis caused by the hypophisectomy. Also, in primary cultures of dog thyroid cells the removal of TSH has a profound effect on thyroglobulin mRNA synthesis which drops to undetectable levels[31]. From these results it is not clear whether TSH modulates thyroglobulin synthesis or whether it is essential for expression of the gene. The different answers collected in several laboratories could reflect differences in the experimental system used. Developmental studies suggest that thyroglobulin synthesis begins before any detectable TSH secretion from the pituitary[32], which indicats that TSH is not an essential requirement for thyroglobulin gene expression. However, it is possible that a TSH dependent mechanism substitutes during development for the primary stimulus which initiated thyroglobulin gene expression. The new technology made available by the manipulation of the mouse embryo may help in solving the issue of the extent of regulation of thyroglobulin gene expression by TSH with the construction of appropriate mouse strains where TSH synthesis is specifically abolished.

The physiological role of IGF-I on thyroglobulin gene expression is not yet clear, although there is a pronounced stimulation of thyroglobulin mRNA synthesis in FRTL-5 cells[30].

CONCLUSION

At day 15 in rat development thyroglobulin synthesis begins[32]. The event is restricted to a group of cells derived from an outpocketing of the primitive pharingeal cavity which are destined to become the follicular cells of the thyroid gland in the adult[33]. What are the molecular event(s) that trigger thyroglobulin production specifically in a few cells of the rat embryo and subsequently maintain it only in the adult thyroid gland? We have begun to address these question using as an experimental model the FRTL-5 cell line, which maintains thyroglobulin expression (and other thyroid specific function) in culture. From our studies we have developed a working hypothesis whereby thyroglobulin mRNA synthesis requires a transcription factor exclusively present in thyroid, which we have called TTF-1. Another thyroid specific transcription factor, TTF-2, is required to achieve full expression of the promoter. We can now move one step backward in the chain of events leading to induction of the thyroid phenotype, by asking how the activity of TTF-1 and TTF-2 are restricted to the thyroid tissue.

The specific expression of genes in tissues different from thyroid has been shown to be dependent on cell type specific transcription factors, but there are several strategies to obtain the tissue specific distribution are van. In the case of the pituitary specific transcription factor Pyt-1, which is necessary for the expression of both the growth hormone and the prolactin genes[34], the regulation is at the level of mRNA, as indicated by the absence of Pyt-1 mRNA in non-pituitary cells. Also in the case of OTF-2, a B cell specific transcription factor necessary for immunoglobulin gene expression[35], the OTF-2 mRNA is restricted to B cells. Curiously, another transcription factor OTF-1[36], which is present in several cell types and is necessary for transcription of many genes, can recognize and bind to the OTF-2 binding site in the immunoglobulin genes but is not able to promote transcription from this promoter. Clearly another type of specificity must be superimposed to the immunoglobulin promoter region, so that does not respond to OTF-1 but only to OTF-2 binding. In the case of immunoglobulin light chain k gene, a factor (NF-kB) binding to its enhancer was exclusively found in B cells[37]. However, it was subsequently demonstrated that the NF-kB protein is present in several cell types in an inactive, cytoplasmic form[38]. The difference in activity and subcellular distribution of NF-kB between B cells and other cell types can be explained by the presence of an inhibitor, specifically absent from B cells, which is tightly associated with NF-kB and keeps it from migrating to the nucleus[39]. In this example the control of the presence of an active transcription factor in B cells is determined by the presence or activity of the inhibitor. Another interesting feature of NF-kB is that while it is required to initiate immunoglobulin synthesis[40] in B-cells, it does not seem to be necessary to maintain expression. Transfection studies have shown that an active form of NF-kB is required to initiate transcription from a immunoglobulin promoter[40], but there are examples where B-cells producing immunoglobulin are devoid of NF-kB activity[41], and another where B-cells producing immunoglobulin are devoid of the NF-kB binding site in the immunoglobulin gene enhancer[42].

In order to address the question of which molecular mechanism allows the exclusive presence of TTF-1 in FRTL-5 cells, we have purified TTF-1 to homogeneity from calf thyroids (Civitareale et al., unpublished). Partial sequencing of the purified protein yielded a peptide of thirteen amino acids. Synthetic oligonucleotides deduced from the amino acid sequence and antibodies against the synthetic peptide are currently being used in order to isolate the gene for TTF-1.

REFERENCES

1. A. Taurog, Hormone synthesis: thyroid iodine metabolism, in: "Werner's The Thyroid," S. H. Ingbar, and L. E Bravermann, eds., J.B. Lippincott Company, Philadelphia (1986).
2. H. Edelhoc, and J. Robbins, Thyroglobulin: Chemistry and Biosynthesis, in: "Werner's The Thyroid," S. H. Ingbar, and L. E. Braverman, eds., J.B. Lippincott Company, Philadelphia (1986).
3. F. S. Ambesi-Impiombato, L. A. M. Parks, and H. G. Coon, Culture of hormone-dependent functional epithelial cells from rat thyroids, Proc. Natl. Acad. Sci. USA. 77:3455 (1980).
4. R. Di Lauro, S. Obici, A. Acquaviva, and C. Alvino, Construction of recombinant plasmids containing rat thyroglobulin mRNA sequences, Gene. 19:117 (1982).
5. V. E. Avvedimento, A. Monticelli, D. Tramontano, C. Polistina, L. Nitsch, and R. Di Lauro, Differential expression of the thyroglobulin gene

in normal and transformed thyroid cells, Eur. J. Biochem. 149:467 (1985).

6. A. M. Musti, V. E. Avvedimento, C. Polistina, M. V. Ursini, S. Obici, L. Nitsch, S. Cocozza, and R. Di Lauro, The complete structure of the rat thyroglobulin gene, Proc. Natl. Acad. Sci. USA. 83:323 (1986).
7. J. Banerji, L. Olson, and W. Schaffner, A lymphocyte-specific cellular enhancer is located downstream of the joining region in immunoglobulin heavy chain genes, Cell. 33:729 (1983).
8. S. D. Gillies, S. L. Morrison, V. T. Oi, and S. Tonegawa, A tissue-specific transcription enhancer is located in the major intron of a rearranged immunoglobulin heavy chain gene, Cell. 33:717 (1983).
9. C. Queen, and D. Baltimore, Immunoglobulin gene transcription is activated by downstream sequence elements, Cell. 33:741-748 (1983).
10. M. D. Walker, T. Edlund, A. M. Boulet, and W. J. Rutter, Cell-specific expression controlled by the 5'-flanking region of insulin and chymotrypsin genes, Nature. 306: 557 (1983).
11. C. Gorman, L. F. Moffat, and B. H. Howard, Recombinant genomes which express chloramphenicol acetyltransferase in mammalian cells, Mol. Cell. Biol. 2:1044 (1982).
12. F. S. Ambesi-Impiombato, and H. G. Coon, Thyroid cells in culture, Int. Rev. Cytol. 12, Suppl. 10:163 (1979).
13. E. M. Volpert, and A. P. Prezyna, Transplantable thyroid tumor in rats - iodoamino acid distribution in successive tumor generations, Acta Endocrinol. 85: 93 (1977).
14. S. P. Nissley, P. A. Short, M. M. Rechler, J. M. Podskalny, and H. G. Coon, Proliferation of buffalo rat liver cells in serum-free medium does not depend upon multiplication-stimulation activity (MSA), Cell. 11: 441 (1977).
15. A. M. Musti, M. V. Ursini, M. V. Avvedimento, V. Zimarino, and R. Di Lauro, A cell type specific factor recognizes the rat thyroglobulin promoter, Nucleic Acids Res. 15:8149 (1987).
16. D. Cristophe, B. Cabrer, A. Bacolla, H. Targovnik, V. Pohl, and G. Vassart, An unusually long poly(purine)-poly(pyrimidine) sequence is located upstream from the human thyroglobulin gene, Nucleic Acids Res. 13:5127 (1985).

17. G. de Martinoff, V. Pohl, L. Mercken, G. van Ommen, and G. Vassart, Structural organization of the bovine thyroglobulin gene and of its 5'-flanking region, Eur. J. Biochem. 164:591 (1987).
18. D. Civitareale, L. Ghibelli, and R. Di Lauro, Partial purification of a thyroid specific protein recognizing the thyroglobulin promoter., in: "Molecular biology approaches to thyroid research," Loos, U.,Wartofsky, L. eds, Georg Thieme Verlag Stuttgart-New York (1987).
19. W. Kramer, V. Drutsa, H-W Jansen, B. Kramer, M. Pflugfelder, and H-J Fritz, The gapped duplex DNA approach to oligonucleotide-directed mutant construction, Nucleic Acids Res. 12:9441 (1984).
20. M. Botchan, W. Topp, and J. Sambrook, The arrengement of simian virus 40 sequences in the DNA of transformed cells, Cell. 9:269 (1976).
21. N. Nakajima, M. Horikoshi, and R. G. Roeder, Factors involved in specific transcription by mammalian RNA polymerase II: Purification, genetic specificity and TATA box promoter interactions of TFIID, Mol. Cell. Biol. 8:4028 (1988).
22. G. Colletta, A. Pinto, P. P. Di Fiore, A. Fusco, M. Ferrentino, V. E. Avvedimento, N. Tsuchida, and G. Vecchio, Dissociation between transformed and differentiated phenotype in rat thyroid epithelial cells after transformation with a temperature sensitive mutant of the Kirsten murine sarcoma virus, Mol. Cell. Biol. 3:2099 (1983).
23. A. Fusco, G. Portella, P. P. Di Fiore, M. T. Berleingieri, R. Di Lauro, A. B. Schneider, and G. Vecchio, A mos oncogene-containing retrovirus, myeloproliferative sarcoma virus, transforms rat thyroid epithelial cells and irreversibly blocks their differentiation pattern, J. Virol. 56:284 (1985).
24. V. E. , Avvedimento, A. M. Musti, M. Bonapace, A. Fusco, and R. Di Lauro, Neoplastic transformation inactivates specific trans-acting factor(s) required for the expression of the thyroglobulin gene, Proc. Natl. Acad. Sci. USA. 85:1744 (1988).
25. S. Kimura, T. Kotani, W. O. McBride, K. Umeki, K. Hirai, T. Nakayama, and S. Ohtaki, Human thyroid peroxidase: complete cDNA and protein sequence, chromosome mapping, and identification of two alternately spliced mRNA, Proc. Natl. Acad. Sci. USA. 84:5555 (1987).

26. S. Kimura, Y. Hong, T. Kotani, S. Ohtaki, and F. Kikkawa, Structure of the human peroxidase gene: comparison and relationhsip to the human myeloperoxidase gene, Biochemistry. in press:(1989).

27. V. E. , Tramontano, D., Ursini, M.V., Monticelli, A. Avvedimento and Di Lauro,R, The level of thyroglobulin mRNA is regulated by TSH both in vitro and in vivo, Biochem. Biophys. Res. Commun. 122:472 (1984).

28. B. Van Heuverswyn, C. Streydio, H. Brocas, S. Refetoff, S. Dumont, J. Dumont, and G. Vassart, Thyrotropin controls transcription of the thyroglobulin gene, Proc. Natl. Acad. Sci. USA. 81:5941 (1984).

29. G. Vassart, A. Bacolla, H. Brocas, D. Cristophe, G. de Martynoff, A. Leriche, J. Parma, V. Pohl, H. Targovnik, and B. van Heuverswyn, Structure, expression and regulation of the thyroglobulin gene, Mol. Cell. Endocrinol. 40: 89 (1985).

30. P. Santisteban, L. D. Kohn, and R. Di Lauro, Thyroglobulin gene expression is regulated by insulin and isulin-like growth factor I, as well as thyrotropin, in FRTL-5 thyroid cells, J. Biol. Chem. 262:4048 (1987).

31. P. P. Roger, B. van Heuverswyn, C. Lambert, S. Reuse, G. Vassart, and J. E. Dumont, Antagonistic effects of thyrotropin and epidermal growth factor on thyroglobulin mRNA level in cultured thyroid cells, Eur. J. Biochem. 152:239 (1985).

32. A. Kawaoi, and M. Tsuneda, Functional development and maturation of the rat thyroid gland in the foetal and newborn period: an immunoistochemical study., Acta Endocrinol. 108:518 (1985).

33. L. Remy, M. Michel-Bechet, A. M. Athouel-Haon, S. Magre, C. Cataldo, and A. Jost, Development of the thyroid gland in the rat fetus in vivo. An ultrastructural and radioautographic study., Anat. Microsc. Morphol. Exp. 69:91 (1980).

34. H. A. Ingraham, R. Chen, H. J. Mangalam, H. P. Elsholtz, S. E. Flynn, C. R. Lin, D. M. Simmons, L. Swanson, and M. G. Rosenfeld, A tissue-specific transcription factor containing a homeodomain specifies a pituitary phenotype, Cell. 55:519 (1988).

35. M. M. Muller, S. Ruppert, W. Shaffner, and P. Mathias, A human lymphoid-specific transcription factor that activates immunoglobulin genes is a homeobox protein, Nature. 336:544 (1988).

36. C. Fletcher, N. Heintz, and R. G. Roeder, Purification and characterization of OTF-1, a transcription factor regulating cell cycle expression of a human histone H2b gene, Cell. 51:773 (1987).
37. H. Singh, R. Sen, D. Baltimore, and P. A. Sharp, A nuclear factor that binds to a conserved sequence motif in transcriptional control elements of immunoglobulin genes, Nature. 319:154 (1986).
38. P. A. Bauerle, and D. Baltimore, Activation of DNA binding activity in an apparent cytoplasmic precursor of the NF-kB transcription factor, Cell. 53:211 (1988).
39. P. A. Bauerle, and D. Baltimore, IkB: a specific inhibitor of the NF-kB transcription factor, Science. 242:540 (1988).
40. M. Lenardo, J. W. Pierce, and D. Baltimore, Protein-binding sites in Ig gene enhancers determine trascriptional activity and inducibility, Science. 236: 1573 (1987).
41. M. L. Atchison, and R. P. Perry, The role of the k enhancer and its binding factor NF-kB in the developmental regulation of k gene transcription, Cell. 48:121 (1987).
42. M. R. Wabl, and P. D. Burrows, Epression of immunoglobulin heavy chain at a high level in the absence of a proposed immunoglobulin enhancer in cis, Proc. Natl. Acad. Sci. USA. 81:2452 (1984).

INDEX